Corneal Topography

David J. Schanzlin Jeffrey B. Robin
Editors

Corneal Topography

Measuring and Modifying the Cornea

With an Introduction by A.E. Reynolds

With 171 Illustrations in 258 Parts, 85 in Full Color

Springer-Verlag
New York Berlin Heidelberg London Paris
Tokyo Hong Kong Barcelona Budapest

David J. Schanzlin, MD
Department of Ophthalmology
St. Louis University
Bethesda Eye Institute
St. Louis, MO 63110, USA

Jeffrey B. Robin, MD
Department of Ophthalmology
University of Illinois
College of Medicine at Chicago
UIC Eye Center
Chicago, IL 60612, USA

Library of Congress Cataloging-in-Publication Data
Corneal topography: measuring and modifying the cornea / [edited by]
David J. Schanzlin, Jeffrey B. Robin.
p. cm.
Includes bibliographical references.

ISBN-13: 978-1-4612-7659-3

1. Cornea—Measurement. I. Schanzlin, David J. II. Robin, Jeffrey B.
[DNLM: 1. Cornea—anatomy & histology. 2. Cornea—surgery. WW 220 C8138]
RE336.C69 1991
DNLM/DLC
for Library of Congress 91-4876

Printed on acid-free paper.

Production coordinated by Chernow Editorial Services, Inc. and managed by Linda H. Hwang.
Manufacturing supervised by Rhea Talbert.
Typeset by TCSystems, Inc., Shippensburg, PA, USA.

9 8 7 6 5 4 3 2 1

ISBN-13: 978-1-4612-7659-3 e-ISBN-13: 978-1-4612-2766-3
DOI: 10.1007/978-1-4612-2766-3

This book is dedicated to our wives, Nancy Schanzlin and MaryAnn Robin, and to our children, Meredith, Michael, and Matthew Schanzlin, and Zachary David and Matthew Joshua Robin.

Introduction: History of Corneal Measurement

A. E. Reynolds

The cornea provides most of the refractive power of the eye's optical system. For the last 150 years, ophthalmologists have tried to determine its topographic characteristics. The oldest method of topographic analysis used the mirror quality of the anterior corneal surface. Several types of images, including straight lines, squares, and concentric rings, were reflected off the corneal "mirror" enabling qualitative assessments of the topography of the anterior corneal surface.

In the 1820s, the French ophthalmologist Ferdinand Cuignet provided the first description of a method for studying images reflected off the anterior corneal surface, calling the technique "keratoscopy." In his system, a light was projected onto a target that was held in front of the patient's eye. The light, target, patient, and observer were positioned so that the observer could visualize the image of the target on the patient's cornea. Distortion of the reflected image, indicating abnormal corneal topography, could then be qualitatively interpreted by the observer. There were several problems with this prototypic technique of keratoscopy. Prime among these was that it was very difficult to properly align patient, observer, target, and lighting so that the image of the target was centered on the patient's visual axis. Additionally, early observers viewed the reflected image on a one-on-one ratio making it very difficult to see minor distortions in corneal shape.

In 1880, A. Placido devised a keratoscopy target that is still in use today. The target was a disk with alternating black and white rings. The disk had a hole in its center through which the observer could visualize the patient's cornea. This was crucial for improving target alignment with the patient's visual axis. Not only could the observer grossly center the target on the patient's cornea, but the patient was able to directly align his or her visual axis with the center of the target disk. If the cornea was grossly spherical, the reflected images (which in reality were the white rings) would appear circular and concentric. Gross distortions of corneal topography could be interpreted as deviations either in the shape of the rings or their concentricity. Although Placido's disk certainly ameliorated the problems with target alignment, the observer still had no magnification capabilities and was thus incapable of detecting small degrees of corneal topographic distortion.

The issue of magnification was addressed in the late 1880s by E. Javal, a pioneer in the development of the keratometer as well as an astute pioneer of corneal topography. He observed that keratoscopy would be greatly benefited by the development of a method for diagrammatically or photographically representing the corneal topography. He stated in his *System of Diseases of the Eye* (p. 152):

> The keratoscopic image would furnish a complete record both of the corneal astigmatism and of the decentration of the visual axis. If only it were practical to fix them by instant photography and measure them under the microscope. Until this shall have been accomplished, we must depend upon the ophthalmometer to obtain an approximate idea of the form of the anterior surface of the cornea. But, whereas the keratoscopic images show the complete topography of the portion of the cornea on which it is reflected, a single measurement made with the ophthalmometer gives information regarding only two points lying in some particular corneal section.

In order to extend the range of observation beyond the area that his ophthalmometer covered, Javal attached to the instrument small disks like Placido's. One of the advantages of this system was that the ophthalmometer had an eyepiece telescope system that magnified the observed images. In 1889, Javal further addressed this problem by placing a large enameled disk behind the arc that carried the ophthalmometric mires. The disk had a black background and concentric white circles. The radius of each of these circles represented the tangent measured from the middle point of the arc that carried the mires. Javal had his subjects look into the center of the ophthalmometer tube; he would then observe the keratoscopic image over the central portion of the cornea. The subject would then look up, down, to the left, and to the right; at each point of gaze, the reflected images would be observed.

A. Gullstrand, realizing the importance of Javal's goal of developing a system for representing the cornea topography, was the first to apply photography to keratoscopy. Keratoscopic photographs ("keratographs") were used by ophthalmologists much as the civil engineer uses photogrammetry. Photogrammetry, simply, can be used to compare the contours of any two objects. For example, to observe a mountain with many cliffs and steep slopes in its entirety, all of its sides must be seen at the same time. A small circle is made on the very apex of the mountain and, at 50-ft intervals, lines are drawn around the mountain. An airplane flying over the mountain takes a photograph of the lines drawn around the mountain; this, in fact, represents a contour map of the mountain. The topography of the mountain can then be determined by examining the photograph. Where the contour lines lie close together, the surface is steep; where they are farther apart, the terrain has a flatter slope.

The cornea is, in many ways, similar to a mountain and its topography can be determined in the same manner. The anterior corneal surface is an ideal reflecting surface and the concentric white rings from the Placido disk can be easily photographed. The rings of the keratograph are interpreted in the same manner as the lines on the contour map. The closer the lines, the steeper the surface; the farther apart the lines, the flatter the surface.

Despite the recognition of Javal and other pioneers that examination of the entire corneal surface was essential to the understanding of corneal topography, keratoscopy never gained significant popularity. The main reason was the purely qualitative nature of the technique. In 1896, following Javal's suggestion, Gullstrand developed a method of using a "dividing engine," a measuring microscope, to determine the distance between two points on a keratoscopic photograph. The measurement was then converted to the radius of curvature. However, the method was very time consuming for the practicing ophthalmologist and not really practical. This is the main reason that, until quite recently, the assessment of corneal topography was almost totally confined to keratometry.

In the 20th century, several attempts have been made to develop methods to quantitatively analyze keratographs. In the late 1940s and early 1950s, keratographs were quantitated by comparing them to photographs of spheres of known radius of curvature. The photograph of the sphere was cut in half and placed over the keratograph. If the corresponding rings matched, that portion of the keratograph had the same radius as the sphere. By using an appropriate number of standards, most keratographs could be quantitated.

Charles Hendricks, in 1961, developed a device known as comparator, in which a keratograph could be analyzed quantitatively. The comparator uses black rings of known radii of curvature, comparing them to the corresponding keratograph rings. By projecting a keratograph on the screen of the comparator and changing the magnification of the projected image to superimpose the rings on the comparator screen, a radius of curvature for each keratograph ring can be determined. A similar instrument was developed by International Diagnostic Instruments in 1972, mainly for the fitting of contact lenses. This instrument enables the practitioner to determine the curvature of approximately 43% of the corneal area; by comparison, a keratometer determines only 6%.

Another method of quantifying corneal curvature from keratographs is to use a method similar to that employed in civil engineering to determine the profile of the earth's surface. Each ring of the keratograph is assigned a given elevation and the rings are placed one upon the other. Using an elevation of 0.1 mm, lines are drawn from each ring to the corresponding elevation. This method can be used to determine the shape of any meridian of the cornea. By connecting the ends of each cord, the profile shape of the cornea can be determined. This method has been helpful for orthokeratology and refractive surgery. In radial keratotomy, profile studies have determined that the meridian receiving the first incisions change shape the most, whereas those receiving the last incisions change least.

Recent developments in contact lenses and corneal surgery have placed even greater emphasis upon knowing the topography of the entire cornea. Most photokeratoscopes on the market today project from 8 to 12 concentric rings onto the cornea. These rings can cover an area from 4 mm to the limbus; the average is a chord of 7 mm to 9 mm. The aspheric contact lens design is based upon the curves in the intermediate portion of the cornea (rings 3 through 5), the area just outside that measured by the keratometer. The aspheric portion of the contact lens must clear the intermediate and peripheral (rings 8 through 12) portions of the cornea in order to be worn comfortably. Additionally, contact lens fitting after radial keratotomy and other refractive surgical procedures is greatly dependent upon knowing the topography of the intermediate cornea.

Perhaps the factor most responsible for the resurgence of interest in corneal topography has been the introduction and development of refractive surgery. As is thoroughly discussed in this book, many of the keratorefractive procedures directly involve the intermediate and peripheral zones of the cornea. Additionally, evaluating the refractive effect of these procedures involves assessing the topography of the cornea far beyond the central 3 mm covered by the keratometer.

For example, the keratograph can be used to observe the changes following radial keratotomy. Lines are drawn from the presurgical keratograph rings to arbitrarily selected elevation points. Using the postoperative keratograph, similar lines are drawn to the same elevation points, always using the outer edge of the ring. These changes, although not quantifiable, are easy to observe and graphically illustrate the alterations in topography induced by this procedure.

Surgeons have realized, however, that simple demonstrations of corneal topographic changes in corneal and keratorefractive procedures do not provide enough information; quantification of the topography of these frequently complex corneal surfaces is necessary. With the explosion of computer technology, it has recently become possible to accurately quantify the curvature of thousands of points on the corneal surface. The details of and applications for these sophisticated instruments are thoroughly described in other chapters.

Because of new contact lens designs, keratorefractive surgical procedures, and sophisticated technology, there is, of late, a great deal of interest in corneal topography. As this chapter has demonstrated, this is actually a renaissance. It appears that the dream of E. Javal is finally being realized.

Contents

Contributors

Robert C. Arffa, MD, Department of Ophthalmology, University of Pittsburgh, Eye and Ear Institute, Pittsburgh, Pennsylvania 15213, USA

Richard F. Beatty, MD, Porter Memorial Hospital, Denver, Colorado 80210, USA

Stephen J. Bogan, MD, Medical Center, Wright-Patterson Air Force Base, Dayton, Ohio 45433-5300, USA

Patrick J. Caroline, American Eye Institute, Los Angeles, California 90048, USA

Kenneth L. Cohen, MD, Department of Ophthalmology, School of Medicine, University of North Carolina, Chapel Hill, North Carolina 27599, USA

Sami G. El Hage, OD, PHD, DSC, Eye Care Associates, Houston, Texas 77056, USA

Joseph F. Fleming, MD, St. John Eye Institute, Tulsa, Oklahoma 74104, USA

Sadeer B. Hannush, MD, Department of Ophthalmology, Jefferson Medical College, Thomas Jefferson University, Philadelphia, Pennsylvania, 19107, USA, and Cornea Service, Wills Eye Hospital, Philadelphia, Pennsylvania, 19107, USA

Stephen D. Klyce, PHD, Ophthalmology Department, Louisiana State University, Medical School Eye Center, New Orleans, Louisiana 70112, USA

Colman R. Kraff, MD, Department of Medicine, University of Illinois College of Medicine, Eye Center, Chicago, Illinois 60612, USA

Maureen K. Lundergan, MD, Department of Ophthalmology, University of Utah, Medical Center, Salt Lake City, Utah 84132, USA

Robert K. Maloney, MD, Jules Stein Eye Institute, Los Angeles, California, USA

Peter J. McDonnell, MD, Department of Ophthalmology, University of Southern California School of Medicine, Los Angeles, California 90033, USA

Timothy T. McMahon, OD, Department of Ophthalmology, University of Illinois College of Medicine, Chicago, Illinois 60612, USA

Craig W. Norman, Department of Ophthalmology, South Bend Clinic, South Bend, Indiana 46617, USA

Paul G. Rehkopf, CCE, Department of Ophthalmology, University of Pittsburgh, Eye and Ear Institute, Pittsburgh, Pennsylvania 15213, USA

A. E. Reynolds, OD, PHD, 5525 East 51 Street, Suite 133, Tulsa, Oklahoma 74135, USA

Jeffrey B. Robin, MD, Department of Ophthalmology, University of Illinois College of Medicine, Eye Center, Chicago, Illinois 60612, USA

David J. Schanzlin, MD, Department of Ophthalmology, St. Louis University, Bethesda Eye Institute, St. Louis, Missouri 63110, USA

John C. Stuart, MD, Department of Ophthalmology, University of Pittsburgh, Eye and Ear Institute, Pittsburgh, Pennsylvania 15213, USA

Nancy K. Tripoli, MA, Department of Ophthalmology, School of Medicine, University of North Carolina, Chapel Hill, North Carolina 27599, USA

Jian-Yi Wang, Department of Biomedical Engineering, School of Engineering, Tulane University, New Orleans, Louisiana 70118, USA

George O. Waring III, MD, Emory Eye Center Ophthalmology, Atlanta, Georgia 30322, USA

Joseph W. Warnicki, BA, Department of Ophthalmology, University of Pittsburgh, Eye and Ear Institute, Pittsburgh, Pennslyvania 15213, USA

Stephen E. Wilson, MD, Department of Ophthalmology, University of Texas Southwestern Medical Center, 5323 Harry Hines Boulevard, Dallas, Texas 75235, USA

1
Quantification and Mathematical Analysis of Photokeratoscopic Images

Steven E. Wilson, Jian-Yi Wang, and Stephen D. Klyce

The need for accurate and precise methods of evaluating the contour of the anterior corneal surface has paralleled the rapid development of keratorefractive surgery. Thus, the suboptimal refractive predictability of procedures such as penetrating keratoplasty, astigmatic keratotomy, and radial keratotomy has provided impetus for the development of techniques for measuring and presenting corneal topography that are essential for understanding changes induced by surgical manipulations of the corneal surface.

Until recently, the keratometer and the keratoscope were virtually the only instruments broadly available for monitoring corneal topography. Although the utility of the keratometer has been established for certain purposes, its usefulness for measuring complex changes in corneal topography induced by keratorefractive procedures is limited. The keratometer measures the distance between two pairs of points reflected from the anterior corneal surface; these distances are converted into radii of curvature in a straightforward fashion.[1] Most clinical keratometers provide a dioptric value of corneal power for a particular radius of curvature by assuming a standard keratometric index (1.3375) or tear index (1.336) for the entire cornea.[1] Using either index combines the negative power of the posterior corneal surface with the positive power of the anterior corneal surface.

Three important factors limit the usefulness of the keratometer. First, it assumes that the cornea is a spherocylindrical surface with a single radius of curvature in each meridian and a major and minor axis of curvature separated by 90.° The normal cornea, however, is aspheric and flattens from the center to the periphery.[2–5] Thus, even for normal corneas, the keratometer provides a curvature that may be flatter centrally and steeper peripherally than the true topography. Second, the keratometer provides no information regarding the shape of the cornea within or outside of the four reference points used for calculating curvature. Finally, even small amounts of irregular astigmatism, frequently associated with anterior segment surgical procedures, distort the keratometer mires and make meaningful measurements impossible.

The keratoscope has been more useful than the keratometer for assessment of the effect of surgery on shape because it provides much greater coverage of the corneal surface. The keratoscope, however, is a qualitative device and subtle, but visually significant alterations of corneal topography are often not discerned. Computerized analysis of keratoscope images, however, can provide quantitative information regarding corneal contour with sufficient detail so that early diagnosis of corneal shape anomalies can be made on a routine basis. These methods will be the subject of the remainder of this chapter.

This work was supported in part by USPHS grants EY03311 and EY02377 from the National Eye Institute, National Institutes of Health, Bethesda, Maryland and the Louisiana Lions Eye Foundation.

Problems in the Reconstruction of Three-Dimensional Topography from Two-Dimensional Keratoscope Data

Several issues must be considered in order to reconstruct accurately the anterior corneal surface from two-dimensional keratoscopic images. The most difficult problem is that there is insufficient information in the keratoscope image to provide a point-by-point, unique solution for reconstructing the three-dimensional shape of the anterior corneal surface. Thus, two surfaces with different radii of curvature placed at different distances from the film plane can project the same single point of light from the keratoscope mires to the same point at the film plane (Fig. 1.1). Therefore, the instantaneous radius of curvature at a specific point on the cornea cannot be uniquely determined from the keratoscope analysis without the presumption of a local or global model for the shape of the corneal surface being analyzed.

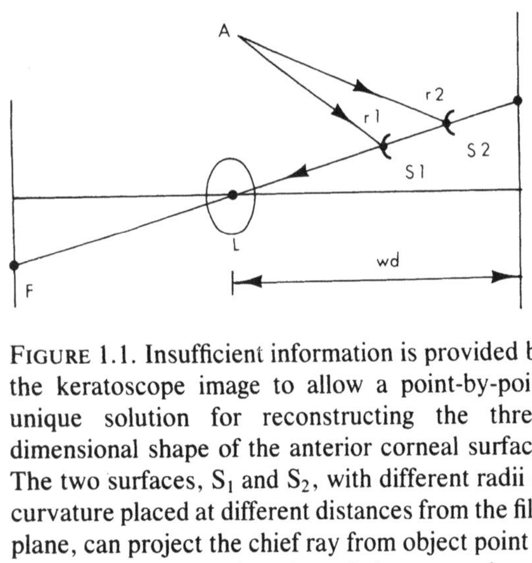

FIGURE 1.1. Insufficient information is provided by the keratoscope image to allow a point-by-point unique solution for reconstructing the three-dimensional shape of the anterior corneal surface. The two surfaces, S_1 and S_2, with different radii of curvature placed at different distances from the film plane, can project the chief ray from object point A on the keratoscope mires through the camera lens L and to the same point at the film plane (F). The virtual image of point A is behind the reflecting convex surface at point I. When focused, the virtual image lies at the fixed working distance (wd) of the camera. Therefore, from the film image, the two surfaces cannot be differentiated. In fact, any point along the line LI can reflect to the same point on the film plane, given the appropriate radius of curvature and surface normal. Assumptions are necessary to make the problem uniquely solvable. (After Wang et al.[17])

Another difficulty in reconstructing three-dimensional surfaces from keratoscope images is that the projected target consists of a series of concentric circles. It is necessary to assume that a light ray arising from one meridian on a particular mire falls on the same meridian at the film plane. This assumption constrains the degrees of freedom of the calculated surface power and produces some error in the reconstruction of the corneal surface. The magnitude of this error is as yet undetermined, although it is thought to be small. It would be possible to ascertain whether this assumption is valid for a particular reflecting surface only if a target with discontinuous punctate mires were used. This, however, would bring with it other problems, such as the accuracy of determination of mire position, that are avoided with the use of continuous rings of light. As the number of discrete points per unit of area increases, it becomes increasingly difficult to identify a specific point at the film plane relative to its origin on the target. As the reflecting surface becomes more irregular, the problem is compounded.

Another major problem in the analysis of keratoscope images is that the accuracy of the reconstruction algorithm is not the only determinant of spatial resolution. The reconstruction algorithm only provides a set of corneal profile elevations from a plane relative to the corneal apex, or other reference point, down to the corneal surface. Other determinants include the geometry of the mire pattern and the density of the surface samples analyzed for reconstruction, which determine the transverse spatial resolution. In general, the more mires that are used, the greater the resolution and the greater the surface area of the cornea that contributes to the surface reconstruction. The ideal target would provide sufficient resolution to detect surface irregularities just large enough to degrade visual function. Unfortunately, this resolution is still to be determined because of imperfect measures of visual performance and an incomplete understanding of the integrative and processing characteristics of the macula, central nervous system, and other components of the visual system in relation to the optical contribution of the cornea.

Related to the topic of spatial resolution is the practical question of the degree of resolution that is needed for the peripheral cornea relative to the central cornea. Under very dim illumination it is possible that the entire corneal surface may contribute to image formation. Under normal ambient lighting, however, the diameter of the virtual pupil in humans is approximately 4.5 mm. Therefore, for tests of macular function it may only be necessary to consider the central region of the cornea in the formation of a crisp image on the retina. Even within the virtual pupil, it is unknown whether all areas of the cornea participate equally in the formation of the retinal image.[6–9] It follows that in determining the level of spatial resolution of the keratoscope necessary to provide accurate reconstruction, the spatial resolution of the measuring system should probably be greatest for the central cornea and may suffer degradation in the periphery without loss of information that is essential for predicting visual function. This empirical reasoning accounts for the design of systems that produce reconstructions from keratoscopes with mires that are spatially denser in the center of the cornea than in the periphery.

Keratoscope Data Acquisition

The initial step in reconstruction of the three-dimensional corneal contour from keratoscope images is to determine and store the positions of all data points on the mires. The resolution of the data capturing technique determines the accuracy of all subsequent data manipulations and ultimately that of the corneal reconstruction. Manual digitization is the method used in the Louisiana State University Corneal Topography System (LSUCTS).[10,11] For keratoscope photographs, 500 lines per frame resolution corresponds with 30 μ of positional accuracy on the corneal surface; 1000 lines per frame, 15 μ; and 2000 lines per frame, 7.5 μ.[11] For a 40-diopter (D) surface, these accuracies correspond with resolutions of 1.2, 0.6, and 0.3 D, respectively. The HIPAD (Houston Instruments, Austin, TX) manual digitizing instrument used with the LSUCTS is capable of a resolution of 2000 lines per frame. Manual digitization is tedious, however, and makes timely clinical application difficult. The Corneal Modeling System (CMS) (Computed Anatomy, Inc., New York, NY) uses an automated digitization system with approximately 500 lines per frame resolution. However, this device employs statistical procedures to achieve subpixel resolution for accuracies of less than 0.25 D. Digitization and mire identification with the CMS are automatic and the process can be monitored by the operator for quality control. As each ring is identified, its position is made to overlay the original image so that the operator can easily observe situations where the mires are too confused for reasonable identification.

Reference System for Keratoscope Image Analysis

In order to transform keratoscope data into three-dimensional representations of the corneal surface, it is necessary to adopt a reference system so that the position of each data point can be mathematically identified and preferably related to an ocular feature such as the visual axis or corneal apex. In most cases, a system has been adopted such that the center of the innermost mire on the keratoscope is the reference point used to specify the position of all other points. Since even normal corneal topography is characterized by asymmetry and asphericity, this reference point is somewhat arbitrary and only coincidentally may approximate the visual axis, the geometric center of the cornea, or the apex of the cornea. Because the geographic area of an individual cornea that participates in the formation of an image consistent with the best spectacle-corrected visual acuity is frequently not centered on any of these landmarks, it would seem to be appropriate to select the most convenient reference point. This central position can conveniently be calculated as the centroid of the corneal surface area enclosed by the first keratoscope mire.[10] A more rigorous approximation involves a repetitive computational procedure that determines the geometrically averaged center of the innermost mire from center coordinates of best-fitting circles for individual 10° arcs around the innermost mire.[11] A more precise determination such as this is essential for accurate approximation of the central corneal power from keratoscope photographs produced with the PKS 1000 (Nidek, Palo Alto, CA) (Fig. 1.2) and the Corneascope (I.D.I., Inc., New York, NY). This is necessary because the central mires of these instruments are relatively large and a central reference illumination spot is absent. Recently introduced autokeratoscopes such as the collimated device used in the CMS (Fig. 1.3) have largely obviated the necessity for computational center approximations by projecting a central mire as small as 0.7 mm in diameter and by providing a reflection of the reference fixation light at the center of the mire pattern. The validity of this fixation light reflection as a reference point depends to a certain degree on accurate fixation by the patient and proper alignment of the instrument. Given these limitations, the reference point determined by each of these methods appears to fulfill the critical requirement for repeatability that allows longitudinal precision in the assessment of corneal shape essential for tasks such as monitoring the stability of corneal refractive manipulations.

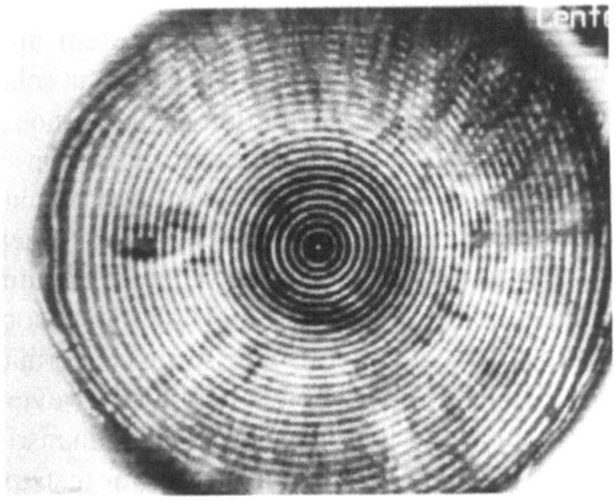

FIGURE 1.3. Videokeratoscope image of the collimated keratoscope of the Corneal Modeling System. Note the relatively small central mires and the reflection of the reference fixation light at the center of the mire pattern.

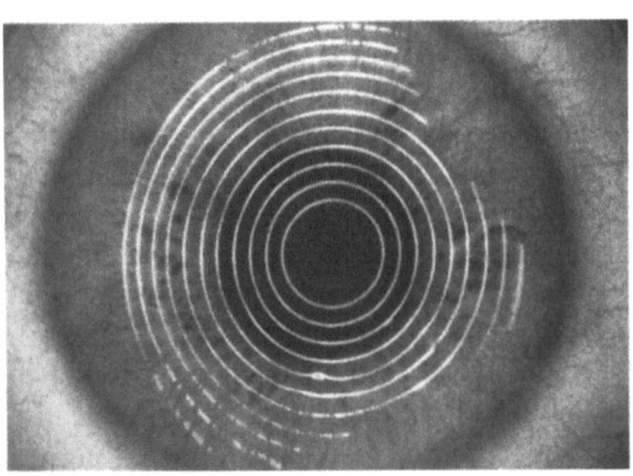

FIGURE 1.2. A Nidek PKS 1000 photokeratoscope photograph. Note the relatively large central mires and the absence of a central reference illumination spot.

Once a reference point has been established, conversion of rectangular coordinates of data points on the keratoscope mires to polar coordinates facilitates corneal reconstruction. For all currently available computer-assisted topography systems, this conversion is performed along hemimeridians extending from the central reference point to the periphery. The LSUCTS and the CMS analyze 180 and 256 equally spaced hemimeridians, respectively. Each data point converted to polar coordinates is determined by the intersection of a hemimeridian with a keratoscope mire. Thus, the theoretical number of data points used in reconstruction is equal to the product of the number of hemimeridians analyzed and the number of mires projected by the keratoscope. In reality, the number of data points included for an individual analysis can be significantly fewer than the theoretical, due to lid positions and gross distortion of mires by surface irregularities.

Reconstruction Algorithms

Once the mire position data have been obtained, the three-dimensional corneal shape is formulated according to a reconstruction algorithm that is specific, device dependent, and nontrivial, although a few generalizations can be made. Two principal assumptions used in algorithms for the reconstruction of corneal shape from keratoscope images have been noted above. These are (1) that the corneal apex coincides with the optical axis of the keratoscope image and (2) that there is no circumferential tilt of the corneal surface, so that light arising from one meridian on the keratoscope target is always reflected at the same meridian in the photograph's virtual image. Although these assumptions are valid only for spherical surfaces and do not yield exact results for the asymmetric and aspheric cornea, they are at present necessary to allow surface reconstruction from keratoscope images without imposing excessive computational burdens on computers that are of a size that is realistic for clinical applications. Yet, as will be discussed in a later section, validation of specific approaches has been a problem. This is primarily because analytical keratoscopy is difficult to verify because the method has a potential resolution far greater than that of industrial techniques for creating defined aspheric surfaces.

Three general approaches formulated for reconstructing the corneal surface from photokeratoscope data are described in the following sections along with the limitations of each method. Different approaches adopted for transformation algorithms require additional assumptions that vary depending on the specific method. In addition, the physical characteristics of the keratoscope that is used influence the algorithm derived to make the transformation to the three-dimensional surface. Detailed analytical expressions are not provided here because they are beyond the scope of this chapter and because they are of necessity dependent on the specific device, but an example for the LSUCTS has been published.[10]

Two-Step Profile Method

Algorithms that compare the diameters of individual keratoscope mires reflected from the corneal surface to mires obtained from calibration spheres were developed by Townsley.[12] For example, if keratoscope ring 4 reflected from the corneal surface has a diameter consistent with the diameter of a 39 D spherical reflecting reference, then the power at that point is designated as 39 D. This method assumed that the images of all the rings are focused at a fixed distance, that the instantaneous centers of curvature for all the reflecting points are on the optical axis, and that the surface is locally spherical. These assumptions are valid only for a globally spherical surface. When evaluating an aspheric surface such as the human cornea, the requirement for sphericity is relaxed for the calculation of the continuous surface. The validity of this method has yet to be verified. The combined effects of the two major assumptions of this approach would be likely to produce a disproportionate amount of error in the final reconstruction and would result in inaccurate modeling of asymmetric and aspheric corneas. It is important to note that many of the earlier attempts to develop corneal surface reconstruction algorithms had less ambitious goals than are currently needed, for instance, to help refine refractive surgical techniques. This aim requires a far greater precision in analysis than might be required, for example, in a difficult case of contact lens fitting.

One-Step Curve-Fitting Method

In this method, the geometry of the reflected mires is fit to a predetermined analytical formula such as a polynomial[13] and the conic curve family.[14,15] This, however, becomes a global constraint that results in a marked degradation of spatial resolution. Real corneas are asymmetric and aspherical, not spherical or ellipsoidal. When a corneal surface altered by surgery is analyzed, the use of a global model is both inappropriate and naive. Thus, algorithms that force the cornea to a shape conforming to such assumptions would lead to inaccurate reconstruction of the corneal surface.

R. Mammone[16] is investigating a refinement of this procedure in which a global geometric model is fit to the corneal shape at each meridian individually with allowance for local nonconformance. This novel approach, however, has not been tested.

One-Step Profile Method

Doss et al.[15] pioneered a potentially more accurate approach to corneal surface reconstruction that incorporates a successive approximation method based on the use of data arising from the central cornea to calculate corneal shape to the periphery in a given meridian. This method assumes that the curvature is constant between two adjacent points and allows a quasicontinuous variation in the corneal shape along a particular meridian. Two assumptions limit the accuracy of the approach[17]: (1) the individual radii of curvature at a point always project to the origin of the coordinate system, and (2) the radius of curvature in the center of the observed cornea is normalized to a standard 7.8-mm radius of curvature. These assumptions produce a system of equations that lacks sensitivity for the detection of variations in curvature normally occurring on the central corneal surface.

The accuracy of this approach was improved by allowing the centers of curvature to be at a point other than on the optical axis and through the use of a range-finding algorithm to calculate rather than assume the power of the innermost keratoscope ring.[10]

Recently, Wang et al.[17] further improved the accuracy of the latter approach for reconstructing radially aspheric surfaces. This new algorithm does not assume that the segment of surface curvature between the central reference point and the reflecting point on a particular mire has a constant curvature nor that the center of curvature of this segment lies at the central reference axis. The limitations of this method are an increase in required computational time and an increased sensitivity to noise, resulting in numerical instability when highly irregular surfaces are analyzed. Nevertheless, Wang et al.[17] found this new algorithm to be much more accurate in the reconstruction of a known ellipsoidal model, especially in the periphery, compared to the original LSUCTS algorithm.

Presentation of Corneal Topography

After the shape of the anterior corneal surface is reconstructed with a specific scheme, it is necessary to present the information in a manner that can be interpreted and applied clinically. Commonly used presentation methods that have been found to be less than optimal have included numerical power plots[18] and three-dimensional wire models.[10] More recently, color-coded topographic maps of corneal surface power have been used for the LSUCTS[11] and have been incorporated into the CMS (Fig. 1-4).[19] These presentation schemes allow the identification of anomalous corneal surface patterns and facilitate understanding of correlations between topography and clinical findings.

Validity of Computer-Assisted Corneal Topographic Analysis

Ultimately, it is necessary that the accuracy of the topographic instrument in producing a reconstruction of the corneal surface be validated. Although this would appear to be straightforward, in reality it is an exceedingly difficult proposition. The difficulty is attributable to the lack of technology for constructing known asymmetric and aspheric reference model surfaces from stable material that adequately simulate the complex surfaces encountered during analysis of corneal shape. Studies using reference spheres[20] are a first step, but these inadequately test the accuracy and precision of the instruments for aspheric surfaces. Corneal topography analysis with the keratoscope has the potential to be an order of magnitude more accurate than models that might be

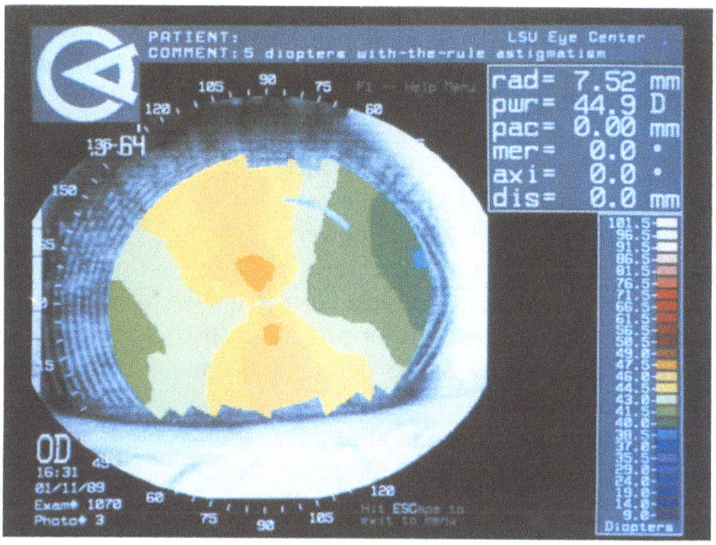

FIGURE 1.4. Color-coded topographic map from a normal cornea with 5 diopters of with-the-rule astigmatism.

machined or molded; therefore ultimate validation is not easily achieved.

Quantitative Descriptors of Corneal Contour

Although color-coded topographic maps 1) allow inspection of a large proportion of the topography from the central to the peripheral cornea, 2) provide information regarding power domains on the corneal surface, 3) facilitate the identification of topographic patterns, and 4) provide an amount of quantitative data, the utility of the analysis could be extended if clinically relevant statistical descriptors of corneal shape were also available. Recently, significant progress has been made in developing useful parameters.[8,9,21,22]

Algorithms have been developed for determining the axis and power of the corneal cylinder. The simulated keratometry value (Sim K)[9] is calculated from an algorithm that determines the power and axis of the steepest and flattest meridians from rings 7, 8, and 9 of the CMS videokeratoscope. These rings were selected because they are at a position on the corneal surface that approximates the location at which the standard keratometer measurement is obtained. The power and axis of the computed values correlate well with keratometer measurements. There is also a good correlation with refractive cylinder and axis in cases where accurate keratometer measurements cannot be obtained due to surface irregularity. Sim K power and axis of the steepest meridian are provided along with both the power of the axis 90° away and the power and axis of the flattest meridian irrespective of the angle between the steepest and flattest meridians.

A parameter of corneal topography predictive of the best spectacle-corrected visual acuity, given an otherwise normal visual system, would be efficacious. The search for such a diagnostic tool led to the development of quantitative predictors. The first predictor was a centrally weighted measure of corneal surface symmetry (surface asymmetry index, SAI) and was found to have significant value in predicting best spectacle-corrected visual acuity in a retrospective study.[22] A more powerful predictor, the surface regularity index (SRI), which considered the localized surface regularity within the central area of the cornea, was subsequently developed.[9] SRI was found, in a prospective study, to have a higher correlation with best spectacle-corrected visual acuity.[9] Outliers in SRI were found, however, in corneas that had pronounced asymmetry with a better spectacle-corrected visual acuity than was predicted by the SRI value. These corneas were usually found in individuals with keratoconus or contact lens warpage. The better-than-predicted visual acuity appeared to be attributable to localized paracentral areas of relatively uniform power on an otherwise irregular corneal surface. With the SRI, potential acuity is correlated with the most frequent population of corneal surface powers. In the prospective study,[9] the correlation between this parameter and best spectacle-corrected visual acuity was higher than for previous estimators of the quality of the corneal surface such as the SAI.

In the near future, quantitative parameters such as these should be incorporated into commercially available corneal topographic instruments such as the CMS.

Alternative Technologies for Corneal Surface Reconstruction

Holography, raster stereo photogrammetry, scanning laser range finders, and optical interferometry have been suggested as alternative methods for making direct measurements of corneal surface contour with high accuracy and precision. Thus far, these alternatives have not been widely used in commercially available instruments, primarily because of limitations in the transverse resolution of the measurements. With time it is possible that these or other methods will be successfully applied to the problem of corneal surface reconstruction, but for the moment traditional keratoscopy approaches with computer reconstruction appear to the only methods generally available.

References

1. Dabezies OH, Holladay JT. Measurement of corneal curvature: Keratometer (ophthalmometer). In: Dabezies OH, Jr., Cavanagh HD, Farris RL, et al, eds. *Contact Lenses: The CLAO Guide to Basic Science and Clinical Practice*. Orlando, FL: Grune and Stratton, 1986; pp 17.1–17.29.
2. Mandell RB, St. Helen R. Mathematical model of corneal contour. *Br J Physiol Opt*. 1971; 26:183–196.
3. Mandell RB. Methods to measure the peripheral corneal curvature. Part two: geometric construction and "computers." *J Am Optom Assoc*. 1962;34:585–589.
4. Mandell RB. *Contact Lens Practice*. 3rd ed. Springfield, IL: Charles C Thomas, 1984; p 62–87.
5. Dingeldein SA, Klyce SD. The topography of normal corneas. *Arch Ophthalmol*. 1989;107:512–518.
6. McDonnell PJ, Garbus J, Lopez PF. Topographic analysis and visual acuity after radial keratotomy. *Am J Ophthalmol*. 1988;106:692–695.
7. Wilson SE, Klyce SD. Topographic analysis and visual acuity after radial keratotomy (Correspondence). *Am J Ophthalmol*. 1989;107:436–437.
8. Klyce SD, Wilson SE, Pittman SD, et al. Estimation of potential visual acuity from corneal shape. *Invest Ophthalmol Vis Sci* (suppl). 1989;30:218.
9. Wilson SE, Klyce SD. Quantitative descriptors of corneal topography. A clinical study. *Arch Ophthalmol* 1991;109:349–353.
10. Klyce SD. Computer-assisted corneal topography: High resolution graphic presentation and analysis of keratoscopy. *Invest Ophthalmol Vis Sci*. 1984;25:1426–1435.
11. Maguire LJ, Singer DE, Klyce SD. Graphic presentation of computer-analyzed keratoscope photographs. *Arch Ophthalmol*. 1987;105:223–230.
12. Townsley GM. New equipment and methods for determining the contour of the human cornea. *Contacto*. 1967;11:72–81.
13. Edmund C, Sjontoft E. The central-peripheral radius of the normal corneal curvature: a photokeratoscopic study. *Acta Ophthalmol*. 1981;99:1261–1265.
14. El Hage SG. Suggested new methods for photokeratoscopy: a comparison for their validities—Part I. *Am J Optom Arch Am Acad Optom*. 1971;26:183–193.
15. Doss JD, Hutson RL, Rowsey JJ, et al. Method for calculation of corneal profile and power distribution. *Arch Ophthalmol*. 1981;99:1261–1265.
16. Mammone RJ, Gersten M, Gormley DJ, et al. 3-D corneal modeling system. *IEEE Trans Biomed Eng*. 1990;37:66–72.
17. Wang J, Rice DA, Klyce SD. A new reconstruction algorithm for improvement of corneal topographical analysis. *Refract Corneal Surg*. 1989;5:379–387.

18. Rowsey JJ, Reynolds AE, Brown DR. Corneal topography. Corneascope. *Arch Ophthalmol.* 1981;99:1093–1100.
19. Gormley DJ, Gersten M, Koplin RS, et al. Corneal modeling. *Cornea*. 1988;7:30–35.
20. Hannush SB, Waring GO. Computer assisted corneal topography: accuracy and reproducibility with three instruments. *Invest Ophthalmol Vis Sci* (suppl). 1988;29:389.
21. Dingeldein SA, Pittman SD, Wang J, et al. Analysis of corneal topographic data. *Invest Ophthalmol Vis Sci* (suppl). 1988;29:389.
22. Dingeldein SA, Klyce SD, Wilson SE. Quantitative descriptors of corneal shape derived from the computer-assisted analysis of photokeratographs. *Refract Corneal Surg*. 1989;5:372–378.

2
The Computerized Corneal Topographer (EH-270)

Sami G. El Hage

The importance of the cornea is that its dioptric power represents about three quarters of the refractive power of the eyeball. In consequence, we can imagine the important role the cornea can play in the formation of the retinal image, and thus we see the necessity of a deeper study of its geometrical form.

With the discovery of the polymers and the diversity of their use, in particular in the field of vision, contact lenses have brought up as many problems as they have been able to resolve. With recent advances in refractive surgery, the predictability of the results remains unknown. It has been at least three centuries since the first attempt to measure the anterior surface of the cornea; however, the exact form of this surface has remained almost unknown.

All the corneal measurements realized so far have been based on the optical property that considers the cornea as a reflective surface (a convex mirror). On the other hand, the proceedings of measurement are numerous and different. They consist generally in measuring the size of an object of a mire reflected from the cornea. The stereophotogrametry is a method of measurement with tridimensional coordinates, similar to the one use for aerial photography, where one draws the lines of the level of the cornea.

In spite of the diversity of the described methods, we can classify them under two large headings: (1) direct optical measurements, and (2) photographic measurements.

Direct Optical Measurements

At the beginning of the 17th century the Jesuit priest Christopher Scheiner[1] tried to measure the cornea by putting several convex mirrors next to the eye of the subject until he found two equal images. Kohlraush[2] in 1839 measured directly the image of the reflected object on the cornea, using the Kepler telescope. Senff[3] in 1846 used a method similar to that of Kohlrausch and found the cornea to be an ellipsoid.

Helmholtz[4] (1854) was the first to introduce the doubling device in his ophthalmometer with fixed mires. Coccius[5] (1867), Landolt[6] (1878), Javal and Schiotz[7] (1881), Sutcliffe[8] (1907), and Hartinger[9] (1935) suggested different measuring devices. Fincham[10] (1925) was the first to measure directly the corneal periphery using an autocollimation microscope. Berg[11] (1929) modified the Javal–Schiotz ophthalmometer by putting in front of it a set of two lenses forming an afocal system of magnification. He was able to explore a zone of 1 mm diameter, from which he measured the corneal periphery.

Mandell[12] (1962) modified the Bausch and Lomb keratometer by drilling apertures into the mire target with a predetermined distance. He put a prism of 2.25 behind the standard doubling system. The fixation points observed by the subjects are located at 2.5 degrees distance. The corneal zone thus explored was approximately 1 mm in diameter.

Bonnet[13] (1960) used an ophthalmometer with the same structure as the Zeiss, where the mire objects are in the focus plan of two symmetric collimators. He modified the doubling system so that the apparatus works in the same manner as a classical ophthalmometer by doubling the image of one mire. In the latter case, he explored a zone 0.5 mm in diameter.

Photographic Measurements

In 1896, Gullstrand[14] opened the era of photokeratoscopy. He used the Placido disk[15] (1880) as an object. His work was followed by Fisher[16] (1927), Berg[17] (1929), Dekking[18] (1930), Amsler and Hartinger[19] (1930), Lenoble[20] (1952), Knoll, Stimson, and Weeks[21] (1952), Reynolds and Kratt[22] (1959), Knoll[23] (1961), Stone[24] (1962), Cochet and Amiard[25] (1966), Mandell[26] (1967), and El Hage[27] (1968). All of these scientists used an object derived from the Placido disk, having modified more or less judiciously its form in space to get more precision as far as the corneal periphery was concerned.

Ergellet[28] (1922) was the first to use photographic restitution in order to measure the corneal surface. He registered the points on the surface by sprinkling a powder. He regularly put through the spatial image of the cornea a parallel section to the plane at different distances.

He determined on each section the coordinates of a certain number of points of equal height. Theoretically, this procedure allows one to find the spatial coordinates of a certain number of points from any shape. This procedure was employed again by Kokott[29], Rzymkowsky[30] (1940), Bertotto[31] (1948), and, more recently, by Bonnet[32] (1959), who gave greater precision to the conditions of the shooting and of the restitution, thus improving the results.

However, in spite of the generality and the theoretical precision of this method, the information given is tarnished with errors due to (1) the anesthesia of the cornea, (2) vaporization of the talcum powder, which may either conceal some deformations or produce other irregularities, and (3) the mechanical separation of the eyelids.

Taking into account the fragile nature and losing of shape of the cornea, one can imagine in advance that the measured surface does not really correspond to the original corneal surface. I think these factors limit the usefulness of the method and make it lose its clinical and experimental value.

Principle of Measurement

In ophthalmometry, it is the normals between the incident and the reflected rays on two successive points on the corneal surface that determine the average curvature in the explored zone. To some extent, the smaller the explored area is, the greater the precision will be. Besides, the Gullstrand formula, which considers the cornea as a sphere, shows it very clearly. The precision of these instruments is determined by calibration on a steel ball of known radius.

In photokeratoscopy, the coordinates (x,y) of a point (incident rays) allow us to measure the photographed corneal element. The precision of the y measurement is of great importance because all the calculations that follow will depend on this experimental datum.

It is necessary to avoid misfocusing and to take into consideration the aberrations that can be present in the optical system and those in the cornea.

From y, one gets x. Having a certain number of x's and y's on a meridian, one can draw the curve of this section.

Analytic Study

Berg reminds us that the points of measurement of the corneal curve cannot be infinitely brought together: this would not make any sense from the experimental point of view in spite of the analytic definition of the ray of curvature. Berg gives practical references on their separation.

For example, Gullstrand, in his measurement of the anterior surface of the cornea by a photographic method, chose a difference of angles between the normals of about 5 degrees. Erickson[33] chose a difference of coordinates of 1 mm in his corneal measurement with the Javal–Schiotz ophthalmometer. Because the validity of the Gullstrand formula cannot be fulfilled exactly, an error is generally associated with such computations. Consequently, to look for the direction and the approximate rates according to the conditions of errors is not without interest.

It is easy to find that for a circle of which the ray of curvature is constant, the Gullstrand formula is valid without approximation even for a finite distance of two successive points:

$$R = \frac{Y_2 - Y_1}{\sin \phi_2 - \sin \phi_1}$$

Berg attached great importance to the study of the errors of measurement, and he showed that the ray of curvature obtained by classical ophthalmometry did not correspond to the real ray of curvature of the explored zone, unless a correction factor was added to the Gullstrand formula. He supposed that the section of the corneal surface was an involute of a circle for the following reasons: (1) the common point between the two surfaces, ie, the increasing of the ray of curvature from the center to the periphery, and (2) the rigorous application of the Gullstrand formula.

Now if we consider the results in the case of a variable curvature through the involute method, the problem would be more complex. It is well known that the analytic expression of the ray of curvature is

$$R = \frac{ds}{dt},$$

where R = ray of curvature; t = angle of the tangent with the abscissa; and s = curvilinear abscissa.

One has for the involute of a circle

$$R = \frac{ds}{dt} = \sqrt{2rs},$$

or

$$dt = \frac{1}{\sqrt{2rs}}\, ds.$$

By integration one gets

$$t = \frac{1}{\sqrt{2r}} \int \frac{1}{\sqrt{s}}\, ds.$$

It would be interesting to take the problem in all its generality where R and r are not constant anymore, introducing the value $1/\sqrt{2r}$ into the integral, that takes then the following form:

$$t = \int \frac{1}{\sqrt{2r(s)}} \cdot \frac{1}{\sqrt{s}}\, ds.$$

At first it is nearly impossible to calculate this integral, which is a function of s (unknown). In this generality we do not possess sufficient information to resolve the equations; otherwise it is indispensable to know one of the two means consisting in finding the involute of the curve and the real form of the curve. But, after all, what interests us is to know the corneal shape. Therefore, I suggest the photokeratoscopic method, which could enable us to determine the corneal topography.

Photokeratoscopy

In photokeratoscopy, the virtual images created behind the cornea are reimaged in the film plane of a camera. From the magnitude of the image on the film, the magnitude of the image behind the cornea can be found. When the keratoscope is composed of several rings, we may compute the curvature of a spheric mirror from the distance of the ring from the cornea, the magnification of the virtual image, and finally the focal length of the camera objective. When the aperture of the objective is stopped down, the rings are imaged by a narrow pencil of rays. The narrow pencil of rays corresponds to the small part of the cornea, which contributes to the images of the ring. The width of the ring's image can be varied by the appropriate choice of the diameter and position of the rings. The method for evaluating the image on the film depends on the position of the aperture stop of the objective.

In this way corneal topography is possible.

The image position in the film plane is a function of the equation of the reflecting surface, the target locus, and camera characteristics. We can write a differential equation for the reflecting surface, but two assumptions are required. One is that the position of the chief ray is determined by the position of the image on the film. When the aperture of the objective is small, the spherical aberrations introduced by the reflecting surface in the meridian utilized lie in one plane. This assumption is valid for surfaces of revolution and in the case of regular astigmatism, in both principal meridians. The intersection of the two principal meridian planes determines the axis of the cornea. To find the differential equation of the cornea in such a meridional plane, meridional rays are traced.

In our system we use as a target a diffused rings keratoscope. The stop of the objective is not near the principal plane, as it is usually, but in the back focal plane. The entrance pupil, is, therefore, at infinity, and the chief rays reflected from the cornea are parallel to the optical axis. This new design has two important consequences.

First, normally the aperture stop is placed at the objective (Fig. 2.1) so that the height y is not recorded directly on the film, and the angle (Ø) that the chief ray forms with the optical axis is a factor in the analysis. In our instrument (Fig. 2.2) we obtain y directly on the film. Although slightly out of focus, it will have negligible effect on the photographed image height.

Second, the new system enables us to give a simpler form of differential equation. Moreover, we propose a numerical method for solving this equation.

The New Differential Equation

The new differential equation was presented in a previous paper.[27] It is

$$\frac{dy}{dx} = -\frac{a - x}{b - y} + \sqrt{1 + \left(\frac{a - x}{b - y}\right)^2} \qquad (2.1)$$

where

a = the distance of the rings from origin 0.0,
b = the distance from the optic axis to the photokeratoscope ring,
y = the distance from the optic axis to image,
x = unknown to be determined (Fig. 2.2)

The differential equation contains, besides the dependent variable x, its first derivative x', and the independent variable y two further magnitudes, a and b. These are two functions, $a\ (y)$, and $b\ (y)$, which must be determined experimentally.

For each ring a_i and b_i we find a ring image on the film y_i. So the experiment gives a number of triples (a_i, b_i, y_i). When a_i and b_i are plotted as a function of y_i, we find two curves $a(y)$ and $b(y)$, for which a polynomial interpolation within the accuracy of the measurement can give an analytical form.

Placing the two functions $a(y)$ and $b(y)$ in the righthand side of equation (2.1) gives a differential equation of the form:

$$x' = f(x,y) \qquad (2.2)$$

The values of the function $f(x,y)$ are determined experimentally. For a spherical surface

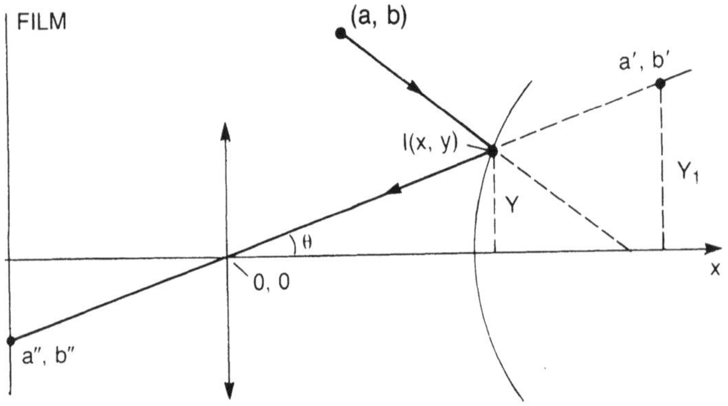

FIGURE 2.1. The diaphragm stop placed at the objective. (From Ref. 34, with permission.)

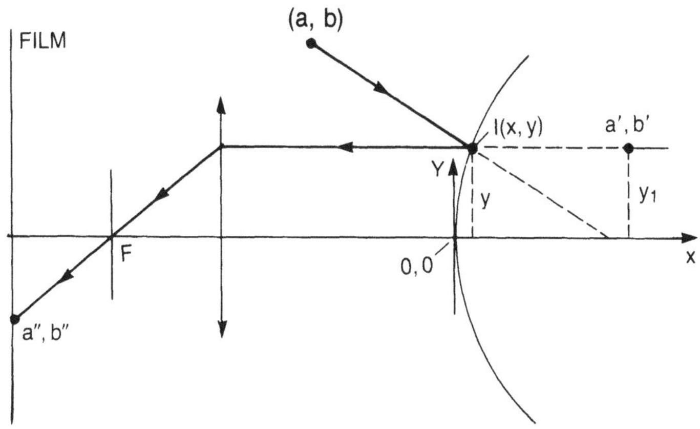

FIGURE 2.2. The diaphragm stop placed in the back focus plane and coordinate system for the differential equation. (From Ref. 34, with permission.)

and for a given radius b, the function $a(y)$ can be calculated. Let R_0 be the radius of the sphere and the angle formed by the normal to the optical axis (Fig. 2.3).

The following formula results:

$$\sin \emptyset = y/R_0$$
$$x = R_0\,(1 - \cos \emptyset)$$
$$a = x - (b - y)\,\mathrm{cotg}\,2\emptyset$$

For certain values of R_0 and b = 75 mm, the function $a(y)$ is plotted in Fig. 2.4.

Solving the New Differential Equation

By construction the position of the keratoscope rings a_i, and measuring y_i the ring images on the film, we obtain a relation between a_i and y_i. The numerical relation can be transformed to an analytical one by fitting a polynomial interpolation $a(y)$ to the measured curve with the least squared method or any other appropriate method. If the keratoscopic ring radii b_c are not equal, the function $a(y)$ and $b(y)$ may be inserted in equation (2.1).

The result is a differential equation of the form $x' = f(x,y)$, where

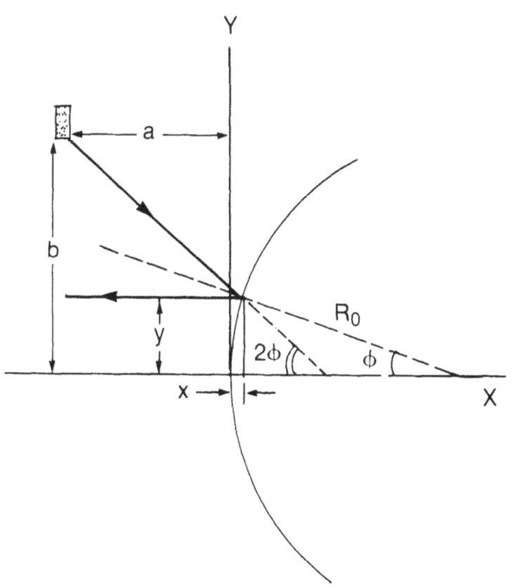

FIGURE 2.3. Chief incident ray from an object (a,b) and reflected from a sphere of radius R_g. (From Ref. 34 with permission.)

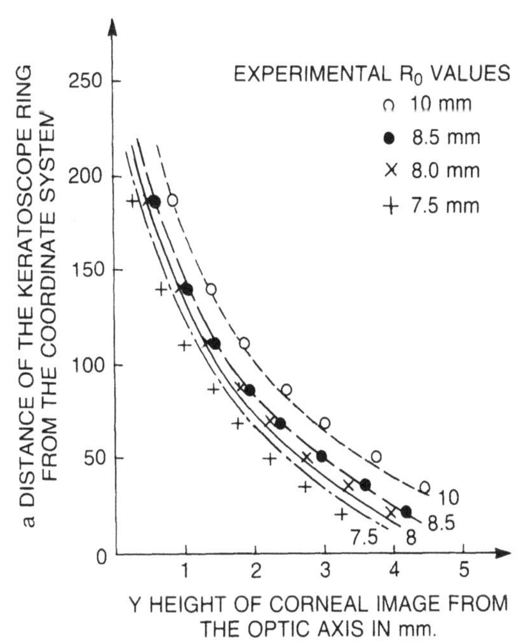

FIGURE 2.4. The experimentally determined $a(y)$ for spheres of radii R_0: 7.5 mm + 8.0 mm × 8.5 mm ● 10.0 mm o and b = 75 mm. The curves are theoretical computer calculated data. (From Ref. 34, with permission.)

$$f(x,y) = \frac{a(y) - x}{b(y) - y} + \sqrt{1 + \left(\frac{a(y) - x}{b(y) - y}\right)^2} \quad (2.3)$$

is a well-defined function.

The function $x(y)$ can be presented in tabular or graphic form.

Equation (2.3) is a first-order differential equation. The solution of such a differential equation contains an arbitrary parameter. One point on the solution curve must be known to start the integration. The point should be in the neighborhood of the vertex of the cornea. This could be done by determining the vertex position of the cornea from the radius of the smallest ring image used (Fig. 2.4). The starting point for integration is then assumed to lie on that sphere.

The Photokeratoscope (EHP)

The photokeratoscope (EHP) was based on a telecentric system. The object was composed of 10 plastic diffusing rings. Although my analysis method did not depend on the image of the rings on the keratogram being equidistant, I preferred to ensure this equidistance in order to obtain regular distribution of the rings over the quasi-totality of the cornea.

An electronic ring flash (type 250w multiblitz) was used as the source. It was positioned between the camera and the first ring. A light was required for photography to reach the posterior surface of the rings. The camera, with an objective corrected for all aberrations, including distortion, was an Alpa type reflex. The distance between the subject's cornea and the camera was calculated so that the keratogram was identical to the object.

The major difficulty was precisely positioning the subject's eye axially as well as transversely. In order to do this, two test projectors were used. They were inclined to the instrument axis so that the two mires were superimposed on the corneal vertex plane, which was the conjugate point of the film. When the cornea was positioned properly, the two mires were coincident. The precision of corneal position was within 0.2 mm. Another difficulty was ensuring that the mechanical axis of the ring support coincided with the optical axis of the camera objective. This was accomplished by centering the ring support mounting on the objective. To maintain coincidence, the complete ring cylinder could be adjusted by means of three screws with the aid of an auxiliary reticle centered on the corneal side of the first ring.

The EHP was mounted on an adjustable base that permitted movements in horizontal, lateral, and vertical directions. The patient was placed in a chin rest and observed a 1 mm fiber-optic luminous point. The fiber optic was placed so that did not interfere with the photographed rings. This photkeratoscope has three major advantages:

1. reduction of geometrical aberrations through the use of a small aperture objective, and correct localization of the corneal vertex plane using the two complementary systems;
2. adjustable fixation point positioned where it does not cause obturation zones; and
3. maneuverability of the apparatus in all three directions (the patient was stationary).

Through continuous research and with the creation of the personal computer, it becomes feasible to fully automate the EHP and come up with a faster, easy-to-use, and on-line real-time corneal topographer.

The Computerized Corneal Topographer (EH-270)

The computerized Corneal Topographer (EH-270) is an on-line, near real-time corneal topography analyzer. It projects 22 rings onto the cornea and covers from 0.37 mm for the smaller central corneal diameter to 10+ mm on the peripheral corneal diameter, depending on the shape of the cornea. It is important to note that by itself, the number of rings has no real value. What is important to know is how many of the projected rings are really imaged, and even more important with what accuracy are these rings measured (Fig. 2.5). Typical measurements are done on 36 semimeridians. One

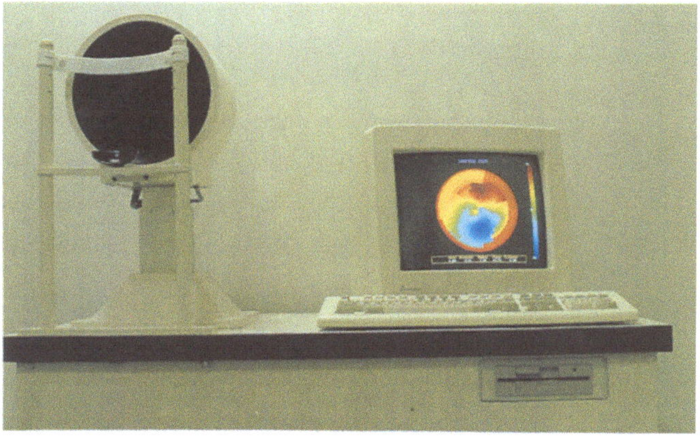

FIGURE 2.5. The computerized Corneal Topographer (EH-270) is an on-line, near real-time instrument. Corneal measurements are obtained in less than 1/2 min.

can measure more semimeridians (up to 360) if need be. Minimally more than 700 data points are calculated and converted into a three-dimensional configuration of the cornea. Tabulation formats can also be obtained and data can also be stored in a memory bank. No assumption is made on the topographical measurements. Auto-positioning is incorporated in the Corneal Topographer to improve accuracy and repeatability of corneal measurements. The reflected image is then enhanced for maximum contrast. The position of the corneal vertex plane is determined; then the data along each meridian are extracted. The positions of each ring for each meridian and the distance of each ring from the corneal center are also determined.

The software consists of a system control program, topographic analysis display system, topographical data, archival and retrieval system, a sophisticated user interface, an operating system, an image digitizer, a graphic controller, a pointing device, and diagnostics. The total software system is menu-driven.

First this data is fit to a high-order polynomial for each meridian. Then each datum is integrated to determine the three-dimensional configuration of the cornea along each meridian. If desired, this can be compared to a sphere for demonstration purpose. The time for the analysis is 21 s and the accuracy of the Computerized Corneal Topographer is ± 0.25 dt as seen in Table 2.1.

Video Displays

Zooming

The photokeratogram can be zoomed by selecting Display/Zoom image from the menu. The practitioner can then scrutinize the cornea by enlarging the corneal image on the screen of the monitor. The cornea may be enlarged two, four, or eight times, so that a small area on the cornea of about 0.5 mm square can be enlarged to fill the entire screen of the monitor. The corneal image may also be panned, or scrolled around the screen of the monitor (Figs. 2.6 and 2.7).

Several displays are available in the main menu. All displays are color-coded to aid in their interpretation. The color code adopted in this instrument is based on the "Visibility Spectrum Color"—that is, the blue color for the short radius of curvature (short wavelength, steep cornea) and red the color for the long radius of curvature (long wavelength, flat cornea). A simple keystroke can reverse this system. Nearly any desired color scheme can be programmed into the displays.

Corneal Contour

The first color-coded display shows the Corneal Contour Map (Fig. 2.8). The graph shows the cornea from the vertex plane. Color at the red end of the spectrum shows areas where this

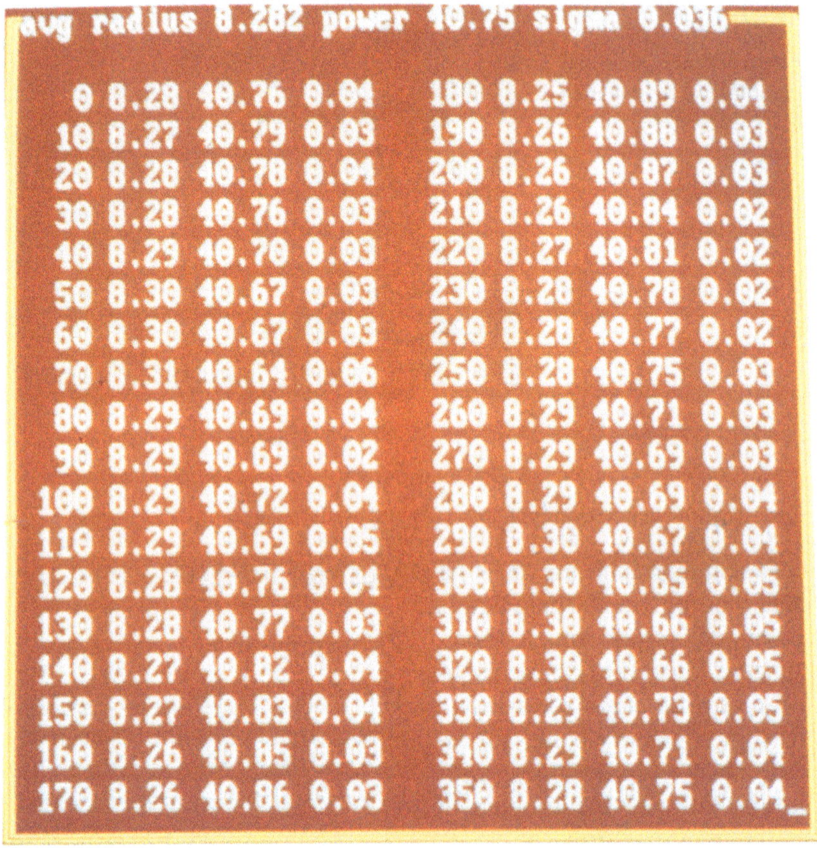

avg radius 8.282 power 40.75 sigma 0.036

0	8.28	40.76	0.04	180	8.25	40.89	0.04
10	8.27	40.79	0.03	190	8.26	40.88	0.03
20	8.28	40.78	0.04	200	8.26	40.87	0.03
30	8.28	40.76	0.03	210	8.26	40.84	0.02
40	8.29	40.70	0.03	220	8.27	40.81	0.02
50	8.30	40.67	0.03	230	8.28	40.78	0.02
60	8.30	40.67	0.03	240	8.28	40.77	0.02
70	8.31	40.64	0.06	250	8.28	40.75	0.03
80	8.29	40.69	0.04	260	8.29	40.71	0.03
90	8.29	40.69	0.02	270	8.29	40.69	0.03
100	8.29	40.72	0.04	280	8.29	40.69	0.04
110	8.29	40.69	0.05	290	8.30	40.67	0.04
120	8.28	40.76	0.04	300	8.30	40.65	0.05
130	8.28	40.77	0.03	310	8.30	40.66	0.05
140	8.27	40.82	0.04	320	8.30	40.66	0.05
150	8.27	40.83	0.04	330	8.29	40.73	0.05
160	8.26	40.85	0.03	340	8.29	40.71	0.04
170	8.26	40.86	0.03	350	8.28	40.75	0.04

TABLE 2.1. Means and standard deviation of a calibrated steel ball of 40.50 D. Note: The accuracy in 99% of the measurements is within one quarter of a diopter.

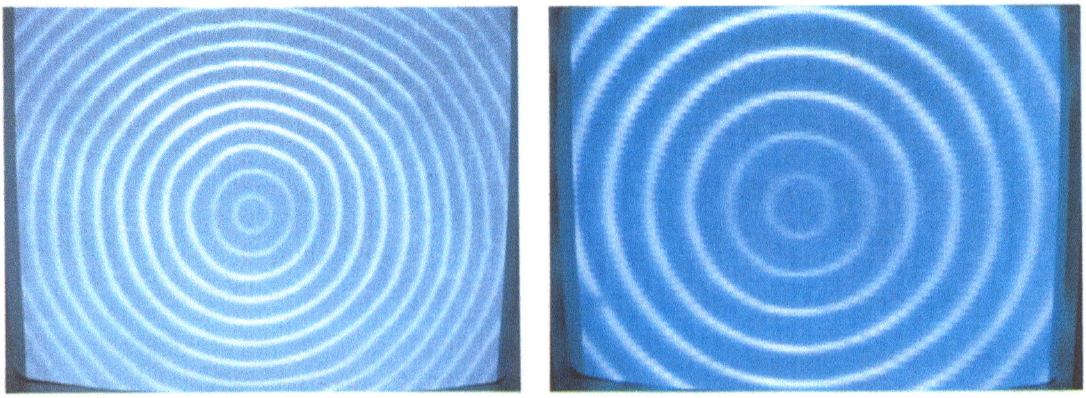

FIGURE 2.6. and 2.7. Zooming and scrolling are other features of the instrument. Practitioners may magnify an area smaller than 1 mm to fill the entire screen.

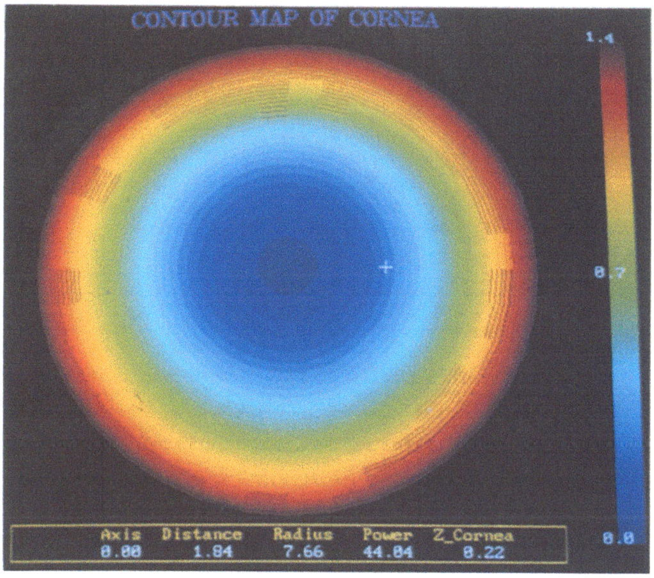

FIGURE 2.8. The color coding used in this display and all others is based on the "Visibility Spectrum Color." This is a plot of the z axis, in which the red shows the area where the distance from the corneal vertex plane, is greatest.

distance is greatest. A white cursor, initially in the center of the graph, may be moved in any direction using the keyboard. The location of the cursor, in terms of distance from the center as well as azimuthial angle, is presented in a box at the bottom of the graph along with the corneal height, radius of curvature, and dioptric power at that location.

Meridional Contour

A cross-sectional view of the cornea through any desired meridian is obtained by selecting the Meridional Contour menu entry. This display will enable the practitioner to choose the desired meridian (eg, 0°–180°). The cursor will then indicate on any given location the dioptric power, the curvature in millimeters, the distance from the center of the cornea, the z value, and the semimeridian on which the cursor is positioned. All this information is displayed on the bottom of the screen (Fig. 2.9).

Astigmatism

Corneal astigmatism can be calculated for any given two meridians, from the center to the periphery. A white cursor, initially in the center of the graph, may be moved to the left or the right of the graph. The box at the bottom of the graph will display automatically the location on the cornea, the amount of astigmatism, and the calculated meridian. The square box in the middle of the screen shows the average astigmatism, the central astigmatism, the astigmatism at 3 mm and at 6 mm from the center of the cornea. Astigmatism is available in both dioptric power and millimeters (Fig. 2.10).

Overlay Image

Another option on the menu is Overlay Image, an overview of corneal astigmatism. By selecting this option, the principal axis of astigmatism for each reflected ring will be overlaid on the corneal image. For each complete ring, 18 ring diameters are calculated and compared. A line is drawn through the minimum diameter as well as the maximum diameter. The angles of these diameters are tabulated along the right-hand side of the screen (for reference, Fig. 2.11). This display demonstrates that corneal astigmatism is not necessarily uniform (as in keratometry) over the entire surface of the cornea, but varies according to the location on the cornea.

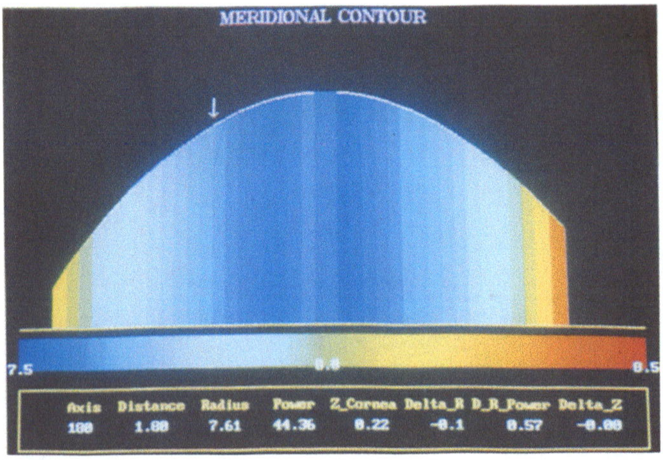

FIGURE 2.9. This is a cross section of the cornea on a particular meridian chosen by the practitioner. In this case, it is the axis 30°–210.° The bottom box shows the axis on which the cursor is located, the distance from the center, the radius of curvature in millimeters, the power of the cornea, and the *z* of the cornea. Also, the difference between the osculatory circle, the radius of curvature, the power, and the *z* of the cornea can be shown.

Three-Dimensional Display

A three-dimensional graph of the cornea may be displayed for an overview. This graph can be rotated in 10° steps, thus practitioners can view the cornea from a different angel (Fig. 2.12).

Dioptric Plot

A dioptric plot of the cornea may be obtained from the main menu. The same white cursor used in all the displays may be moved in any direction using the keyboard. The location of the cursor, in terms of distance from the center as well as azimuthial angle, is presented in a box at the bottom of the graph along with the difference the cornea makes with the oscullatory circle at any given location. The color code of the plot can, at a glance, show the practitioner where the steep and flat areas are located on the cornea. For example, in a normal cornea the central portion will be blue, the intermediate yellow/green, and the periphery red (Fig. 2.13).

Inflection Graph

The inflection point graph of the cornea may also be displayed. The dioptric value differential between two points on a given meridian can be changed to the practitioner's needs, so

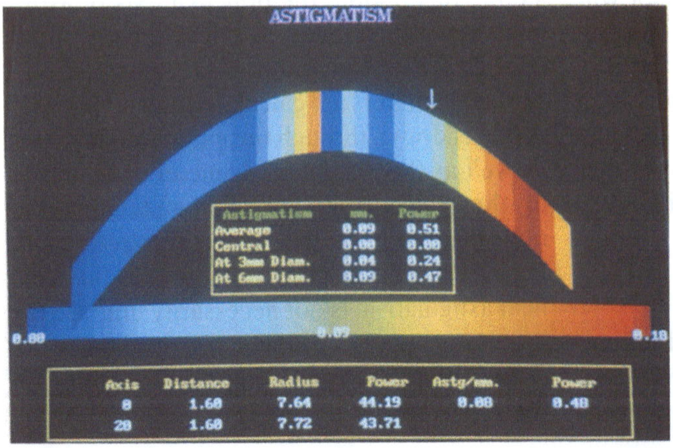

FIGURE 2.10. The practitioner has the option to select any two meridians on the cornea to determine the astigmatism along the axis of the meridian, ie, from the center to the periphery on any position. In this particular case, the meridians are 0–180° and 20°–200.° The central box shows the average astigmatism along these meridians, the central astigmatism, at 3 mm and at 6 mm from the center. The lower box shows the axis on which the measurements are taken, the position of the measurements (how far from the center), the radii of curvature in millimeters, the surface powers in diopters, and the astigmatism both in millimeters and diopters.

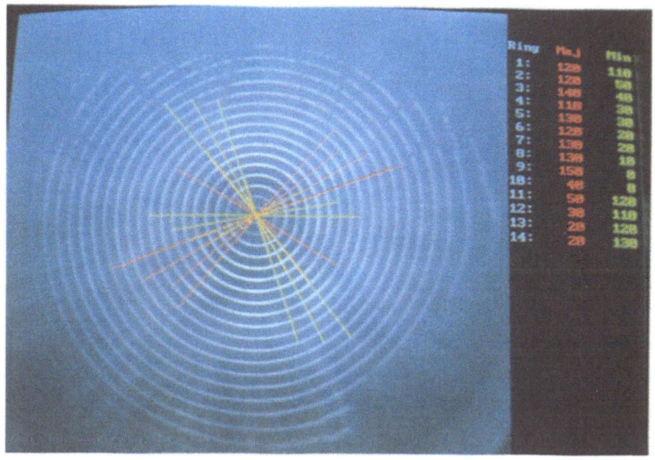

FIGURE 2.11. The overlay display shows at a glance the axis of astigmatism for different locations on the cornea. The smallest area measured is less than 0.5 mm depending on the shape of the cornea. This figure shows that corneal astigmatism is not necessarily uniform over the entire surface of the cornea.

that many configurations can be seen and the desired one chosen. This display may have a particular use in relaxing incisions and in identifying positions on the surface of the cornea where the changing curvature is the greatest (Fig. 2.14).

Clinical Applications

The following are few of many clinical applications of corneal topography

1. The data are in a format that can be a part of the information presented in the treatment plan to the patient. Corneal topography can be recorded for comparative change before and after surgery. The storage of this information can be on a hard disk, a floppy disk, or in a tabulation format on a print-out.
2. New laser techniques used in refractive surgery will require the accurate knowledge of corneal topography.
3. Surgeons who perform refractive proce-

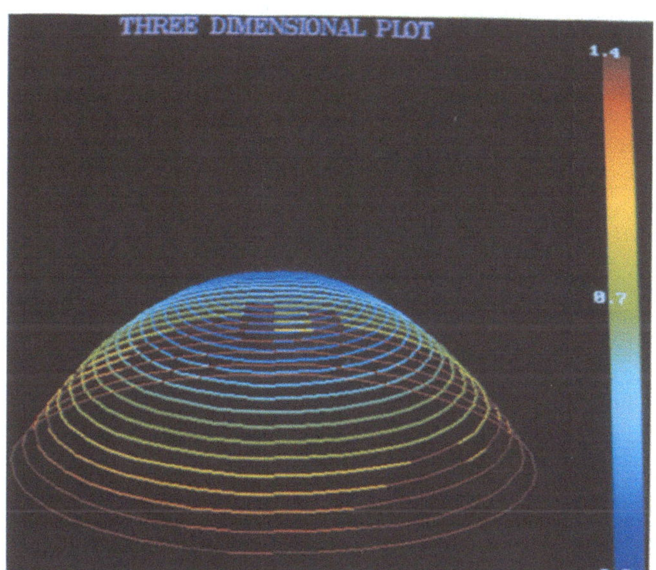

FIGURE 2.12. A three-dimensional graph of the cornea can be displayed and rotated in 10° increments for general observation.

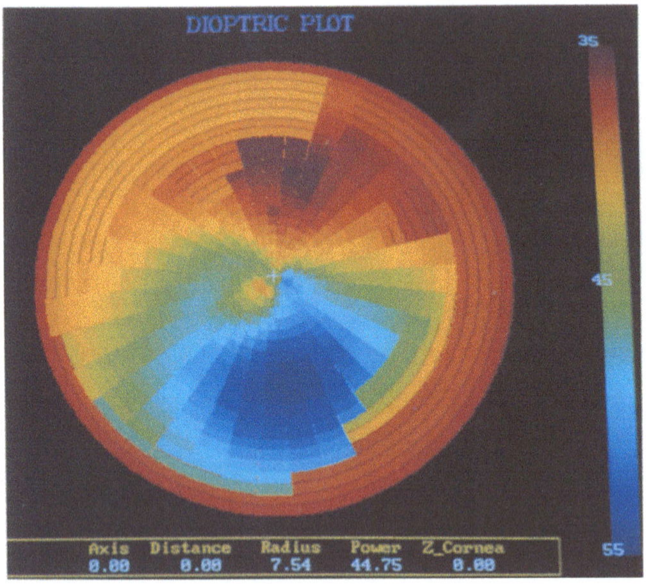

FIGURE 2.13. The dioptric plot is color-coded so steep and flat areas on the cornea can be easily visualized. The cursor can also show precisely the dioptric value on any location on the cornea. The lower box shows the axis, the distance from the center, the radius in millimeters, the dioptric power, and *z* value for each position on the cornea.

dures will be able to better help their patients by understanding corneal topography. The accuracy of their procedures (radial keratotomy, myopic keratomileusis, epikeratophakia) in some degree will be dependent on the accuracy of the original corneal topography.

4. The intraocular lens can be calculated for aphakic patients. Conventional keratometry takes one measurement on an average of a 3- to 4-mm area, to be used in calculating the intraocular lens (IOL). The Corneal Topographer is capable of providing more than one power reading for the same 3- to 4-mm area. The surgeon has more than one power from which to choose, and hence improves the predictability of the intraocular lens (IOL) power.
5. Reduction of postoperative astigmatism after corneal transplant or intraocular sur-

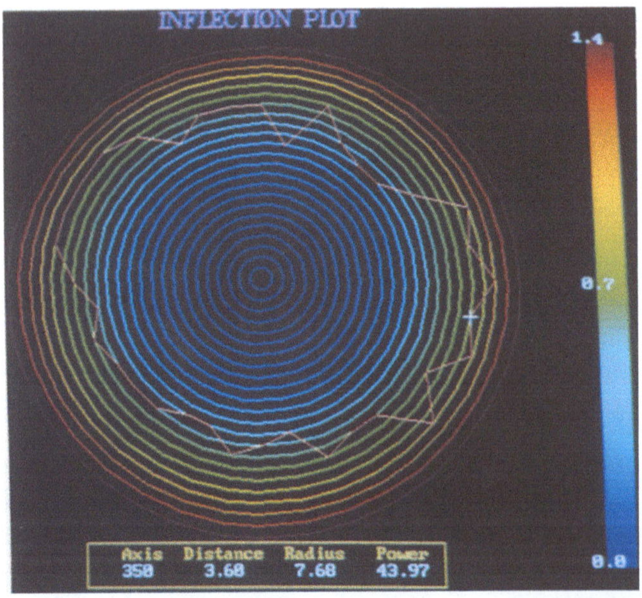

FIGURE 2.14. This display can identify points on the corneal surface where the changing curvature is the greatest. The amount of dioptric change can be preset to the practitioner's needs.

gery through suture manipulation is made possible.
6. Corneal topography is useful for fitting postoperative radial keratotomy patients. In this case the central and peripheral corneal relationship is reversed; that is, the cornea becomes flat in the center and steep at the periphery.
7. The practitioner's personal technique for fitting contact lenses can be programmed into the computer, thus providing contact lens parameters, customized, if desired, for each patient. The same can be applied to the synthetic epikeratoplasty.
8. The instrument reduces the time spent fitting patients by trial and error using a diagnostic set of contact lenses and fluorescein pattern. The Corneal Topographer can provide the parameters of an aspheric contact lens, based on an optimum tear layer relationship between the cornea and the contact lens. This is to say, the instrument removes the guesswork in these kinds of fittings, both saving time and preventing mistakes.
9. This instrument can be used by clinician and contact lens manufacturer so that ordered lens design, no matter how complex (like the new generation of bifocal contact lenses), can be verified with common device.
10. The instrument can be used for study of the long-term effect of creeping myopia.

Conclusion

The purpose of the instrument described in this chapter is to improve the accuracy and repeatability of corneal measurements. With the advancement of computer technology and the use of a computerized near real-time system we are able to make a more detailed, accurate, comprehensive, and rapid analysis of corneal topography. I feel this will improve the success rate of surgeons presently using the various techniques of keratoreformation. After working for so long on the problem of corneal topography measurement, I hope I have contributed to the solution.

References

1. Scheiner C. Occulus Hoc est: fundamentum opticum. Innsbruck, 1619.
2. Kohlrausch, Über die Messung des Radius der Vorderfläche der Hornhaut am libenden menschlichen Auge. *Okens Isis Jahrg* 1840;5:886.
3. Senff. In Wagners R. *Handworterbuch der physiol.* Bd. III. abt. 1. Art.: Schen, 1846;S. 271.
4. Helmholtz H. In: *Graefe's Archiv für Ophthalmologie.* Vol. 2. 1854; 3.
5. Coccius A. Über den Mechanismus der Akkommodation des menschlichen Auges. Leipzig, 1867. Ophthalmometrie und Spannungsmessung am kranksen Auge. Leipzig, 1872.
6. Landolt E. L'ophthalmomètre, compte réndu at mèmoires du Congrès international de Geneve. 1878.
7. Javal E, Schiotz, Un ophthalmomètre pratique, Trans. International Medical Congress VIII. Session London 1881. III. p. 30. *Annales d'Oculistique.* 1881;87:5.
8. Sutcliffe JH. One-position ophthalmometry. *Optician Photographic Trades* Rev (suppl). 1907;33:8.
9. Hartinger H. In: Le Grand Y, ed. *Optique Physiologique, Revue d'Optique,* 1935;ch. 2, p. 154.
10. Fincham EF. The changes in the form of the crystalline lens in accommodation, *Trans Opt Soc, Lond* 1925;26 (5):239–269.
11. Berg F. Bemerkungen zur Theorie der ophthalmometrischen Messungen von Flächenkrümmungen, *Acta Ophthalmologica.* 1929;7:225–243.
12. Mandell RB. Reflection point ophthalmometry, a method to measure corneal contour, Am J Optom Arch Am Acad Optom. 1962;39(10):513–537.
13. Bonnet R. Contribution à l'étude de la topographie cornéenee, *L'Opticien Lunetier.* 1960.
14. Gullstrand A. Photographish-ophtalmometrishe und klinische Untersuchungen über die Hornhautrefraktion, *Kungl So Vet Akad Handl.* 1896; 28.
15. Placido A. Novo instrumento de Esploracao da Cornea. *Periodico d'Oftalmologica Practica, Lisbon.* 1880;5:27–30.
16. Fisher, In: *Vers O G Heidelberg.* 1927;Blz 31 en 429 ef in *Zentralbl,* f.g.o. 1927; XVIII, Blz. 342 en 349.
17. Berg F. Vergleichende Messungen der form der vorderen Hornhäutflache mit Ophtalmometer und mit photographischer Method. *Acta ophtalmologica* 1929;7:386–423.

18. Dekking HM. Fotografie der Cornea opperwlakte Assen. Van Gorcum, 1930, in 8^{cm}, 91, 360 (1930) No. 2, 71 p. *Groningue th med* 1930;no. 2.
19. Amsler, Hartinger, Ber d'Deutsch. *Ophthalm* Ges. 1930.
20. Lenoble J. Méthode Optique pour étudier la forme d'une surface réfléchissante, *Rev Opt.* 1952;31:393.
21. Knoll HA, Stimson R, Weeks CI. New photokeratoscope utilizing a hemispherical object surface, *J Opt Soc Am.* 1957;47(3):221–222.
22. Reynolds AE, Kratt HJ. The photo-electronic keratoscope, *Contacto.* 1959;3(3):53–59.
23. Knoll HA. Corneal contours in the general population as revealed by the photokeratoscope. *Am J Optom Arch Am Acad Optom.* 1961;38(7):389–397.
24. Stone J. The validity of some existing methods of measuring corneal contour compared with suggested new methods, *Br J Physiol Optics.* 1962;19(4):205–230.
25. Cochet P, and Amiard H. La photokératoscopie élément de biométrie cornéenne, *Bulletin des Sociétés d'Ophtalmologie de France.* 1966;66:1094–1104.
26. Mandell, RB. Corneal contour of the human infant. *Arch Ophthalmol.* 1967;77(3):345–348.
27. El Hage S. Recherche de l'quation mathématique de la cornée a partir d'une méthode photokératoscopique, En Conference Faite Au l'Congres National D'Optione de Contact, Tours 1968. *Opticien Lunetier.* 1969; No. 192, Jan.
28. Ergellet H. Bericht über die 48 Tagung der Deutsch. *Ophthalische Gesellschaft, Jena.* 1922.
29. Kokott W. Stereoskopische Photokeratoskopie, *Klinische Monatsblätter für Augenheilkunde.* 1938;100:191–195.
30. Rzymkowsky J, Schumann WP. Stereophotographic and stereophotogrammetric reproduction of the cornea and sclera of the living eye. *Am J Optom Arch Am Acad Optom.* 1954;31(8):416–422.
31. Bertotto EV. The stereophotogrammetric study of the anterior segment of the eye. *Am J Ophth.* 1948;31(5):573–579.
32. Bonnet R. Stéréophotogrammétrie de la cornée humaine, *Revue d'Optique.* 1959;38:(9–10): 447–460.
33. Eriksen, Hornhinnmaalinger. Aarhus, 1983.
34. El Hage S. Differential equation for use of the diffused ring photokeratoscope. *Am J Optom Physiol Opt.* 1972;49(5):423–425; © The Am. Acad. of Optom.

3
Corneal Topography Using a Projected Grid

Joseph W. Warnicki, Paul G. Rehkopf, Robert C. Arffa, and John C. Stuart

This chapter describes a new rasterstereographic method that can utilize either a modified slit lamp or operating room microscope. A grid is projected onto the cornea through a cobalt blue filter, and the tear film is stained with sodium fluorescein. The fluorescein is excited by the blue light, causing a grid pattern to become visible on the surface of the cornea. This corneal surface grid pattern is imaged by a video camera attached to the slit-lamp operating microscope. The video image is digitized by a digital image processor that utilizes the grid pattern to calculate the corneal topography. Unlike methods based on the Placedo disk, this system provides information across the full corneal diameter, including the optical axis, and extending onto the sclera, and this method is not affected by corneal surface or stromal defects.

With the accelerated interest in keratorefractive procedures, there has also been an increased realization that both quantitative and qualitative measurements of corneal topography may be significant in evaluating the effects of these procedures. Rowsey and colleagues,[1,2] Maguire and colleagues,[3] and Binder,[4] have described the usefulness of corneal topography in radial keratotomy, evaluating the design of epikeratophakia lenticules for myopia, the diagnosis and staging of keratoconus, and as a guide to suture removal after corneal transplantation.

A keratoscopic method for visually assessing corneal topography was developed by Antonio Placido and refined by Gullstrand.[5] This keratoscopic system consists of a series of alternating black-and-white concentric rings on a circular disk. When this disk is placed in front of the eye, the rings are reflected by the corneal surface, where their position, size, and spacing in the reflected image are determined by the corneal shape. The observer views these reflected rings on the corneal surface through a hole in the center of the disk. The current commercial systems use illuminated concentric circular rings surrounding a viewing port through which photographs are taken. When viewing the reflected image of the Placido disk, if the cornea is spherical, the rings appear round and regularly spaced (Fig. 3.1A). If the cornea is oval or astigmatic, the rings are oval and the spacing varies in different axes (Fig. 3.1B). These techniques, while providing a visual representation of the corneal surface, do not provide any quantitative information. Doss et al.[6] have described computer programs that calculate the corneal profile and the optical power distribution on the corneal surface from the Placido disk images. Klyce[7] has developed computerized methods for deriving quantitative information about the corneal shape from keratoscopic photographs and displaying the results both numerically and graphically in easily understood forms.

Placido disk techniques for recording and quantifying the corneal surface have certain limitations that reduce their clinical usefulness. These limitations arise from the fact that as attempts are made to extend the reflected rings on the corneal surface toward the periph-

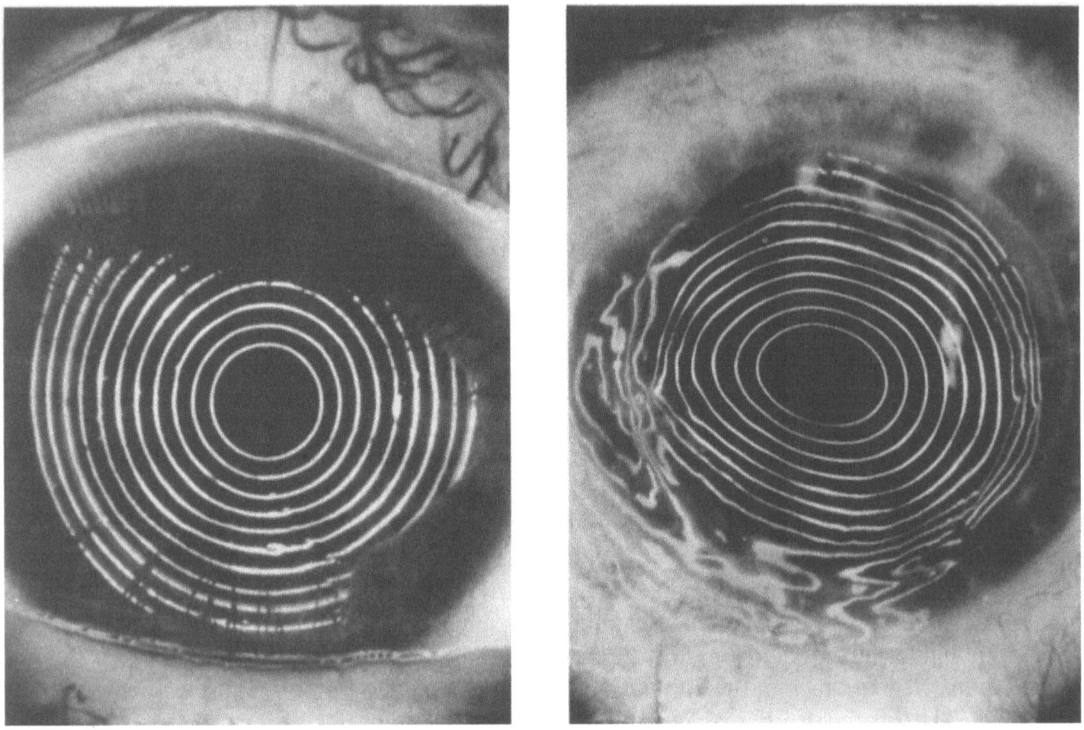

A

FIGURE 3.1. (A) Placido disk photograph of a spherical cornea. (B) Corneal transplant with astigmatic central cornea and irregular periphery. (From Ref. 10, with permission.)

ery, the lighted rings of either the Placido disk must move closer to the cornea or the disk must become larger in diameter. One of the disadvantages of moving the disk closer or increasing the diameter is that portions of the cornea become shadowed by the nose, brow, and lids, with no reflected ring segments visible in these shadowed areas (Fig. 3.1A). Another disadvantage of the Placido disk is that corneas with epithelial defects, or stromal ulcers, typically do not exhibit the reflective properties necessary to make the rings visible on the corneal surface. In addition, corneas that are highly irregular in shape cause the reflected rings to run together, making it difficult or impossible to obtain quantitative information (Fig. 3.1b).

Grid Projection

The use of a projected grid system is an adaptation of a technique known as stereorasterography,[8] as a method of obtaining contour or topographic information. One of the cameras in a stereo pair is replaced with a light source that projects a grid of vertical parallel lines and reference points onto a subject. Previously, rasterography was used medically for measuring large body surfaces in reconstructive plastic surgery and assessing the degree of spinal curvature.[9] Industrial applications include the sizing of machine parts and depth perception in robotics. A grid projected onto the corneal surface eliminates the problem caused by shadowing, does not require an intact epithelium, and is affected very little by highly irregular or steep keratoconus corneas.

In corneal rasterography a grid is projected onto the corneal surface (Fig. 3.2), rather than reflected by it. The projected image covers the full cornea, including the central optical zone and the limbus, and by changing the magnification of the optical system it can include the sclera and the lids. The image of the cornea is acquired electronically, then digitized and analyzed by a computer imaging system. The data obtained by analyzing these images are dis-

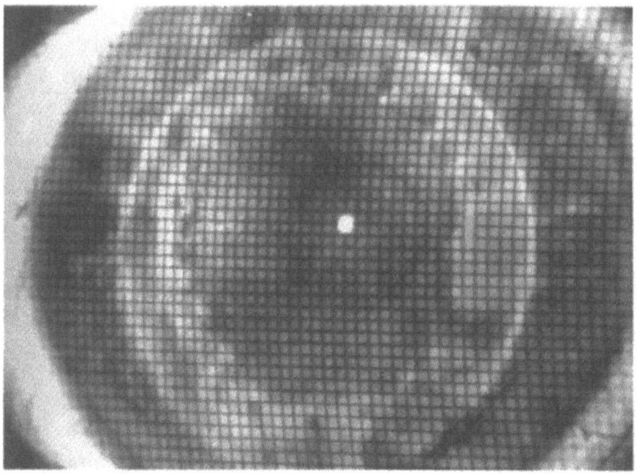

FIGURE 3.2. Grid pattern of horizontal and vertical lines projected on a cornea.

played in easily interpretable formats, which are described later.

Optical System and Computer Image Acquisition

The optical system described by Warnicki et al.[10] consists of a stereo slit lamp, either a Zeiss or Topcon, which has been modified to be both a camera and projection system (Fig. 3.3). This modification requires that two cine elbows be mounted on the accessory beam splitter. Attached to one of these elbows is a black-and-white video camera, and to the other elbow a coaxial illuminator/flash system that has been modified so that the focusing illuminator and the flash project through a grid of horizontal and vertical rulings mounted at the focal plane of the optical system. This grid pattern is projected through the slit-lamp optics onto the corneal surface.

When acquiring rastergraphic images of the cornea, the operator moves the slit-lamp optical system until the grid is in focus on the corneal surface in the same manner as when taking slit-lamp photographs. The illumination required for this focusing operation is provided by the illuminator/flash unit. When the system is in focus, the operator triggers the flash, which provides sufficient intensity for the video camera to acquire an image of the projected grid on the corneal surface.

The normal cornea has a transparent nondiffusing surface; therefore a projected grid will not be visible unless a diffusing material is used to provide a surface on which an image can be visualized. Bonnet[11] in 1962 sprayed talcum powder on anesthetized corneas in order to obtain stereo photographs of the corneal surface. In the projected grid method, sodium fluorescein is used to stain the tear film and obtain corneal surface detail. A cobalt blue excitation filter (Zeiss SB40) in the flash illumination pathway causes the corneal tear film to fluoresce in a checkered pattern corresponding to the grid. Occasionally tear film is insufficient or the fluorescein stain disperses too rapidly, making for an uneven distribution of the fluorescein across the corneal surface. To overcome this problem, the fluorescein can be mixed with a solution of methycellulose and artificial tears; this mixture persists long enough for images of the corneal surface to be acquired. The image produced during the flash exposure is viewed by the video camera through a yellow barrier filter (Zeiss SB50) that is placed in the viewing optical pathway. The image is then digitized by the processor and stored for analysis.

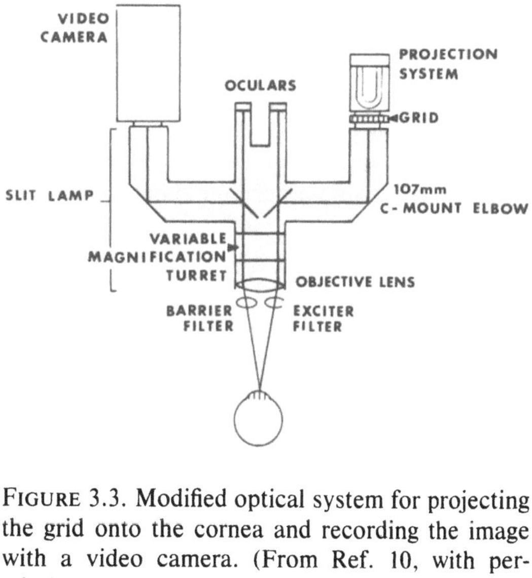

FIGURE 3.3. Modified optical system for projecting the grid onto the cornea and recording the image with a video camera. (From Ref. 10, with permission.)

Image Processing System and General Operation

The acquisition and processing computer is an IBM PC AT based system that incorporates a matrix imaging board, a 40 megabyte hard disk for program and temporary image storage, and a $3\frac{1}{2}$ in. floppy disk drive for image archiving and program transfer. A digital laser disk with a capacity of 700 megabytes may be added to the system for mass storage and retrieval of images. All system control functions can be performed at the keyboard. However, most functions can also be controlled from a touch panel on the display screen, making the system more user friendly and easier to use by untrained personnel in the examination or operating rooms. This image processing system is calibrated for each individual slit lamp or operating room microscope optical system on which it will be mounted. Because each slit lamp and microscope has a slightly different stereo base, magnification, and optical distortion, it is necessary to perform this initial calibration on each optical system. During the calibration process, the computer analyzes and compensates for these variables and saves the results for recall when the system is moved from one optical system to another. The analysis system also provides a means of entering patient identification information, which is attached to each image. The system also provides a method of filing the results of analyses with the original image for retrieval at a later time to make comparisons with images acquired in the future.

During image acquisition, the operator can view the image and determine whether the image is in focus, whether it has proper illumination, and whether the fluorescein is spread evenly in the tear film. If any one of these criteria is not met, the image can be rejected, adjustments made, and another image acquired. When the operator is satisfied with an image, the computer is instructed to process the image and display the results.

The position and spacing of the grid lines on an acquired corneal image provide the information necessary for determining corneal topography. The computer calculates the corneal surface elevation trigonometrically, by comparing the horizontal and vertical displacement of the grid pattern on the cornea to the position of the pattern when it was projected onto a flat plane placed perpendicular to a line midway between the projection and acquisition optical axes. A two-dimensional matrix of elevation points is created from these data. The matrix size is approximately 55 horizontal points by 55 vertical points, for a total of 3000 elevation points at any magnification on the corneal surface. Since both the slit lamp and the operating room microscope have multiple magnification capabilities, it is possible at low magnification to acquire and analyze images of the full cornea including the sclera. Then, by increasing the magnification to visualize the most central or visual axis of the cornea, a highly detailed analysis of that area can be obtained.

Computer Processing

The image of the grid varies widely in contrast across the various anatomical areas of the eye (Fig. 3.4), with low-contrast areas typically on the sclera, and high-contrast areas on the cornea over the iris and pupil. Only contrast variation of the vertical lines is shown. To compensate for this variation in contrast, the image is

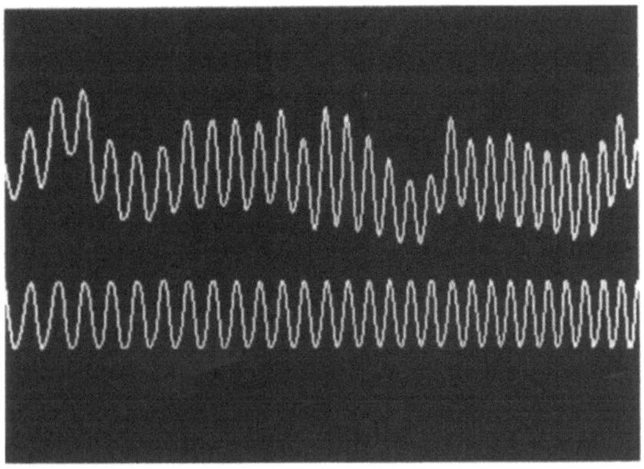

FIGURE 3.4. Intensity contrast pattern horizontally across the cornea through optical zone top tracing, normalized pattern shown bottom. (From Ref. 10, with permission.)

normalized in intensity over the entire image. This normalization is performed by computing the maximum and minimum pixel intensity values in pixel neighborhoods along each horizontal analysis line, with the neighborhood being slightly larger than one grating cycle. The maximum intensity for the pixels measured in each neighborhood is then substituted for the original intensity value. Pixels in the vertical direction are not used in this calculation, because the data are mostly duplicates of the horizontal data; their inclusion does not significantly aid calculation and increases the processing time. Each pixel is then rescaled as follows to make a uniform intensity plot across the entire line:

$$\text{New value} = (\text{LpREV} - \text{Lmin}) * (256/\text{Lmax} - \text{Lmin}),$$

where LpREV is the original value of a pixel, Lmin is the lowest value in a processing neighborhood, Lmax is the highest value in a neighborhood, and 256 is the desired contrast range.

The system then determines the position of the center of each grid by computing a high-value intensity profile across each grid line. The precise location of this point is determined by finding the horizontal position of a sine wave (the image of the grating contains only small amounts of higher order harmonics), which provides the minimum root mean square error. This technique locates the center of each projected grid line with an accuracy greater than a single pixel. The computer then registers and displays each of these identified points in a graphics overlay. It also analyzes the intensity pattern of the points to ensure that each point falls within a normal range, compared to its neighboring pixels. If several points fall outside these parameters, the system indicates that the confidence threshold has been exceeded and the image is discarded and another acquired.

Calculations and Display Methods

The elevation for each matrix point is calculated by using the formula:

$$\text{Elevation} = \frac{\left(\dfrac{\text{deviation of grid}}{\text{sine alpha} * \cos(\text{B})\text{beta}}\right)}{\text{Magnification Ratio}}$$

where alpha equals the angle between the projected grid and the viewing optics, (B) beta is one-half the angle of alpha, and the magnification is the number of pixels per millimeter in the image. This relationship is shown schematically in Figure 3.5. To simplify the drawing, only vertical projection lines are shown.

As the radius of the corneal curvature decreases, the relative elevation of the central cornea increases, and the grid lines in the acquired image deviate toward the projection optical pathway, as shown in the schematic diagram. This calculation is repeated for all

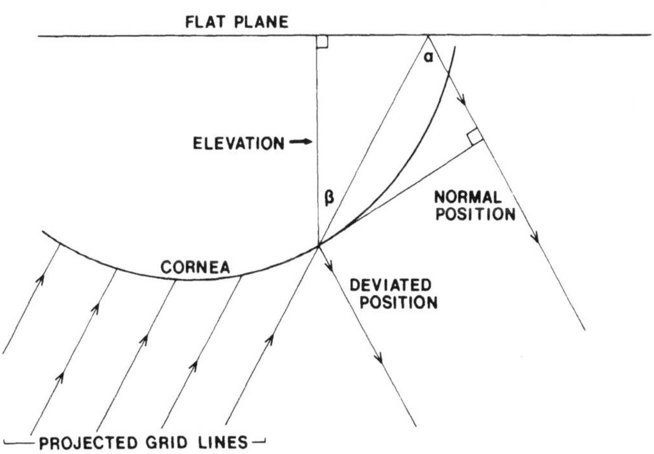

FIGURE 3.5. Schematic diagram showing lines on the cornea that have been displaced from the assumed normal position and the trigonometric relationship of these lines to elevation. (From Ref. 10, with permission.)

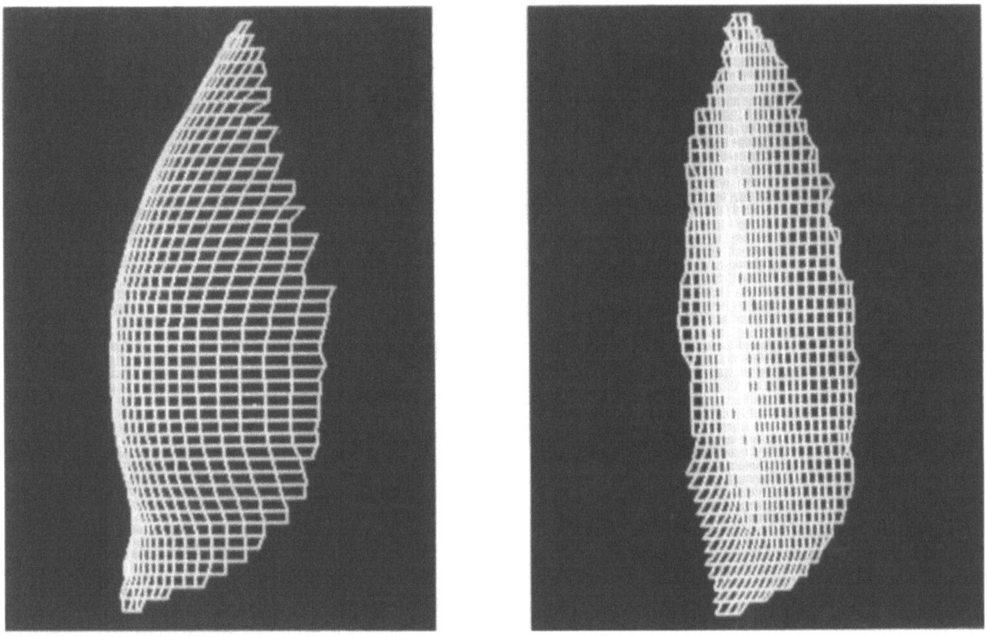
a b

FIGURE 3.6. (a) Orthogonal view of normal cornea (side view). (b) Same cornea with common curve removed. (From Ref. 10, with permission.)

analysis points on the corneal surface. This matrix of elevation values can be processed immediately or stored for future analysis. The computer has the capability of displaying a cross-sectional view of the cornea along any axis. The radius of curvature is calculated by using the simplex computer algorithm described by Caceci and Cacheris,[12] which plots a best fit curve to the elevation points. Using this method, curvatures can be determined for any axis of the cornea or for a small portion of a curve along any of the axes.

The accuracy of these measurements is 0.3 diopters (D) for a diameter of 7 mm through the central visual axes. Using the matrix file, the image can be represented in several forms. Standard graphics processing techniques[13] can be used to develop an orthogonal display that can be rotated around the x or y axis. Figure 3.6a shows the cornea rotated 80° to the right,

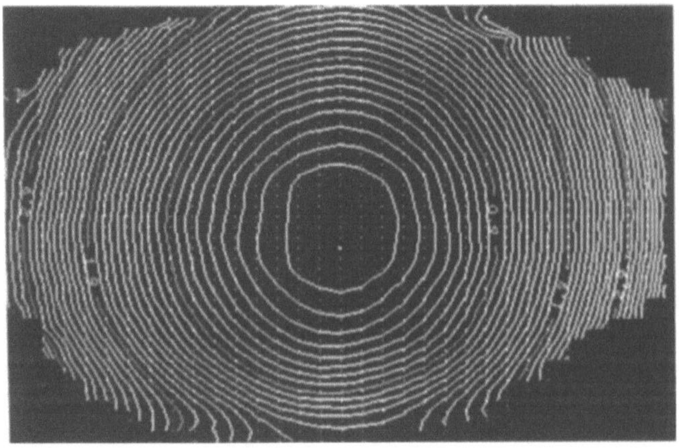

FIGURE 3.7. Contour plot of cornea. Each line represents a 0.1 mm change in elevation. (From Ref. 10, with permission.)

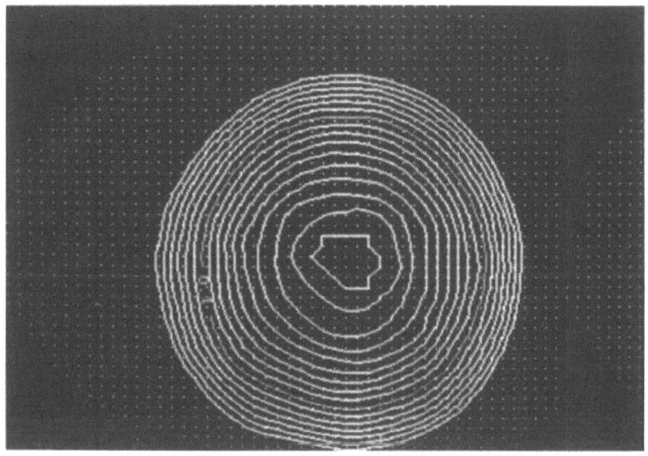

FIGURE 3.8. 2.5 × optical magnification of the center of the cornea shown in Figure 3.7. Each line represents 0.0125 mm difference in elevation. (From Ref. 10, with permission.)

which simulates a view of the cornea across the bridge of the nose. In this view, the tear film meniscus is clearly visible at the juncture of the lower lid and cornea. Figure 3.6b shows the same cornea with the common curve of the cornea subtracted to accentuate the deviations from a spherical shape, as reported by Klyce.[7] Contour plots of the cornea are shown in Figures 3.7 and 3.8. Although these plots appear to be similar to Placido disk photographs, unlike the Placido disk each line represents an area of equal height on the corneal surface. The analysis system requires approximately 1.25 min from the time an image using the slit lamp is acquired until the contour plot is displayed. The color coding of elevation in millimeters as referenced to the apex of the cornea presents an easily interpretable display (Figs 3.9 and 3.10). This standardized color coding makes possible the comparison of images acquired at different times, such as before and after a surgical procedure. Precise elevation values at any location on the cornea can be obtained by positioning a graphics marker at the area of interest. The analysis system then displays the numerical value for that location.

The image used to obtain the data in Figure 3.8 was magnified 2.5 times greater than in Figure 3.7. At this magnification, only the central 3 mm of the cornea is analyzed and the elevation detail has increased proportionately.

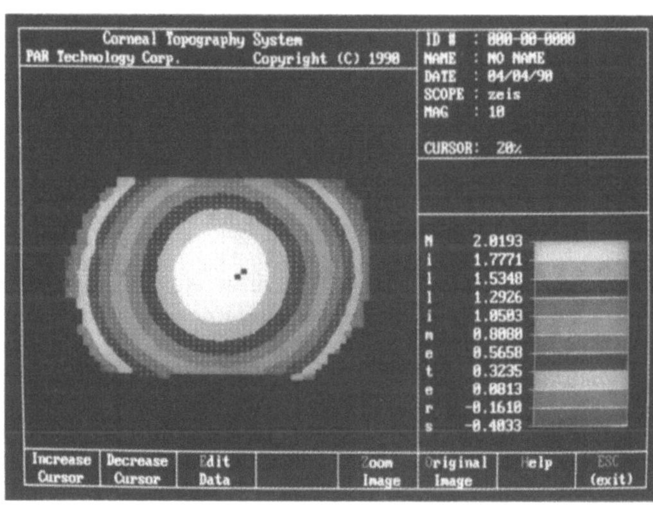

FIGURE 3.9. Color-coded map of corneal topography.

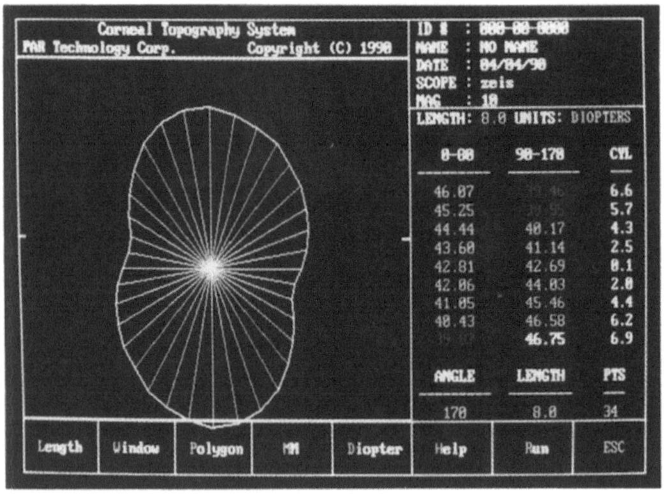

FIGURE 3.10. Diopter vector map.

Summary

Determining corneal topography using rasterstereographic images is a new technique that has several advantages over the more traditional systems currently used. Full corneal measurements are obtainable as well as more detailed measurements of the central cornea or other areas. Images can be obtained from corneas with irregular or nonreflective surfaces. This method also does not require an intact corneal epithelium but allows it to be used when corneal defects are present.

The system currently employs the optics of a Zeiss or Topcon slit lamp for grid projection and image acquisition. The camera and projection system are mounted on the standard beam splitter normally used for photography. This system adapts easily to a parallel optic operating microscope with a beam splitter, making it possible to obtain images during surgery without cumbersome attachments.

References

1. Rowsey JJ, Gelinder H, Krachmer J, et al. PERK corneal topography predicts refractive results in radial keratometry. *Ophthalmology.* 1986;93(8) (suppl):94.
2. Rowsey JJ, Reynold AE, Brown R. Corneal topography. *Arch Ophthalmol.* 1981;99:1093–1100.
3. Maguire LJ, Klyce SD, Singer DE, et al. Corneal topography in myopic patients undergoing epikeratophakia. *Am J Ophthalmol.* 1987;103:404–416.
4. Binder PS. Selective suture removal can reduce postkeratoplasty astigmatism. *Ophthalmology* 1985;92:1412–1416.
5. Duke-Elder S, Abrams D. The dioptic imagery of the eye. In: *System of Ophthalmology: Ophthalmic Optics Refraction.* Vol. 5. St. Louis: CV Mosby, 1970; Ch3, p 128.
6. Doss JD, Hutson RL, Rowsey JJ, et al. Method for calculation of corneal profile and power distribution. *Arch Ophthalmol.* 1981;99:1261–1265.
7. Klyce SD, Computer-assisted corneal topography: high-resolution graphic presentation and analysis of keratoscopy. *Invest Ophthalmol Vis Sci.* 1984;25:1426–1435.
8. Frobin W, Hierholzer E. Rasterstereography: a photogrammetric method for measurement of body surfaces. *J Biolog Photog* 1983;51,1:11–18.
9. Koepfler JW. Moire topography in medicine. *J Biolog Photogy.* 1983;51, 1.
10. Warnicki JW, Rehkopf PG, Curtin DY, et al. Corneal topography using computer analyzed rasterstereographic images. *Applied Optics.* 1988;27:1135–1140.
11. Bonnet R. New method of topographical ophthalmometry, its theoretical and clinical applications. *Am J Opt.* 1962;39:227–251.
12. Caceci MS, Cacheris WP. Fitting curves to data. *Byte.* 1984; 340–348 May.
13. Foley JD, Van Dam A. *Fundamentals of Interactive Computer Graphics.* Reading, MA: Addison-Wesley, 1982.

4
Normal Corneal Topography

Colman R. Kraff and Jeffrey B. Robin

Topographical analysis of the cornea has recently emerged as an important part of the ophthalmologist's diagnostic and therapeutic repertoire. This has occurred for a number of reasons, the most prominent being the recent advances in keratorefractive surgery. To accurately understand and perform this type of surgery, ophthalmologists found that central keratomery alone was insufficient; it was necessary to examine the shape of the entire cornea. This realization has led to a renaissance of Gullstrand's original technique of photokeratoscopy. With the development of sophisticated microchip technology, computerized videokeratoscopic instruments now allow accurate quantitative and qualitative analysis of the entire corneal surface, far beyond the central 3 mm measured by the standard keratometer. The goal of this chapter is, in light of these new developments, to explore in detail the topography of the normal cornea.

General Structure and Function

The cornea is truly a complex and geometric structure. The basic anatomic components of the cornea account for its thickness, radius of curvature, and surface regularity, all of which play a role in its anterior topography. It is appropriate to begin any discussion of corneal topography with an analysis of these structural characteristics.

The cornea is not uniformly thick throughout. It is typically thinnest centrally, measuring about 0.5 mm, with a general trend of increasing thickness as the limbus is approached. The average thickness at the limbus measures about 1.2 mm. The difference in thickness from the center to the periphery determines, in large part, the difference in radius of curvature between these two regions,[1] with the average radius of curvature of the anterior surface of the cornea being about 7.8 mm while that of the posterior surface is about 6.7 mm (Fig. 4.1).

The difference between the anterior and posterior radii of curvature yields an average of 43 diopters (D) of convergence, with the anterior surface contributing 49 D of convergence and the posterior surface 6 D of divergence. In actuality, the air–tear film interface, the interface having the greatest change in index of refraction in the eye's optical system, is responsible for the majority of this D of convergence. Because the tear film assumes the shape of the anterior corneal surface, for all practical purposes the curvature of the anterior tear film is that of the anterior cornea. As the crystalline lens only contributes about 20 D of convergence, the anterior surface of the cornea is the major topographic determinant of the eye's optical system and is thus a critical factor in proper visual function.[1]

The anterior surface of the cornea is lined with an epithelial layer which is five to eight cells thick and approximately 50 to 100 μm in depth. The superficial cells of this epithelial layer are polyhedral in shape and, under normal circumstances, do not keratinize. Their

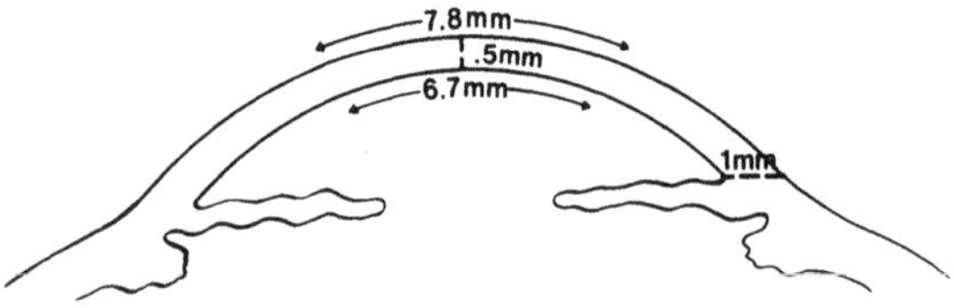

FIGURE 4.1. Cross section through the center of the cornea demonstrating the increasing thickness of the cornea from the center to the periphery. Also, note the difference between the anterior and posterior radii of curvatures.

nuclei are flat and are projected posteriorly. These qualities combine to create for a very smooth anterior surface, an essential component for pinpoint refraction of light rays onto the fovea and thus for maximal visual acuity.[2]

Disorders of these three basic components—thickness, radius of curvature, and surface regularity—can directly affect the topography of the cornea. The actual topographic effects created by these disorders will be discussed elsewhere in this book.

Topographical Zones

The topography of the normal cornea can be arbitrarily broken down into three zones (Fig. 4.2).[3] Although the precise boundaries of each zone are controversial, the recent introduction of sophisticated computerized keratoscopes

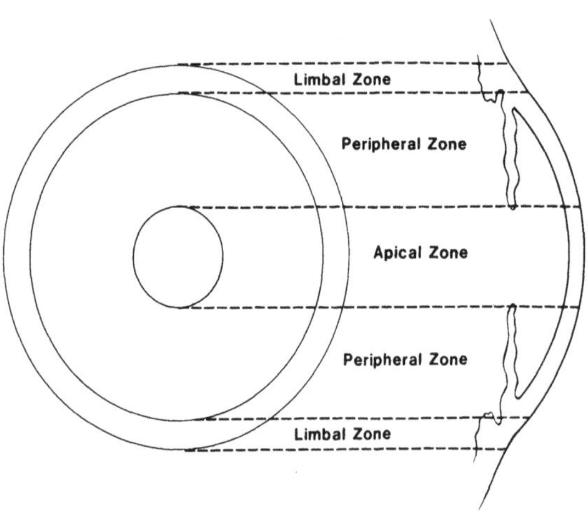

FIGURE 4.2. Three arbitrary topographic zones of the anterior corneal surface and their relationship to the anterior segment.

has enabled us to better understand these areas.

Topographically, the central area of the cornea is generally referred to as the apical zone. This can be defined as the area surrounding the corneal apex that does not vary in curvature by more than 1 D. Various investigators have defined this zone differently.[4] Mandell defined the apical zone as being that area which the central refraction differed by less than 0.25 D.[4,5] Others have defined it as the region around the apex where the radius of curvature differs by less than 0.05 mm.[6–8] With the advent of more sophisticated instruments to assess corneal topography, most authors now believe that the apical zone does not have a distinct boundary and that it varies in size from person to person.[9] For purposes of this discussion, we will broadly define the apical zone as the central region of the cornea that has the least variability of change in dioptric power.

The peripheral zone (sometimes referred to as the intermediate region) is defined as the area from the peripheral margin of the apical zone to the central border of the limbus. Topographically, the general tendency is for this region to show progressive flattening resulting in an aspheric surface.[3,7,8] This peripheral zone is of great importance when fitting contact lenses because it is this area of the cornea that supports the greatest area of the contact with the lens. It is a maxim in contact lens fitting that the peripheral radius of curvature of the lens should approximate the radius of curvature of the peripheral zone. Thus, it is not surprising that many of the developments in keratoscopy and photokeratoscopy have come from individuals associated with contact lens practice or industry; keratometry alone cannot provide any information regarding the topography of the peripheral zone. In addition to contact lens fitting, the peripheral zone also plays an important role with regard to refractive surgery. As a result, new interest in both of these areas has fueled the resurgence in keratoscopy.

The third zone, called the limbal zone, is defined as the junction between the cornea and the sclera. Because the cornea has a generally steeper radius of curvature than does the rest of the globe, there is an apparent sulcus at this juncture that defines the end of the cornea and the beginning of the sclera.[1] This region is of significance because it is involved in many peripheral corneal thinning disorders, as well as being the site of numerous surgical procedures. Surgical procedures or disease processes involving this region can directly alter its shape, and thus indirectly change the central corneal topography and thus affect visual acuity.

In the ideal situation, the apical zone of the cornea would be perfectly spherical. In actuality, the majority of corneas are spherocylindrical lenses with the axis of highest power separated from the axis of lowest power by 90.° Because of the pressure applied by the blinking eyelids, in most individuals the horizontal meridian is the flattest and the vertical meridian the steepest (a condition referred to as "with-the-rule astigmatism"). In certain situations, such as high congenital astigmatism, the meridins may not be perpendicular to each other.[9]

A few other definitions need to be addressed. The "visual center" of the cornea is the point through which the visual axis passes. The "geometric center" is the point at which the longest horizontal and vertical surface arc lengths intersect.[3] The distance from the apical center to the visual center varies from person to person. Although the locations of the visual center and the apical centers are rarely identical, most instruments that measure the corneal surface make this assumption and center their measurements about the patient's visual axis.

Quantitative Analysis of Corneal Topography

Recently, computer-assisted topographic analysis has enabled the development of a more accurate and more complete picture of the topography of the normal cornea (Fig. 4.3). The

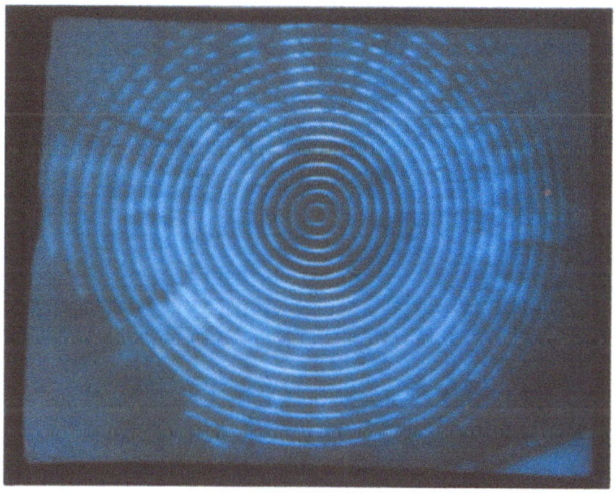

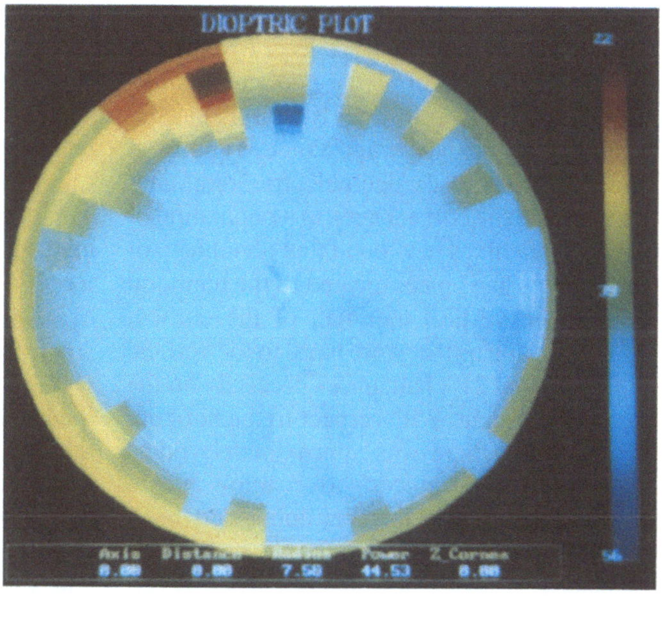

FIGURE 4.3. Color-coded dioptric plot of normal cornea using computer-assisted, digital videokeratoscopy (unit EH-270, Visioptics, Houston, TX).

different types of systems are discussed in detail elsewhere in this book.

Dingledein and Klyce recently used a color-coded, computer-assisted, topographical analysis system to quantitatively determine the surface contour of normal corneas.[10, 11] Previously, our understanding of normal corneal topography was limited to the central 3 mm as assessed by the keratometer. Even this information was not a true reflection of the central topography, because the standard keratometer merely averaged the curvature between its two points of measurement. Therefore, the studies by Dingledein and Klyce have provided new insights into some previously held concepts about the topography of normal corneas.

First, it appears that the arbitrary division of the cornea into the central and peripheral topographic regions is far too simplistic. Although these concepts may be useful when fitting contact lenses, in reality one can only state with certainty that the normal cornea is steeper centrally and flatter in the periphery. Dingledein and Klyce found that the existence of a definable apical region could not be confirmed.[11] Their data suggest that a definitive apical area probably does not exist, but rather the central region blends homogeneously with the rest of the cornea.

The exact location of the geographic corneal apex has also been a subject of much investigation over the years. In the past, its clinical importance related mainly to contact lens fitting. Now, with the emergence of refractive surgery, the location of the geographic apex and its relationship to the visual axis has acquired greater clinical importance. Tomlinson and Schwartz[12] used photoelectric keratometry to locate the corneal apex in a population of normal patients. They found that about 63% of the patients had apices located to the temporal side of the vertical meridian of the cornea, 16.3% had apices that were nasal to the vertical meridian, and 21% had apices precisely on the vertical meridian. With respect to the horizontal meridian, there was approximately equal distribution of the apices above, below and on the horizontal meridian. They concluded that it was four times more likely for the apex to be displaced nasally. They also found, however, that the corneal apex was within 0.5 mm of the visual axis in 62% of the eyes. Other authors have found similar temporal displacement of the corneal apex.[13, 14] Dingeldein and Klyce,[11] although they did not precisely attempt to locate the corneal apex, did find that the area of greatest dioptric power (ie, steepest corneal curvature) was at the central visual axis in 52% of the eyes, but in a significant percentage was often displaced temporally with respect to visual line of sight.

Computerized keratoscopy has also revealed information about the topography of the normal peripheral cornea. Several investigators have found that peripheral flattening was found to be asymmetric in the majority of eyes.[12–15]

Normal Variations in Corneal Topography

Corneal topography, although relatively stable with respect to maintaining accurate visual acuity, appears to undergo diurnal fluctuations. These changes appear to be dependent on a number of physiologic and anatomic conditions, including eyelid pressure, time of day, tear film tonicity, and hormonal levels. Corneal topographic abnormalities caused by mechanical pressure applied to the cornea by the eyelids was first observed by Snellen in 1869.[16] More recently, this topic was discussed by Gullstrand.[17] The theory that the eyelids influence the shape of the cornea is widely accepted in the optometric literature. Masci was able to demonstrate that when the eyelids are retracted there is a shift toward "against-the-rule" astigmatism, suggesting that the pressure of the eyelids causes a with-the-rule astigmatism.[18] Wilson et al. found that not only was there a shift toward against-the-rule astigmatism, but the shift was a result of a steepening in the horizontal axis and not a flattening in the vertical axis.[19, 20] In addition to these studies, which demonstrated changes in the corneal shape after eyelid retraction, there have been reports of bilateral monocular diplopia following extended periods of visual tasks at short distances.[21] It was suggested that, because of a progressive ptosis that occurs during reading, the resulting pressure on the cornea from the upper eyelid may have caused an alteration in the corneal shape resulting in monocular diplopia.[21, 22]

In addition to the long-term influence of exogenous structures such as the eyelids on corneal topography, there are a variety of diurnal corneal changes that can alter normal topography. The most common of these occurs nightly during sleep. A number of investigators have attempted to measure the effect of sleep on the cornea.[23, 24] Most have found that during sleep there is a 3 to 8% increase in anterior corneal thickness. Following exposure during waking hours the increased thickness returns to baseline within 1 to 12 hours.[23–25] About 75% of this thinning process occurs within the first 2 hr with a gradual thinning over the rest of the day. Although the reason for increased corneal thickness during sleep is not completely understood, it is believed that it may result from a change in the tonicity of the tear film. Another theory[23] suggests that there may be relative tear film hypoxia that occurs when the eyes are closed, causing a dysfunction of the epithelial pump and subsequent anterior edema. The interesting fact is that despite this corneal swelling, most patients with normal corneas are unaware of any difference in visual acuity when first arising in the morning. However, in some patients with marginally compromised endothelial function, such as in bullous keratopathy or Fuchs's dystrophy, we have observed that visually significant corneal edema may occur during sleep.

Other factors that may influence the topography of the normal cornea seem to be hormonal in origin. Although there is conflicting evidence, some data suggest that fluctuations in corneal topography may occur during the menstrual cycle. Kiely studied the changes in corneal topography and corneal curvature through the complete menstrual cycles of several women.[25, 26] Even though their patient population was small, keratometric steepening of both the horizontal and vertical meridia was found to occur at the beginning of the cycle with a tendency toward flattening after ovulation. The changes in corneal thickness during menstruation tended to be quite variable throughout the cycle. Much of the variation in measurement in these studies was believed to be dependent upon variabilities in the length of the ovulatory cycle, thus making it difficult to assign any statistical significance to these changes.

Finally, it has been well documented that the cornea does change shape during the course of each day.[23, 25] Most of this diurnal shift appears to be related to the effect of lid pressure on the cornea during sleep. As mentioned above, lid pressure on the cornea by the superior tarsus has a tendency to cause flattening in the horizontal meridia. Manchester[23] found that there was an average increase in corneal steepening from morning to evening of 0.12 D in the horizontal meridian and 0.15 D in the vertical meridian. The flattening in the morning was attributed to the lid effect during sleep (Fig. 4.4). These diurnal variations in corneal topography have not been noted to cause clinically significant changes that have been noted in normal patients.

Summary

The cornea is a unique geometric and biomechanical structure. The recent development of computer-assisted, digitalized videokeratoscopy systems has resulted in a more com-

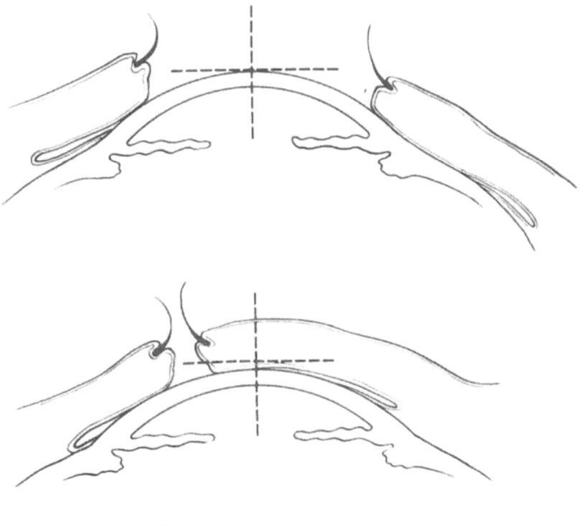

FIGURE 4.4. Artist's rendition of the flattening effect of the upper lid of the cornea while the lids are closed during sleep.

plete understanding of the complexity of the topography of the normal cornea. It is this complexity of shape that enables us to see with great precision and accuracy. In addition, the topography of the normal cornea is not a static function but appears to be constantly changing. Understanding the qualities of normal cornea topography will become more important as newer surgical techniques requiring precise resculpting of the anterior surface become popular.

References

1. Smith TW. Corneal topography. *Documenta Ophthalmologica*. 1977;43:249–276.
2. Klyce SD, Beurman RW. Structure and function of the cornea. In: Kaufman HE, Barron BA, McDonald MB, Waltman SR, eds. *The Cornea*. New York: Churchill Livingstone, 1988; pp 5–55.
3. Rowsey JJ. Corneal topography. In: Dabezies OH, ed. *Contact Lenses: The CLAO Guide to Basic Science and Clinical Practice*. Boston: Little, Brown, 1984; 4.1–4.8.
4. Mandell RB, St Helen R. Stability of the corneal contour. *Am J Optom*. 1968;45:797–806.
5. Mandell RB. *Contact Lens Practice*. Springfield, IL: Charles C Thomas, 1974; p 65.
6. Clark BA. Mean topography of normal corneas. *Aust J Optom*. 1974;57:107–114.
7. Clark BA. Topography of some individual corneas. *Aust J Optom*. 1974;57:65–69.
8. Ludlam WM. Photographic analysis of the ocular diopteric components: Part 3. *Am J Optom Arch Am Acad Optom*. 1967;44:276–296.
9. Maguire LJ. Corneal topography. In: Kaufman HE, Barron BA, McDonald MB, et al eds. *The Cornea*. New York: Churchill Livingstone, 1988; ch 34, pp 897–909.
10. Dingeldein SA, Klyce SD. The topography of normal corneas. *Arch Ophthalmol*. 1989;107:512–518.
11. Dingeldein SA, Klyce SD. Imaging the cornea. *Cornea*. 1988;7:170–182.
12. Tomlinson A, Schwartz C. The position of the corneal apex in the normal eye. *Am J Optom Phys Optics*. 1979;56:236–240.
13. Edmund C. Location of the corneal apex and its influence of the stability of the central corneal curvature. *Am J Optom Phys Optics*. 1987;64:11,846–852.
14. Mandell RB, St Helen R. Position and curvature of the corneal apex. *Am J Optom Arch Am Acad Optom*. 1969;46:25–29.
15. Knoll HA. Corneal contours in the general population as revealed by the photokeratoscope. *Am J Optom Arch Am Acad Optom*. 1961;33:389–397.
16. Snellen H. Die Richtung der Hauptermeridiane des astigmatischen Auges. *Albrecht von Graefes Arch Ophth*. 1869;2:199.
17. Gullstrand A. The cornea. In: Southhall JPC, ed. *Helmholtz's Treatise on Physiological Optics*, vol. 1. New York: Dover, 1962; pp 320–321.
18. Masci E. Sull'astigmatismo of talmometrico: modificazioni della curvatura corneale in rapporto alla attivta' palpebrale ed alla rigidita sclerale. *Bolletino d'Oculistica*. 1965;44:755–763.
19. Wilson G, Bell C, Chotai S. The effect of lifting the lids on corneal astigmatism. *Am J Optom Phys Opt*. 1982;59:670–674.
20. Vihlen FS, Wilson G. The relationship between eyelid tension, corneal toricity and age. *Invest Ophthalmol Vis Sci*. 1983;24:1367–1373.
21. Bowman KJ, Smith G, Carney LG. Corneal topography and monocular diplopia following near work. *Am J Optom Phys Opt*. 1978;55:818–823.
22. Mandell RB. Bilateral monocular diplopia following near work. *Am J Optom Arch Am Acad Optom*. 1966;43:500–504.
23. Manchester PT. Hydration of the cornea. *Tr Am Ophth Soc*. 1970;68:425–461.
24. Mertz GW. Overnight swelling of the human cornea. *J Am Optom Assoc*. 1980;51:211–213.
25. Kiely PM, Carney LG, Smith G. Diurnal variations of corneal topography. *Am J Optom Phys Optics*. 1982;59:12:976–982.
26. Kiely PM, Carney LG, Smith G. Menstrual cycle variations of corneal topography and thickness. *Am J Optom Phys Optics*. 1983;60:822–829.

5
Topography of Corneal Disease Processes

Colman R. Kraff and Jeffrey B. Robin

In the chapter on normal corneal topography, we discussed the anatomic and physiologic aspects of the cornea that contribute to its surface topography. In this chapter we consider the effects of pathologic processes upon corneal topography. Surgically and traumatically induced topographic changes are covered elsewhere in this book.

There are essentially three fundamental ways in which corneal topography can be altered by pathologic processes: (1) abnormalities in the epithelium, (2) changes in stromal thickness, and (3) external compression by either a lid or limbal mass. These three variables can alter surface topography independently or in conjunction with one another.

Epithelial Abnormalities

Any irregularity in the epithelial surface of the cornea can result in altered corneal topography. The mechanism by which epithelial disorders can induce irregular astigmatism has not been well elucidated. It is known that the normal refraction of light rays entering the eye is dependent upon a smooth and regular interface between air and the anterior refracting surface of the eye.[1] This surface, which is actually the anterior layer of the tear film, has a curvature that is directly related to that of the underlying anterior surface of the cornea.[1] It is conceivable, therefore, that focal depressions or elevations in the anterior corneal surface—such as could occur with epithelial cell death or edema—could be directly reflected in the height of the overlying tear film. In these situations, this would result in focal areas of the tear film being either steeper or flatter than adjacent areas overlying unaffected cornea, thus causing irregular astigmatism. If this irregular astigmatism involves or is close to the visual axis, a resultant decrease in visual acuity will occur.

There are numerous disorders of the corneal epithelium that can cause visually significant surface irregularity.[2] These can be the result of either inflammatory or noninflammatory processes (Fig. 5.1). Examples of inflammatory disorders that can cause epithelial surface abnormalities include infectious keratitis (bacterial, fungal, viral, and parasitic), Thygeson's punctate keratopathy, and any of the toxic epitheliopathies.[3, 4] Additionally, systemic inflammatory processes that cause severe keratitis sicca (eg, rheumatoid arthritis, mixed connective tissue disorders, and Sjogren's syndrome) can indirectly cause surface irregularity via nutritional deprivation and eventual death of epithelial cells.[5, 6]

Surface irregularity can also result from disorders that cause epithelial edema. These may be an indirect result of an endothelial disorder (such as Fuchs's dystrophy or aphakic bullous keratopathy) or the direct result of nutritional deprivation of the epithelium (such as contact-lens induced hypoxia).[7, 8]

In addition to inflammatory epithelial disorders, several noninflammatory processes can cause epithelial surface irregularities. Prime among these are the anterior corneal dystro-

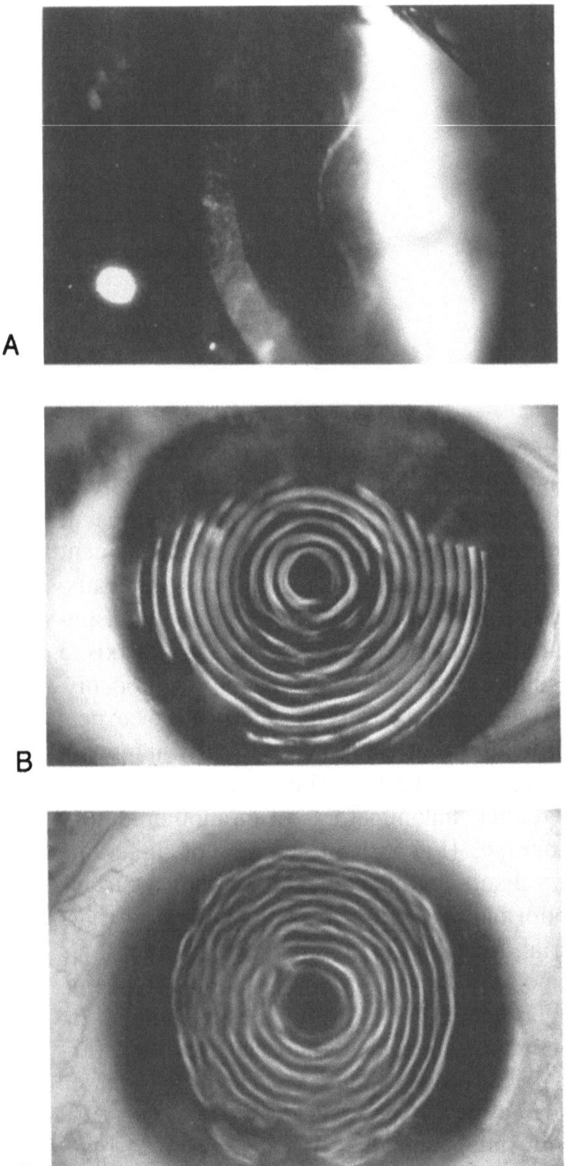

FIGURE 5.1. (A) Slit-lamp photograph demonstrating superficial amyloid deposits in lattice dystrophy. (B) Corneascope photograph of the same patient demonstrating marked irregularity of the circular mires secondary to superficial amyloid deposits. (C) Epithelial irregularity secondary to epithelial keratitis from herpes simplex virus.

phies, such as map-dot-fingerprint, Meesman's, and Reis–Bucklers's dystrophies.[9] Map-dot-fingerprint (or basement membrane) dystrophy is the most common of these three disorders. Because of the production of an anomalous basement membrane there is an abnormal accumulation and thickening at the subepithelial level.[9, 10] In the majority of patients, these abnormalities cause no significant problems. However, some individuals with this disorder are prone to recurrent epithelial erosions.[9, 11] In some cases, multiple erosions can lead to fine, focal scarring at the level of Bowman's layer and anterior stroma; this can result in focal topographic alterations (usually flattening over the area of scarring) and irregular astigmatism. Additionally, topographic abnormalities may simply result from the focal surface elevations overlying the areas of abnormal basement membrane accumulations.[9] These changes can be exquisitely subtle and are difficult to perceive with routine biomicroscopy alone. We have found that with the use of photo- or videokeratoscopy (in coordination with retroilluminated slit-lamp biomicroscopy) the appropriate diagnosis can usually be made. Although the other anterior corneal dystrophies have different pathophysiologies, associated topographic alterations can occur and are similarly the result of either focal elevation of the epithelium over the dystrophic tissue or subepithelial scarring from previous epithelial erosions.

Visual loss in cases of epithelial abnormalities is almost always the result of topographic abnormalities. However, it can be difficult to appreciate these abnormalities, particularly in those cases in which there are minimal degrees of surface irregularity. On routine slit-lamp biomicroscopy, epithelial changes can be very subtle. Keratometry may or may not reflect these subtle epithelial changes, depending upon their degree of severity and their proximity to the central cornea. In order to best illustrate topographic abnormalities resulting from epithelial disorders, we have found photokeratoscopy to be invaluable (Fig. 5.2). Even subtle changes in the epithelial surface are well reflected as irregularities in the keratoscopic rings. Also, the large area covered by the photokeratoscope can illustrate abnormalities far removed from the visual axis. Additionally, in order to confirm the effect of any anterior surface irregularities on visual acuity, we have found it extremely helpful to perform a rigid

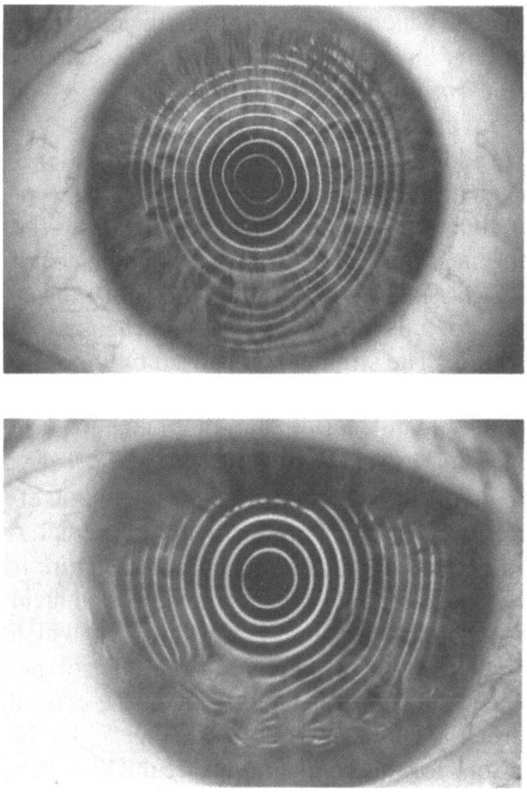

A

B

FIGURE 5.2. (A) Corneascope photograph of a patient with map-dot-fingerprint dystrophy. Note the marked irregularity of the inferior mires due to accumulation of abnormal basement membrane material. (B) Corneascope photograph of a patient with exposure keratitis secondary to lag ophthalmus. Note the irregularity of the rings, particularly inferiorly. Also, the central mires demonstrate the minimal amount of irregularity that can account for a reduction in visual acuity.

contact lens refraction. The rigid contact lens will provide a smooth anterior refracting surface, thus neutralizing any surface irregularity. If the irregular astigmatism is the sole reason for the decreased vision, the patient's visual acuity should improve upon placement of the contact lens.

Epithelium-induced changes in corneal topography are generally self-limited and subside when the epitheliopathy resolves. However, in rare cases, these processes can permanently alter surface topography by causing subepithelial scarring at the level of Bowman's layer and anterior stroma.

Stromal Abnormalities

The second fundamental class of pathologic processes that can result in corneal topographic abnormalities involves alterations in the integrity of the corneal stroma. Until recently, there has been very little published information describing the effects of stromal disorders on corneal topography.

Loss of stromal tissue is a common sequela of many inflammatory and noninflammatory disorders of the cornea.[12] The mechanisms by which these disorders alter surface topography are frequently quite complex and depend, in part, on both the depth and breadth of stromal loss as well as its location on the cornea. Commonly, a mixture of flattening and steepening will occur over the thinned area. Furthermore, the topographic effects of the stromal thinning will also involve adjacent (and even distant) areas of unaffected cornea, making it almost impossible to predict the final topographic pattern.

Classically, thinning of the corneal stroma causes flattening in the area of tissue loss and steepening as the borders of unaffected tissue are approached. This type of configuration, not unlike that of a canyon, is commonly seen with peripheral thinning disorders, such as Terrien's marginal degeneration (Fig. 5.3).[13] In rare cases, the thinning may be advanced enough to allow for anterior protrusion of the affected area; topographically, the thinned area may then be steep Fig. 5.4).

In addition to the direct topographic effects in the area of stromal thinning, indirect changes are produced in the remainder of the cornea. Particularly in the case of peripheral stromal thinning disorders, secondary alterations in the central corneal topography ultimately account for most visual abnormalities. It is, therefore, appropriate to consider separately the topographic effects of peripheral and central stromal thinning disorders.

It is an axiom that loss of peripheral corneal stroma results in flattening of the central topography in the meridian perpendicular to the tangent of the thinned area. For example, in Terrien's marginal degeneration (which classically results in a band of thinning in the

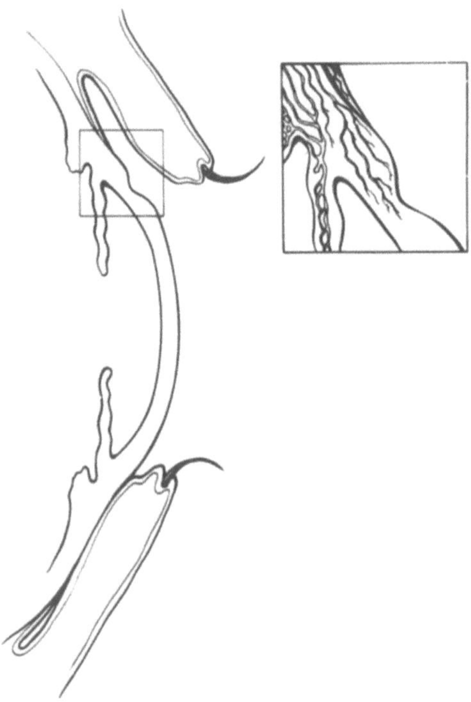

FIGURE 5.3. Artist's rendition of Terrien's marginal degeneration. Note the superior canyon-like thinning of the superior limbal region.

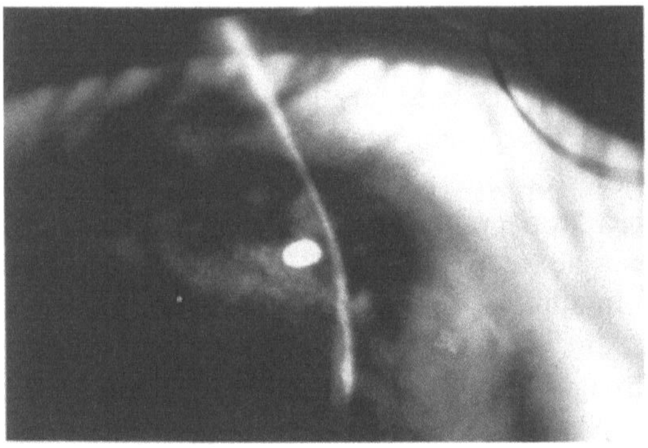

FIGURE 5.4. Slit-lamp photograph demonstrating anterior protrusion in a markedly thin region of Terrien's marginal degeneration.

superior corneal periphery centered around the 12:00 limbus), the most frequently observed central topographic finding is vertical flattening, most significantly in the 90° (12 o'clock to 6 o'clock) meridian.[13] Conceivably, this topographic pattern occurs because the thinning involves destruction of the collagen lamellae which are running from the inferior to superior limbus; the result is an increase in the radius of curvature—and thus flattening—in the involved meridians.

In addition to the noninflammatory Terrien's degeneration, this pattern of flattening centered about the meridian perpendicular to the tangent of the peripheral corneal thinning band also classically occurs in inflammatory disorders, such as Mooren's ulcer and rheumatoid arthritis. The stromal loss caused by these inflammatory disorders is prone to extend circumferentially and/or centrally. Obviously, in this case, increasingly complex vector forces are involved and the resultant topographic effects become much more difficult to predict.

Another complicated topographic picture is produced by the noninflammatory pellucid marginal degeneration. In this disorder, which produces corneal thinning in the inferior periphery, a "tabletop" flattening of the central cornea is classically observed (Fig. 5.5). The reasons for this configuration are unclear. Perhaps this pattern occurs because the inferiorly directed pressure of the upper lid on the central cornea causes the central wall of the thinned area to rotate inferiorly, in effect "stretching" (and thus flattening) the central cornea (Fig. 5.6).[14]

These basic principles for topographic alterations resulting from peripheral thinning lesions can be applied to any disorder, regardless of whether the underlying process is inflammatory or noninflammatory. Although the exact mechanisms for these topographic alterations are not completely understood, factors such as width and depth of thinning, location of the thinning, and the effect of upper lid pressure, all appear to contribute to the topographic changes.

Processes that cause central stromal thinning characteristically cause visually significant topographic abnormalities. Keratoconus is a prime example. This disorder is discussed in more detail elsewhere in this book. There are however, other disorders that cause central corneal thinning. Most of these are the result of infectious or immunologic processes that result in the production of collagenases or other proteases.[15] The stromal loss that occurs as a

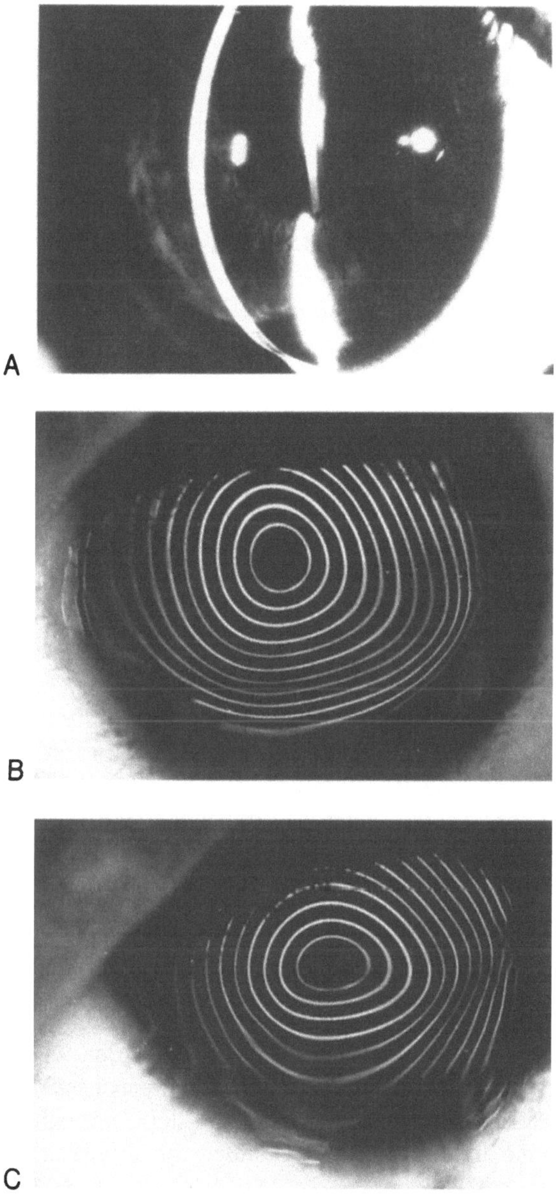

FIGURE 5.5. (A) Slit-lamp photograph demonstrating inferior band of thinning in a patient with pellucid marginal degeneration. (B) Corneascope photograph of the same patient with pellucid marginal degeneration. The photograph is taken with the patient looking in primary gaze. Note the inferior steepening as demonstrated by narrowing of the mires. (C) Same patient with the photograph taken in upgaze. Note the change in mire configuration.

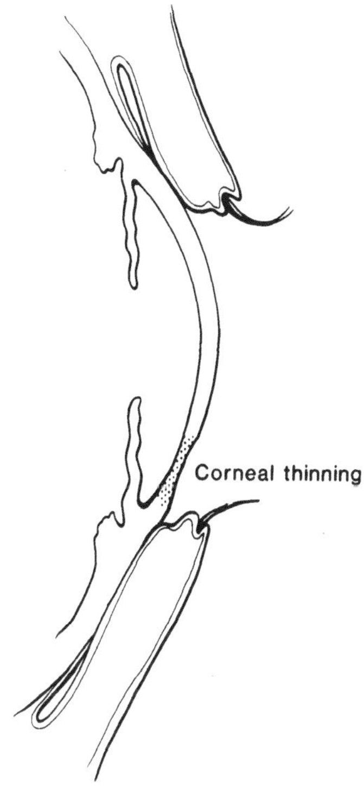

FIGURE 5.6. Artist's rendition of the peripheral band of thinning in pellucid marginal degeneration. Note the effect the upper lid may play in contributing to the "tabletop" configuration of the central and inferior cornea.

result of these disorders can alter normal corneal topography by two basic mechanisms.

The first mechanism has to do with the fact that the underlying cause of the tissue loss is most commonly a necrotizing keratitis (secondary to collagenase or other protease production) that typically destroys the corneal stroma in an anterior-to-posterior direction.[15] This type of tissue destruction commonly leaves a rough irregular surface that eventually reepithelializes as the inflammatory process subsides. Because of the irregular stromal thickness, the surface topography of the healed cornea is markedly irregular. Generally, these topographic effects can be easily appreciated by slit-lamp biomicroscopy, keratometry, and photokeratoscopy (Fig. 5.7). The visual effects of these topographic changes can be confirmed by rigid contact lens refraction. It is important to bear in mind that, in most cases of central stromal keratitis, the resultant topographic abnormalities may account for as

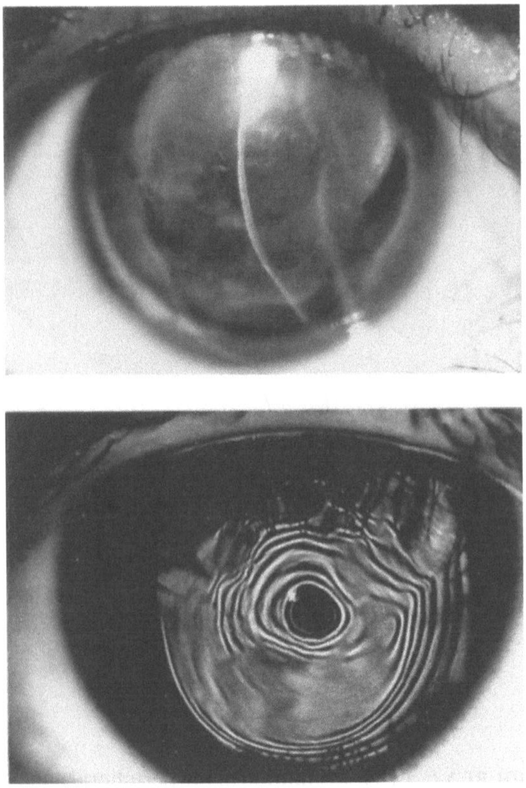
A
B

FIGURE 5.7. (A) Slit-lamp photograph and (B) corneascope photograph of a patient with necrotizing stromal keratitis secondary to herpes simplex virus. Note the marked irregularity of all the mires secondary to stromal tissue loss in (B).

much or even a greater amount of visual loss than does stromal opacification. This fact has obvious therapeutic implications. In cases of healed central stromal keratitis, rigid contact lens fitting may improve visual acuity to useful levels, thus obviating the need for penetrating keratoplasty. If, on the other hand, the visual loss cannot be improved by a rigid contact lens overrefraction, it should be assumed that the stromal opacity is primarily responsible for the visual reduction; a penetrating keratoplasty is usually then necessary for visual rehabilitation.

The second mechanism by which central thinning processes can alter surface topography relates to the depth of thinning. If the primary necrotizing tissue loss is deep enough (80 to 90%), an ectasia may occur in this thinned region. On photokeratoscopy, the ectatic region will typically appear as an area of steepening with adjacent areas of flattening. As one might expect, significant visual loss will usually occur in these cases because of marked irregular astigmatism.

Alteration Due to External Compression

The third fundamental nonsurgical process by which corneal topography can be altered is related to external compression on the cornea by either an eyelid or limbal mass. Regardless of whether the mass lesion is in the lid or located at the limbus, the manner in which it alters topography is the same. The compressive effect of the mass causes a flattening of the cornea directly under the area of compression.[16] For eyelid lesions that compress the midperipheral or central cornea, there is steepening peripheral to this central region. A prime example of this compressive effect is seen in a child who develops a capillary hemangioma of the upper eyelid.[16] These large lid masses can cause a significant amount of astigmatism, usually manifested centrally as with-the-rule (90° axis) steepening. The clinical significance of these lesions is that, in the pediatric population, the resultant astigmatism may result in amblyopic visual reduction.

Limbal masses can similarly cause significant alterations in surface topography. A classic example of these perilimbal processes in a limbal dermoid. Typically, a dermoid will cause flattening directly under the involved area with steepening centrally.[16, 17] This is easily demonstrated on photokeratoscopy (Fig. 5.8). Another example of a limbal process that frequently causes topographic abnormalities is a pterygium. A pterygium may alter surface topography by two processes.[18, 19] The first alteration in topography results from the irregular astigmatism that is produced on the epithelial surface as the head of the pterygium progresses onto the cornea. The second factor that may contribute to the topographic changes is related to the fact that, as the pterygium grows, stromal scarring and contracture may result, producing further flattening over the lesion and central steepening. The mechanism of

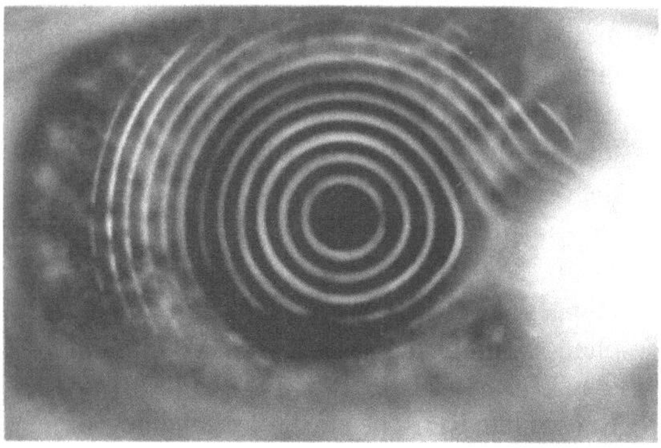

FIGURE 5.8. Corneascope photograph of a limbal dermoid demonstrating widening of the mires—flattening under the dermoid.

this topographic change is similar to that of a limbal suture that is tied too tightly, producing flattening under the suture and steepening central to the suture.[20] Pterygium-related topographic changes can be easily identified with photokeratoscopy and frequently account for visual loss associated with these lesions (Fig. 5.9). Other perilimbal mass lesions can produce similar types of topographic changes.

Summary

Essentially, there are three fundamental pathologic processes that can produce abnormal corneal topography. These include abnormalities of the surface epithelium, alterations in stromal thickness, and external compression by either a lid or limbal mass. Even though it was well known that these processes are capable of to altering surface topography, it has taken the recent advent of sophisticated photo- and video keratoscopy to fully illustrate the degree of these surface changes. Additionally, these technologies have enabled investigators to begin to understand the mechanisms by which these changes occur. In the future, our understanding of the topographic effects of corneal disorders will be further advanced by the development of even more sophisticated technology for the analysis of corneal topography, as well as the development of animal models that accurately depict these disease processes.

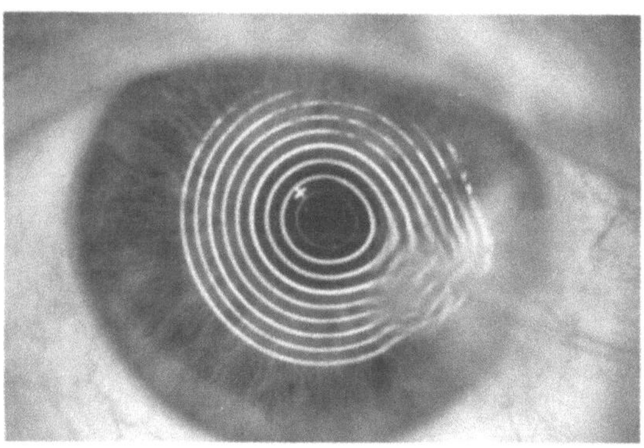

FIGURE 5.9. Corneascope photograph of a pterygium demonstrating resultant irregular astigmatism.

References

1. Duke-Elder S, Abrams D. Ophthalmic optics and refraction. In: Duke-Elder S, ed. *System of Ophthalmology*. St Louis: CV Mosby, 1970; pp 93–119.
2. Coster DJ. Superficial keratopathy. In: Duane TD, Jaeger EA, eds. *Clinical Ophthalmology*. Philadelphia: Harper & Row, 1985; ch 17, pp 1–9.
3. Leisegang TJ. Bacterial and fungal keratitis. In: Kaufman HE, Barron BA McDonald MB, et al, eds. *The Cornea*. New York: Churchill Livingstone, 1988; pp 217–270.
4. Tygeson P. Further observations on superficial punctate keratopathy. *Am J Ophthalmol*. 1966;61:1346.
5. Bron AJ, Mengher LS. The ocular surface in keratoconjunctivitis sicca. *Eye*. 1989; 3:428–437.
6. Lamberts DW. Keratoconjunctivitis sicca. In: Smolin G, Thoft RA, eds. *The Cornea*. Boston: Little Brown, 1987; pp 387–404.
7. Doughman DJ. Corneal edema. In Duane TD, Jaeger EA, eds. *Clinical Ophthalmology*. Philadelphia: Harper & Row, 1985; ch 16A, pp 1–17.
8. Lohman LE. Corneal epithelial response to contact lens wear. *CLAO J*, 1986;12:153–156.
9. Kenyon KR, Fogle JA Grayson M. Dysgenesis, dystrophies and degenerations of the cornea. In: Duanes TD, Jaeger EA, eds. *Clinical Ophthalmology*. Philadelphia: Harper & Row, 1985; ch 16, pp 1–56.
10. Waring GO, Rodrigues MM, Laibson PR. Corneal dystrophies I. Dystrophies of the epithelium, Bowman's layer and stroma—*Ophthalmol*. 1978;23:71.

11. Fogle JA Kenyon KR, Stark WJ, et al. Defective epithelial Adhesion in anterior stromal dystrophies. *Am J Ophthalmol.* 1975;79:925.
12. Robin JB, Schanzlin DJ, Verity SM, et al. Peripheral corneal disorders. *Survey Ophthal.* 1986;31:1, 1–36.
13. Wilson SE, David TC, Klyce SD, et al. Terriens marginal degeneration; corneal topography. *refract corneal surg.* 1990;6:15–20.
14. Maguire IJ, Klyce SD, McDonald MB et al: Corneal topography of pellucid marginal degeneration. *Ophthalmology* 1987;94:519–524.
15. Wilson LA. Bacterial corneal ulcers. In: Duane TD, Jaeger EA, eds. *Clinical Ophthalmology.* Philadelphia: Harper & Row, 1985; ch 18, pp 1–19.
16. Bogan S, Simon JW, Krohel GB, et al. Astigmatism associated with adnexal masses in infancy. *Arch Ophthalmol.* 1987;1368–1370.
17. Cuttone JM, Druso F, Miller M, et al. The relationship between soft tissue anomalies around the orbit and globe and astigmatic refractive errors: a preliminary report. *J Ped Ophthalmol Strab.* 1980;17:29–36.
18. Hansen A, Norus M. Astigmatism and surface phenomena in pterygium. *Acta Ophthalmologica.* 1979;58:174–181.
19. Bedrossian RH. The effect of pterygium surgery on refraction and cornea curvature. *Arch Ophthalmol.* 1960;105–109.
20. van Rij G, Waring GO III. Changes in corneal curvature induced by sutures and incisions. *Am J Ophthalmol.* 1984;98:773.

6
Classification of Corneal Topography with Videokeratography*

George O. Waring III, Sadeer B. Hannush, Stephen J. Bogan, and Robert K. Maloney

The topography of the cornea has been imaged for over a century. The popularity of refractive corneal surgery in the past decade has emphasized in a practical way the need for accurate and reproducible methods of measuring the power of the entire corneal surface. The comparative usefulness of keratometry, photokeratography, and videokeratography are now matters of active study. We have used videokeratography to study the topography of normal corneas and of those that have undergone radial keratotomy and penetrating keratoplasty. We summarize our findings in this chapter.

Measurement of Corneal Curvature and Shape

We propose the following conventional terminology to foster improved communication.[1]

Corneal Light Reflection

The image formed by light reflected from the convex anterior corneal surface was first called the first Purkinje image, the corneal light reflex, or the corneal light reflection. This virtual, erect image is viewed during keratometry and keratoscopy and is located approximately 4.0 mm posterior to the anterior surface of the cornea at the level of the anterior lens capsule. Because the reflected image size is determined by the curvature of the cornea (the greater the curvature, the smaller the image), it is used to quantify the anterior corneal curvature and power.

Keratometer (Ophthalmometer)

This is a good example of how colloquial usage can set linguistic standards. "Keratometer" is the trade name of the Bausch and Lomb device, but like "Xerox" and "Kleenex," the commercial term has taken on a generic use. The original designation by von Helmholtz (1853) for an instrument that measures the central corneal curvature was "ophthalmometer," a term still used outside the United States.

Keratometry (Ophthalmometry)

A keratometer measures corneal curvature in designated meridians by reflection of a mire from small areas along an annulus 3 to 4 mm in diameter, centered around the apex of the cornea.[2, 3] Small-mire keratometry is done with special instruments that reduce the size of the reflected image. Keratometry done outside the central cornea must be designated as paracentral or peripheral, using instruments such as the Soper topogometer or the American Opti-

* The authors acknowledge the valuable contributions of Kenneth L. Cohen, James M. Coggins, Susan Crawford, Carolyn Chortkoff Drews-Botsch, Mary C. Gemmill, Osama Ibrahim, Michael J. Lynn, Azhar Nizam, and Nancy Tripoli. Supported by a grant from Computed Anatomy, Inc.

cal keratometer, neither of which is currently marketed.

Radius of Curvature and Refractive Power of the Cornea

The radii of curvature of the anterior and posterior corneal surfaces affect its refractive power (Fig. 6.1). A shorter radius of curvature creates a steep arc and greater refractive power. Conversely, a longer radius of curvature creates a flatter arc and less refractive power. All keratometers and keratoscopes measure the size of the image reflected from the anterior surface of the cornea and calculate the radius of curvature and the refractive power of the whole cornea, using 1.3375 as the "keratometric" index of refraction for the cornea instead of the true index of 1.3376.

Keratoscope

An instrument that presents a series of mires, most commonly rings, to the anterior corneal surface is a keratoscope. Keratoscopes fitted with a still film are called photokeratoscopes; those fitted with a video camera are called videokeratoscopes. Corneascope is the trade name used by the Kera Corporation.

Keratoscopy

Direct observation of the images of mires reflected from the anterior surface of the cornea is keratoscopy, in the same sense that examination of the ocular fundus with an ophthalmoscope is ophthalmoscopy.

Keratography

The term "keratography" denotes a record or portrayal of the cornea in the same sense that angiography records the pattern of vessels. Currently, there are two methods of recording pictures (keratographs) of the mires reflected from the anterior corneal surface: (1) With photographic film, one uses a photokeratoscope to produce a photokeratograph, a process called photokeratography (in the same sense that one uses a photomicroscope to take a photomicrograph), and (2) with video recording, one uses a videokeratoscope to produce a videokeratograph, a process called videokeratography.

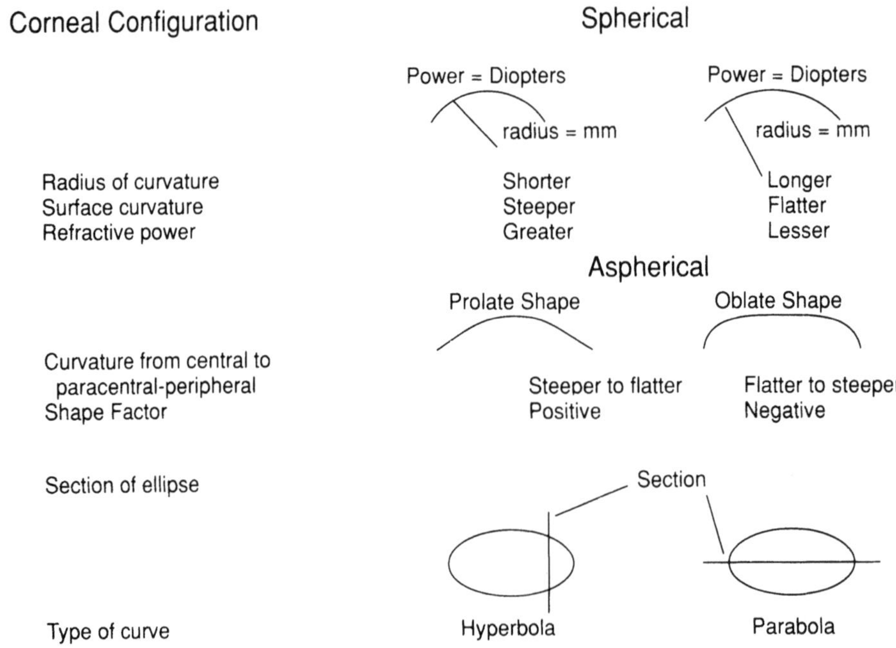

FIGURE 6.1. Terminology used in describing corneal configuration topography for both spherical and aspherical surfaces. (With permission of ref. 1.)

A keratograph can be interpreted qualitatively or quantitatively. A qualitative interpretation is done by visual inspection of the shape and spacing of the mires and has practical value in diagnosing corneal disorders such as keratoconus or in adjusting sutures after penetrating keratoplasty.[4] Quantitative keratography is done by assigning numerical coordinate values to points on the mires and describing mathematically the curves that the points form. Complex formulas and algorithms are required for accurate quantitation of corneal topography. Quantitative keratography is usually done with the assistance of a computer that uses image-analysis programs. The computer may be located in a separate instrument (as in the Kera and Nidek systems, both photokeratoscopes) or in the keratoscope itself (as in the Computed Anatomy and EyeSys systems, both computer-assisted videokeratoscopes).

Topography

Topography refers to the shape of the surfaces, whether they be the surface of the earth or the surface of the cornea. The most common representation is one in which the relative elevations of the surface are delimited by contour lines.

The mires used to study corneal topograhy and shape have many configurations: circles, arcs, parallel lines, interference fringes, steps, and grids. The most commonly used are circular rings. The concentric ring mires are commonly called Placido rings, but strictly speaking, that designation should describe only Placido's flat disk with equally spaced, circular black rings. Modern keratoscope rings are designed differently. By convention, however, the rings are numbered from innermost to outermost. This can be confusing, because a specific ring (eg, ring 3) in different instruments may cover a different location on the same cornea. Therefore, it is important to designate the diameter of a projected ring and indicate the area on the cornea that it covers.

There are four basic methods of displaying corneal topographic information: (1) the keratograph, (2) representation of the radius of curvature or dioptric power at various locations on the surface of the cornea, either in a fixed pattern on a "face plate" or at any location identified by a cursor in a computer-assisted videokeratoscope, (3) graphic three-dimensional figures often with exaggerations to show changes in curvature, and (4) color-coded maps using colors to designate areas of uniform radius of curvature and refractive power. In the most widely used color coding scheme,[5] reds and oranges indicate steeper areas with greater refractive power, and greens and blues indicate flatter areas with less refractive power (LSU Topography System, Computed Anatomy Corneal and Topographic Modeling Systems, and EyeSys Corneal Analysis System). A quantitative scale indicates the values corresponding to each color.

Shape of the Anterior Corneal Surface

Corneal Asphericity

The anterior corneal surface is asymmetrically aspheric; that is, the radius of curvature changes from the center to the limbus and does so at a different rate along different semimeridians. Such a complex shape is difficult to measure mathematically, difficult to represent graphically, and difficult to understand and treat optically. Therefore, we have customarily simplified matters by conceiving of the cornea as a spherocylindrical lens or as a section of an ellipse, a practical assumption as proven by generations of wearers of spectacles and contact lenses. This simplification will some day be replaced by more accurate "shape factors," mathematical indices, or ray tracing diagrams.[6]

A useful simplification to understand the overall topographic pattern of the cornea is to consider the corneal curvature as a section of an ellipse.[7] In most normal corneas, the central zone is steeper than the paracentral and peripheral zones, a configuration referred to as having a positive shape factor (positive because the radius of curvature becomes larger from the center to the periphery), and a prolate shape (the shape of a section across the steep end of an ellipse). The opposite topographic pattern occurs rarely in normal eyes but commonly after radial keratotomy: the central zone is flatter than the paracentral and peripheral zones, a configuration referred to as having a negative shape factor and an oblate shape (the shape of a section across the flatter side of an ellipse) (Fig. 6.1).

Surface Zones of the Cornea

A similar oversimplification takes place when the cornea is divided into surface zones ("optical zone," "apical zone"). None of these areas is discrete, because the cornea forms continuous curves. Nevertheless, for practical optical and anatomic purposes we can divide the surface of the cornea into two overall regions: the central optical zone and the remainer of the cornea (sometimes called the periphery).[8] The optical zone forms the foveal image through the entrance pupil of the eye; its size, shape, and curvature vary among individuals. The rest of the cornea serves three purposes: a refracting surface for peripheral vision and for the foveal image when the pupil is widely dilated, a mechanical structure, and a source of cells during normal turnover and repair.

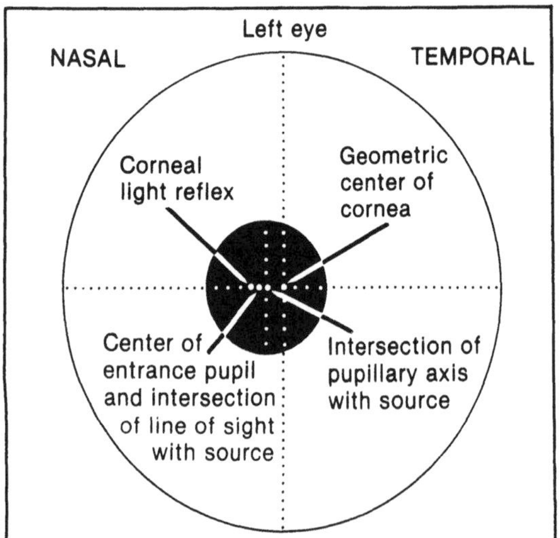

FIGURE 6.2. Terminology describing topographic regions of the cornea, including the circular central zone and the three concentric annular zones. (With permission of ref. 1.)

Conventionally, four concentric anatomic zones are recognized: central optical zone, paracentral intermediate zone, peripheral transitional zone, and limbal zone (Fig. 6.2).

Central Zone

The central zone is approximately 4 mm in diameter and has been called the apical zone, the corneal cap, the optical zone, and the central spherical zone—all terms intended to designate this region of the cornea as the more spherical, symmetrical, and optically important. Now that corneal topography is requiring more careful definitions, we must distinguish among four designations: (1) the anatomic central zone, which is the area that overlies the entrance pupil, (3) the "spherical" central part of the cornea, which is present in a minority of normal corneas, and (4) the apex of the cornea, which is highest spot on the cornea (as discussed subsequently).

The center of the optical zone can be defined in one of five ways, depending upon the optical circumstances: (1) the anatomic center of the cornea equidistant from the limbus, (2) the optical axis, which connects the center of the curvature of the cornea and centers of curvature on the crystalline lens, (3) the pupillary axis, which connects the center of the entrance pupil and the center of curvature of the cornea, (4) the line of sight, which connects the fixation point with the center of the entrance pupil, and (5) the visual axis, which passes from the foveola through the nodal points of the eye (Fig. 6.3). Detailed discussion of these often confusing axes can be found in most standard ophthalmic and physiological optics textbooks. For practical purposes, the center of the optical zone should be considered the intersection of the pupillary axis with the cornea because the entrance pupil determines the image-forming bundle of rays that reach the fovea.

The term "optical zone" is used with four different meanings in the context of refractive surgery. The first meaning is that just defined, the central, more spherical portion of the normal cornea overlying the entrance pupil. The second meaning refers to the portion of a keratomileusis lenticule, epikeratoplasty lenticule,

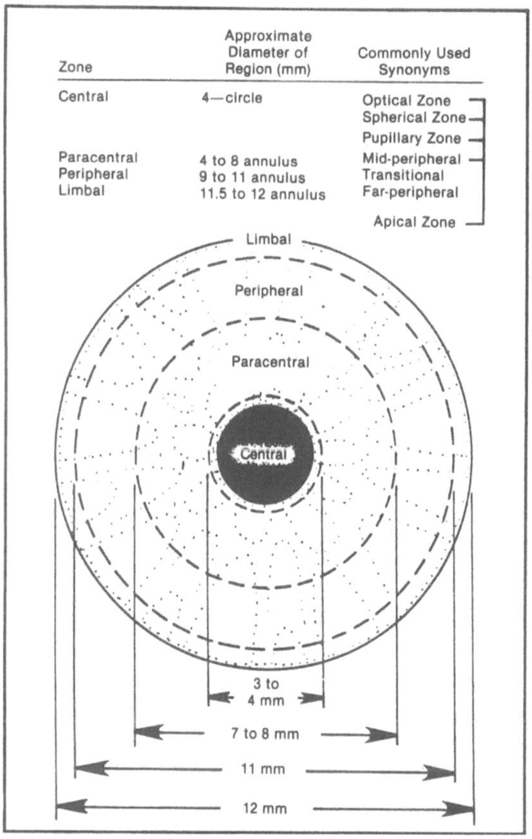

FIGURE 6.3. Drawing shows intersection of various axes with cornea. (With permission of ref. 1.)

or excimer laser surface ablation that creates the major refractive change; in this context, it is possible to decenter the "optical zone." The third meaning is to designate the central uncut clear zone in radial keratotomy; the term "optical zone" (OZ) is so engrained in the radial keratotomy literature that it is not likely to disappear, even though the preferred designation is "clear zone." The fourth meaning is the diameter of any circular mark on the cornea, for example, a "7-mm optical zone" used for transverse incisions; in this context, "optical zone" is truly a misnomer, and should be replaced by the simple designation "zone," or "zone mark" (eg, "the transverse incisions were placed at the 7-mm zone").

The apex of the cornea is the high spot of the cornea, and location of the greatest sagittal height on the anterior corneal surface. It is from this point that the corneal light reflection emanates, and, therefore, it is the point around which the keratoscopy rings center. The apex or high point of the normal cornea is close to the optical axis. However, in pathological states such as keratoconus and after corneal surgery, the apex may be displaced so that the keratoscopy rings no longer center around any clearly identifiable point or axis on the cornea or over the entrance pupil. Thus, the patient may be looking through an area of the cornea eccentric to that in the center of the keratography mires.

Paracentral Zone

The paracentral zone is an annulus approximately 4 to 7 mm in diameter and has been called the "mid," "intermediate," or "midperipheral" cornea. The term "midperipheral" is a misnomer, because this zone does not occupy the middle of the periphery (eg, a transverse incision made at the 6 mm zone is not "midperipheral," because it is still within the central half of the cornea). The central and paracentral zones together compose what contact lens fitters call the apical zone. Normally, the paracentral zone has a flatter radius of curvature than the central zone. After radial keratotomy, this is the region where a marked change in curvature—the paracentral knee—between the new, flatter, central zone and the new, peripheral, steeper cornea occurs.

Peripheral Zone

The peripheral zone is an annulus of approximately 7- to 11-mm diameter. This is the area in which the normal cornea flattens the most and becomes more aspheric. For this reason it has also been called the transitional zone.

Limbal Zone

The limbal zone is the rim of cornea approximately 0.5 mm wide that abuts the sclera. Its extent varies depending on the amount of sclera override and it is usually covered by the limbal vascular arcade. A focal steepening occurs here adjacent to a small furrow known as the scleral sulcus.

Directions on the Cornea: Meridians, Semimeridians, and Axes

Locations on the surface of the cornea are designated as meridians, lines that span the diameter of the cornea from one point on the limbus to a point on the opposing limbus. The meridians are designated from 0° to 180°, proceeding counterclockwise starting at 3 o'clock for both the right and left eyes (Fig. 6.4).

The term "axis" designates the direction in a cylindrical lens along which there is no power; it is parallel to the focal line. Because clinicians align the axes of cylindrical lenses with meridians in the cornea, it is common practice to substitute the term "axis" for "meridian" when referring to directions on the cornea. Thus, clinicians commonly refer to the steep "axis" of the cornea when they mean steep "meridian," a habit that is unlikely to change. The clinician who says that a correcting cylindrical lens is placed at a certain axis is simply using a shortened way of saying that the axis of the cylinder is placed along a certain corneal meridian; this shorthand is used so commonly as to be acceptable.[9, 10] However, when clinicians refer to the "steep axis" or the "flat axis" of the cornea, the term "axis" is used incorrectly; the term "meridian" should be used when referring to the direction of corneal refractive power.

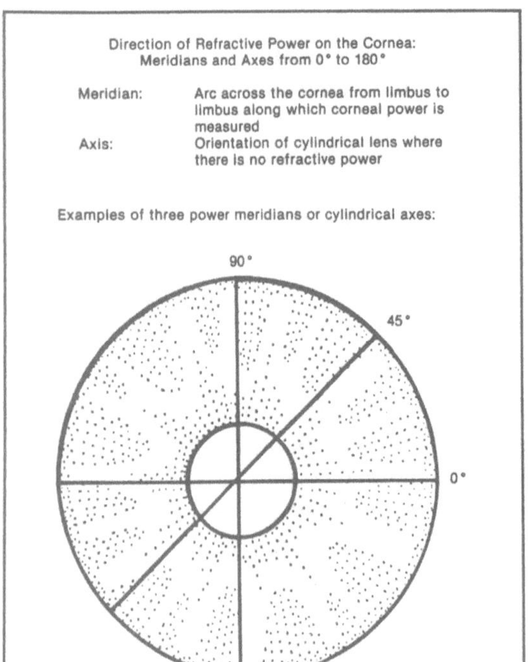

FIGURE 6.4. Terminology describing meridional directions on the surface of the cornea and axes of correcting cylindrical lenses. (With permission of ref. 1.)

Designating the meridians as 0° to 180° is conventional, but, unlike geographers, opthalmologists have no north-south longitude lines to indicate a point along a meridian. Thus, if one refers to making a transverse incision or removing a tight corneal suture in the 90° meridian, it is not clear whether the activity occurs in the 12 o'clock direction or in the 6 o'clock direction. Therefore, directions from the center of the cornea are designated in semimeridians. (The term "semimeridian" is preferred because both components of the word are derived from Latin. The term "hemimeridian" is a Greek and Latin hybrid, which etymologic purists eschew.) The semimeridians are located around the 360° circumference of the cornea in degrees, such as the "225° semimeridian." Another convention is to consider the cornea as the face of a clock; for example, 7:30 o'clock indicates the 225° semimeridian. This clock-hour system is too crude for refractive surgery, which requires more accuracy.

A specific point on the surface of the cornea is designated by indicating its location in millimeters from the center of the cornea along a semimeridian (ie, polar coordinates). For example, at 3 mm from the center along the 225° semimeridian, the corneal power may be 41.00 D. The location of a transverse incision could be accurately described as follows: it was placed 3 mm from the center at the 6 mm zone perpendicular to the 225° semimeridian (in current jargon: "A T cut was made at the 6 mm optical zone at 7:30 o'clock" (Fig. 6.5).

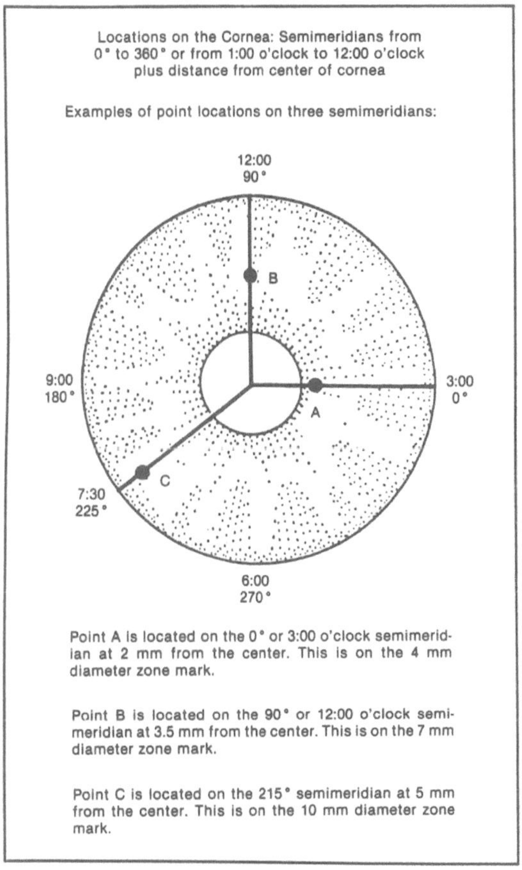

FIGURE 6.5. Terminology describing locations on the cornea. (With permission of ref. 1.)

Comparision of Keratometry, Photokeratography, and Videokeratography

We have compared three instruments—the Bausch and Lomb Keratometer, the Kera Corneascope, and the Computed Anatomy Corneal Modeling System—on both calibrated steel balls and normal human eyes.[11,12]

Surface Area of Cornea Measured

The area of the corneal surface measured by the three instruments differed markedly (Fig. 6.6). The Keratometer projected a mire onto the corneal surface and images only two points on the ring, approximately 3 mm apart. Thus, the Keratometer does not directly measure any identifiable surface area on the cornea, but derives its values from calculations based on the size of the single reflective image. This is adequate for the measurement of the surface of a spherical steel ball, but on an asymmetrical aspheric surface, such as the human cornea (particularly after refractive surgery), the Keratometer gives no useful topographic information, although it can estimate the overall central corneal curvature.

Both the Corneascope and the Corneal Modeling System project Placido rings onto the surface of the cornea, the 12-ring Corneascope covering approximately 70% of the available surface and the Corneal Modeling System approximately 95% of the available surface. The Corneascope does not directly measure the apex or periphery of the cornea, whereas, the Corneal Modeling System covers almost the entire cornea. Each instrument measures only that part of the corneal surface directly beneath the projected rings; therefore, the greater the number of rings and the closer they are together, the greater the ability to detect perturbations in the corneal topography.

A reflected ring image, however, is not enough—it must be read accurately and precisely. We did not perform a ring-to-ring analysis of the 12 rings on the Corneascope, but we observed frequently that the surface area quantified was closer to 40% of the cornea. With the Corneal Modeling System, the first ring and rings 27 through 31 were read inaccurately or not at all, so that the readable rings on the steel balls covered approximately 70% of the surface. Currently, the formulas and algorithms used by each instrument to compute the radius of curvature of the corneal surface assume that the cornea is spherical. In fact, the cornea is asymmetrically aspherical.

Comparision of Instruments on Steel Test Balls

Surgical manipulation of corneal shape requires an accurate and reproducible method of

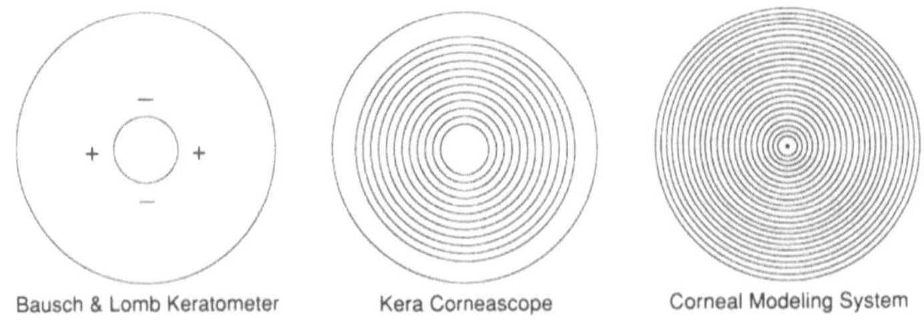

FIGURE 6.6. Drawings show area covered by mires of Bausch and Lomb Keratometer, Kera 12-ring Corneascope, and Computed Anatomy Corneal Modeling System. Outer circle represents limbus of cornea. Keratometry mires measure only two points approximately 3 mm apart. Twelve-ring Corneascope mires cover approximately 70% of the surface, omitting central and peripheral zones. The Corneal Modeling System covers approximately 95% of the surface. (With permission of *Arch Ophthalmol.* 1989; 107: 1235–1239. © 1989 American Medical Association.)

measuring anterior corneal curvature from apex to limbus. We evaluated the accuracy and reproducibility of the three instruments by measuring comparable locations on four calibrated steel test balls. Comparable locations on the surfaces of the test balls were determined for each of the three instruments. For the 42 D ball, the keratometer images were located on a circle 3.15 mm in diameter, the Corneascope ring number 3 was closest to this location, and the moving cursor on the Corneal Modeling System was placed to obtain values around a 3.0 mm circle (which was approximately on ring 8). The dioptric powers at two points on the 0° and 90° were average for comparision among the three instruments. The Keratometer and Corneal Modeling System were more accurate and precise than the Corneascope. No statistically significant difference was found between the Keratometer and the Corneal Modeling System with respect to accuracy and reproducibility.

Because the Corneal Modeling System projects rings that cover the entire surface of the cornea, we were especially interested in evaluating the accuracy and reproducibility of the measurements made by all of the rings, 1 through 31. The instrument was not programmed to measure rings 27 through 31, so these were omitted. Measurements for ring 1 yielded large deviation scores. Therefore, we chose rings 2 through 26 for detailed study.

The measurement values were within a clinically acceptable range of ± 0.25 D for balls 43 D, 42 D, and 38 D; those balls had dioptric powers that fell within the range of the central and peripheral normal cornea (38 to 46 D) (Figs. 6.7 and 6.8). Less accurate measurements were obtained for the 50 D ball. This suggests that the Corneal Modeling System software may need to be adjusted to measure more accurately corneas that are steeper than normal. Inaccuracies in the measurement of ring 1 were probably the result of greater error in the application of the proprietary corrective computer algorithms to that ring with a smaller diameter. Since ring 1 is often read inaccurately, it could be omitted from interpretation by the computer program without loss of clinical utility. The clustering of deviation score values on the positive side of zero for balls 43 D, 50 D, and 38 D suggested a systematic error in the interpretative computer programs that probably could be corrected.

Comparision of Instruments on Normal Human Eyes

Comparisons on normal human eyes made among the three instruments at the significance level of 0.05 indicated that the keratometer was more reproducible than the Corneal Modeling System and the Corneascope, and the Corneal Modeling System was more reproducible than the Corneascope. Of the 31 rings projected on the surface of each cornea by the Corneal Modeling System, rings 2 through 13 were read "reasonably reproducibly" in that 76% of the measurements on these rings differed by no more than 0.5 D. The Corneal

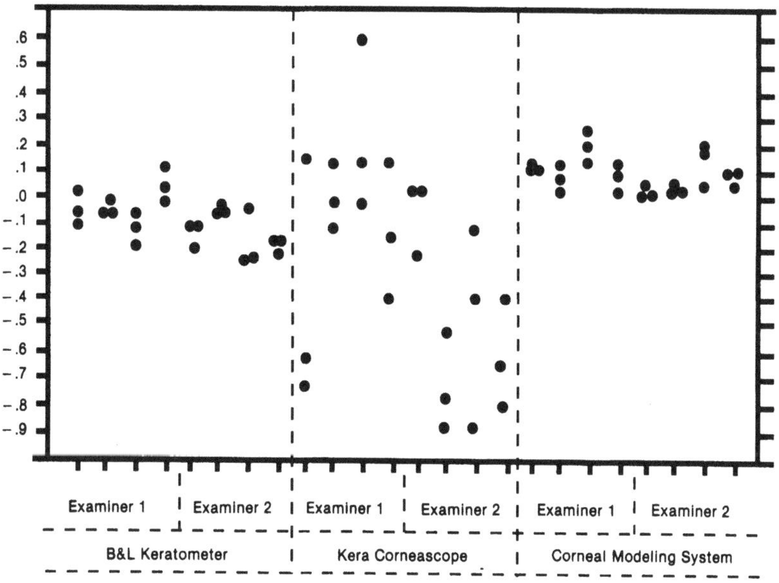

FIGURE 6.7. Scattergram shows accuracy of reading of the Keratometer, Corneascope, and the Corneal Modeling System in the form of deviation scores (difference between actual and measured values as indicated on the *y*-axis in diopters). Two examiners performed three readings on each of four test steel balls (A, 43.00D; B, 42.52 D; C, 50.14 D; and D, 38.66 D). The Keratometer and the Corneal Modeling System were more accurate than the Corneascope. (With permission of *Arch Ophthalmol.* 1989; 107:1235–1239. © 1989 American Medical Association.)

Modeling System (software version 1.16) is 83% as reproducible as a Keratometer reading at approximately the edge of the 3-mm central zone on normal human corneas and provides information about corneal topography in a more reproducible and visually useful manner than the other two instruments (Fig. 6.9, Table 6.1).

Because the Corneal Modeling System potentially can image the entire surface of the cornea, we analyzed separately the precision of the measurements of all rings for this instrument, omitting rings 28 through 31. The instrument did not consistently read rings 21 through 27. The instrument could consistently quantify rings 1 through 20, but its reproducibility on these rings was less than desired, because only rings 2 through 13 could be read with a reproducibility of 0.50 D (maximum difference scores of less than or equal to 0.50 D for 76% of measurements, as contrasted to our finding that 9% of the measurements for ring 8 alone were less than, or equal to, 0.50 D (Table 6.2).

Thus, at the time of this study, there was not available to clinicians an instrument that could reproducibly quantify the curvature of the peripheral cornea. The presumed reason for the greater variability in the analysis of rings 21 through 27 was that the algorithms written to analyze the keratographs assumed that the cornea is a sphere. This assumption is approximately correct for the central zone, but not for the aspheric paracentral and peripheral zones. Rewriting of the algorithms to take into account the aspheric optics of the cornea may improve the reproducibility of these measurements.

We did not do a similar analysis across the rings of the Corneascope and, therefore, do not know the precision of readings for any rings other than ring 3.

Clinical Factors that Affect Use of Instruments

Cooperation of the patient was important. Patients had to maintain fixation to achieve re-

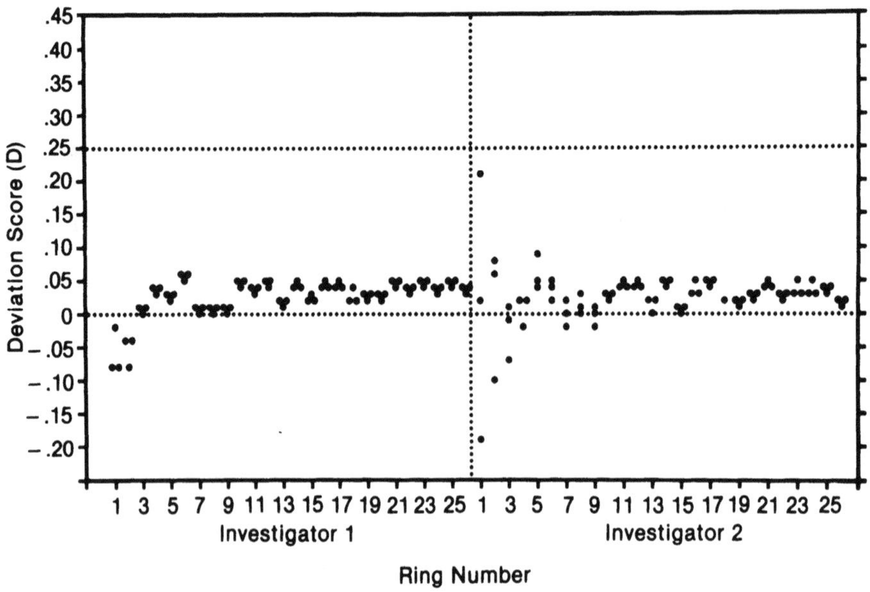

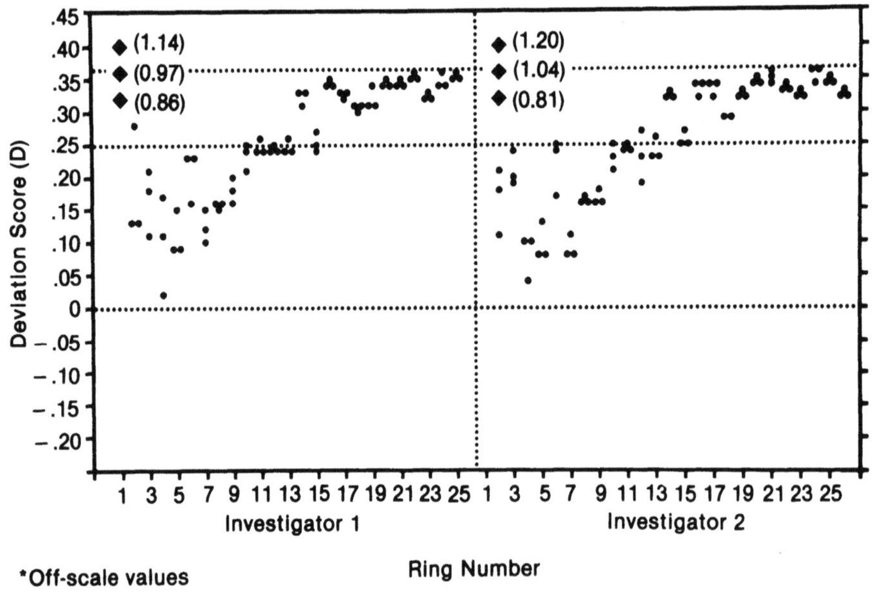

FIGURE 6.8. Accuracy of rings 1 through 26 of the Corneal Modeling System. The deviation score (difference between actual and measured values) is represented on the *x*- axis. On the *y*-axis are the results of readings from 1 through 26 by two investigators, with three readings taken per ring. Except for ring 1, deviation scores for the 43.00 D ball (top left) and the 42.52 D ball (top right) were within ± 0.1 D. However, for the 50.14 D ball (bottom left), readings were less accurate, particularly those from rings 13 through 26. For the 38.66 D ball (bottom right), readings were consistently read too steeply, but not by more than 0.2 D. (With permission of *Arch Ophthalmol.* 1989; 107:1235–1239. © American Medical Association.)

producible measurements and blink frequently to keep a good corneal reflecting surface. Focusing the instruments was also important; all three instruments were focused by visual inspection of an image on the cornea. The Keratometer was the easiest to focus, because the two circular mires created by the doubling prism could be superimposed exactly. The

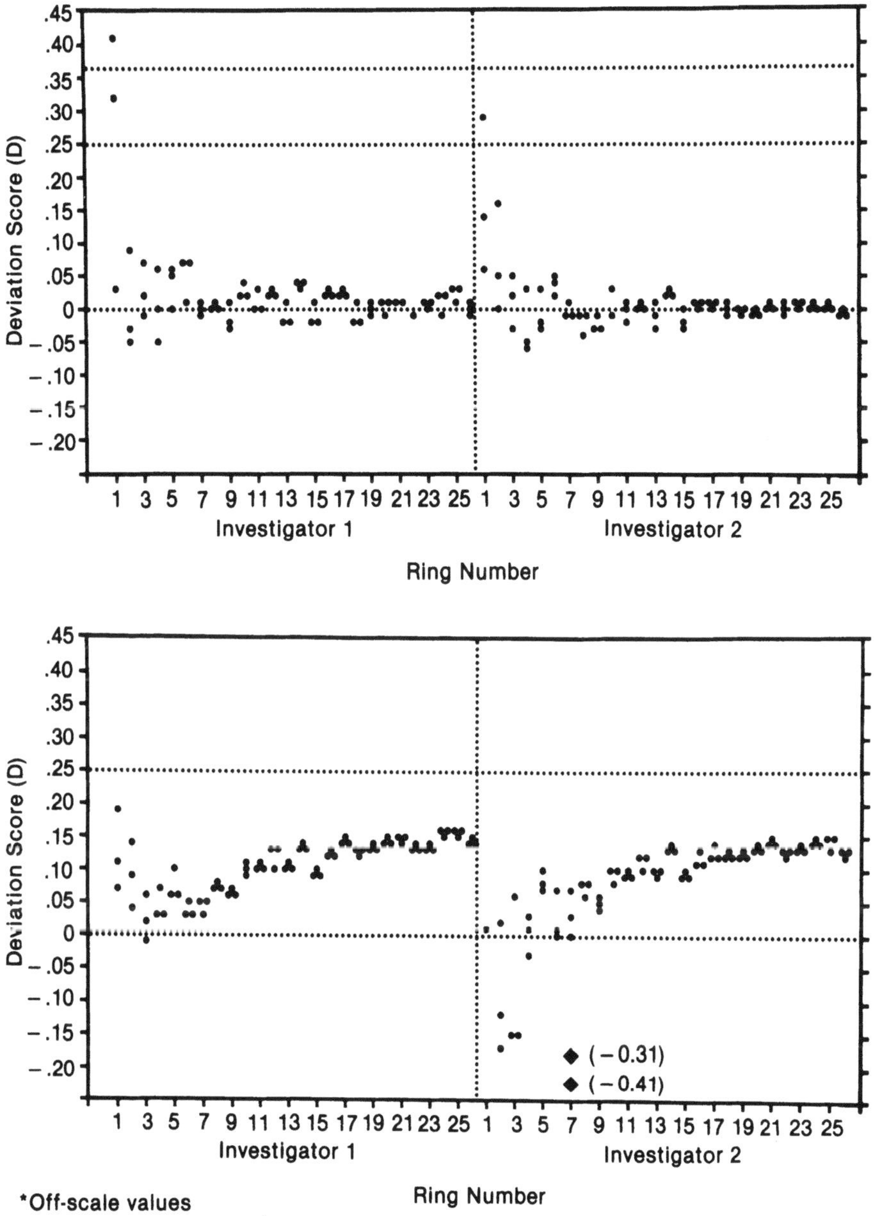

FIGURE 6.8. *Continued.*

Corneal Modeling System required an overlap of two helium-neon laser (HeNe) slit-beam images, without an exact endpoint. The newer topography modeling system has an improved method for focusing that centers the cornea horizontally and vertically by placing a cross image within a small box and then focuses by overlapping two HeNe spots within the box. The Corneascope focused a single image of a cross, without a second image to superimpose. We think that the subjective judgment of the examiner required for focusing was a major factor that contributed to the difference in the precision of the instruments, particularly when it was made more difficult by patient movement, improper alignment of the eye because of brow or eyelid obstruction, and the patient's inability to maintain ocular fixation. Improved

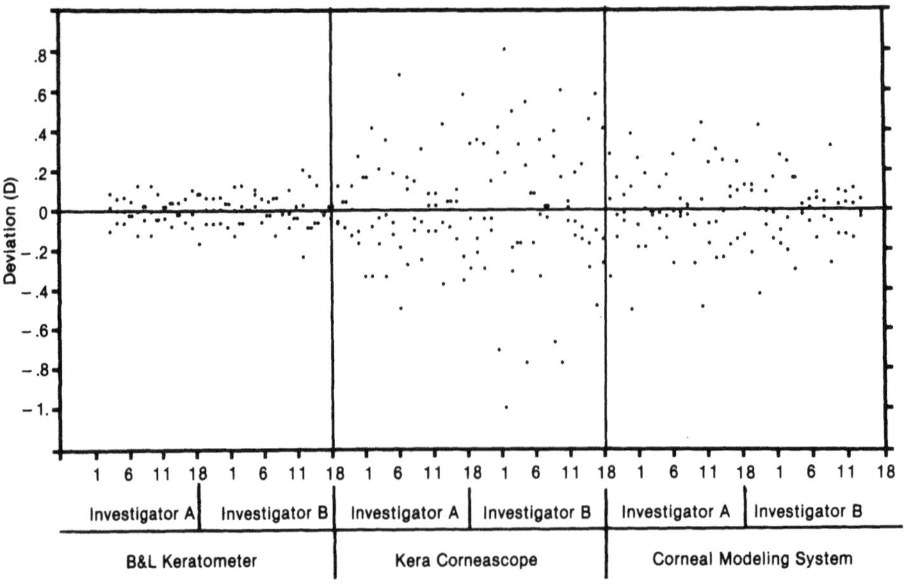

FIGURE 6.9. Comparison of the reproducibilty of measurements at approximately the 3-mm diameter zone by three instruments on 18 normal human corneas. The scattergram shows the deviation from the mean of each of the three measurements of the corneal vertical axis obtained by one investigator with each instrument. The 18 normal eyes, the two investigators (A and B), and the three instruments are indicated across the horizontal axis. D indicates diopters. (With permission of *Arch Ophthalmol.* 1990; 108:539–544. © 1990 American Medical Association.)

sophisticated designs for photokeratoscopes and videokeratoscopes might include an autofocus feedback mechanism that would allow keratography only when the image is in focus.

At the time of this writing, we are comparing two newer videokeratoscopes, the Computed Anatomy Topographic Modeling System (TMS) and the EyeSys Corneal Analysis System. Data on comparative accuracy and reproducibility of the two are not yet available, but we present some comparative features (Table 6.3).

TABLE 6.1. Comparison of three instruments using the deviation of each measurement from the mean corneal power in 18 normal corneas.*

Range of deviation, diopters	Percent of 54 measurements by each investigator					
	Bausch and Lomb keratometer		Kera Corneascope		Computed Anatomy Corneal Modeling System	
	A	B	A	B	A	B
±0.25	100	100	69	54	78	89
±0.50	—	—	96	83	98	100
±1.00	—	—	100	100	100	—

*Three measurements were taken on each cornea by each investigator with each instrument. These three measurements were averaged for each instrument. The deviation score was calculated as the difference of each individual measurement from the mean of the three for that instrument. A and B indicate the two investigators.

From Hannush SB, Crawford SL, Waring GO, Gemmill MC, Lynn MJ, Nizam A. Reproducibility of normal corneal power measurements with a keratometer, photokeratoscope, and video imaging system. With permission of *Arch Ophthalmol.* 1990;108:539–544. © 1990 American Medical Association.

TABLE 6.2. Reproducibility of the Corneal Modeling System as measured by distribution of maximum difference scores across the cornea (Rings 1 through 27) in 18 normal human corneas.*

Maximum difference score (range, diopters)	Percent of maximum difference scores within each range		
	Rings 1–27	Rings 2–13	Rings 3–9
≤0.25	26	42	50
≤0.50	54	76	84
≤1.00	78	97	98
≤1.50	86	100	100
≤2.00	87	—	—

*We calculated the maximum difference between any two of the three measurements taken by an examiner on a ring and used this value to estimate the reproducibility for that ring. A maximum difference of less than 0.5 D was selected as acceptable.

From Hannush SB, Crawford SL, Waring GO, Gemmill MC, Lynn MJ, Nizam A. Reproducibility of normal corneal power measurements with a keratometer, photokeratoscope, and video imaging system. With permission of *Arch Ophthalmol* 1990;108:539–544. © 1990 American Medical Association.

Normal Corneas

Based on keratometric and keratoscopic data, we know that the cornea has an aspheric, radially asymmetic anterior surface and that the size, shape, and the position of the assumed central "spherical zone," as well as the rate and amount of peripheral flattening, are highly variable.[13–18]

Qualitative description of normal corneal topography with videokeratography is important for many reasons: (1) to systematically describe and characterize the variability of normal corneal topography, (2) to develop a basis for the interpretation of color-coded keratographs of the cornea, (3) to develop a framework for differentiating pathologic corneal topography from variants of normal corneal topography, (4) to facilitate investigation and the effects of corneal surgical procedures such as radial and transverse keratotomy, and (5) to understand the relationship between corneal topography, refractive error and visual acuity.[19]

We evaluated the topography of 399 normal corneas in 212 subjects with computer-assisted videokeratography (Computed Anatomy Corneal Modeling System) using the normalized scale. The mean subject age was 37 years (range 8 to 79 years). Mean spherical equivalent manifest refraction was −1.00 D (range +5.50 to −8.37 D). A qualitative classification system for corneal topography was derived based on patterns seen on color-coded topographic maps, and the corneas were classified into groups by three independent masked ophthalmologists, based on criteria published elsewhere.[20] Patterns included round (22.6%), oval (20.8%), symmetric bow-tie (17.5%), asymmetric bow-tie (32.1%), and irregular (7.1%) (Fig. 6.10). All corneas were steeper centrally and flatter peripherally. There was a satistically significant difference among patterns for keratometric astigmatism (Table 6.4), but not for spherical equivalent refraction, mean keratometric power, or age of subject.

Interestingly, we did not detect a statistically significant difference in astigmatism between the round and oval patterns, each having a mean keratometric astigmatism of about 0.5 D. Why does the increased radial asymmetry in the corneal radius of curvature represented by the oval pattern not translate into clinically significant astigmatism? One expla-

TABLE 6.3. Technical comparison of two videokeratoscopes.*

Components	Computed Anatomy Inc. Topographic Modeling System	EyeSys Laboratories Corneal Analysis System
Year of first clinical use	198-	1988
Computer components		
IBM AT compatible 386-based computer	Yes	Yes
High-speed computer upgrade	Yes	Yes
101 key enhanced keyboard	Yes	Yes
Hard disk drive	Yes	Yes
Floppy disk drive	Yes	Yes
High-resolution CCD video camera (512 × 512 pixel)	Yes	Yes
Monitors	Two: 14-in. high-resolution color (for viewing), 5 in. black and white (for taking image)	14 in. color monitor, multisync (for taking image and viewing)
Motorized table	Yes	Yes
Polaroid camera	Yes	Yes
Ink-jet color printer	Yes	Yes
Keratoscope	Solid-state light cone,™ no nose-brow shadow	Placido conical, some nose shadow
View of patient by examiner	Minimally restricted	Moderately restricted
Change of keratoscope for greater coverage	Yes; requires cone replacement	No
Approximate light level (LUX)	800	1400
Number of rings	TMS: 25 CMS: 32	8 (16 edges)
Approximate area of coverage (diameter)	TMS: 0.5 to >8 mm, CMS: 0.5 to 11 mm for 42D cornea	0.7 to 9.6 mm at 42.50 D
Number of points available	256 on each of 25 rings	360 on each of 16 edges
Diopter range	10 to 100D	9 to 99D
Accuracy (steel ball)	± 0.2D**	± 0.2D***
Fixation light	Blinking white light	Green light
Focusing and centering	1. Fixation light 2. Cross hairs in box-central 3. Solid-state diode laser range finder can focus on irregular cornea	1. Focusing optical cross hairs—limbal 2. Video centering box-center 3. "X" on Placido image
Sequential images	May take 4 before processing; minimal between images—5 sec.	Process after each picture; minimal time between images = 50 sec.
Displays		
Color map of dioptric power	Shows only areas with data that can be analyzed; fail safe prevents plotting missing or false data; continuous edges	Missing data not plotted; edit function allows manual override; edges jagged
Time to process and display one color map	55 sec.	33 sec.
Proprietary software	Superresolving	Subpixel resolution
Cursor movement	Arrow keys	Mouse
Normalized and absolute scales	Yes	Yes
Selectable scales (change range)	Yes	Yes
Tabular data	Ring average	Zone average semimeridian
Numerical map	Yes	Yes
Profile graph	No	Yes, at 1° increments
Map data subtraction	Yes	Yes

(*continued*)

TABLE 6.3. *Continued.*

Components	Computed Anatomy Inc. Topographic Modeling System	EyeSys Laboratories Corneal Analysis System
Multiple maps	Two to three on screen	Two to four on screen
*Pupil detection algorithm	Yes—in development	Yes—in development
**Display options	1. Overlay of rectangular and/or polar coordinates 2. Overlay of color maps on rings 3. Klyce statistics a. Predicted best visual acuity b. Surface assymetry index c. Surface regularity index d. Simulated keratometry, min. K	1. Torque profile astigmatism maps
Base system price	$24,950	$21,500

* Information provided by manufacturer in June, 1991. Table does not compare all features of each instrument.
** Hannush SB, Crawford SL, Waring GO, Gemmill MC, Lynn MJ, Nizam A: Accuracy and precision of keratometry, photokeratoscopy, and corneal modeling on calibrated steel balls. *Arch Ophthalmol.* 1989;107:1235–1239.
*** Williams CA, Hannush SB, Reynolds DR, Menduke H: Reproducibility of normal corneal power measurements with a keratometer and a video keratoscope. *Invest Ophthalmol Vis Sci* 1990; 2(suppl):999.

nation might be that the area of the cornea measured by the keratometer (central 3 to 4 mm), or by refraction (the entrance pupil), was within the central area, so that paracentral ovality was not detected.

The bow-tie patterns, both symmetric and asymmetric, had a statistically significant and clinically meaningful greater amount of astigmatism than the round and oval patterns. Somewhat surprisingly, however, was the difference in astigmatism between the symmetric bow-tie and the asymmetric bow-tie patterns, which was highly significant for both refractive and keratometric astigmatism. Possible explanations for the occurrence of the asymmetric bow-tie pattern include (1) eccentric fixation, (2) different locations of the corneal apex and the intersection of the line of sight with the cornea, (3) radial asymmetry in the rate of change of corneal radius of curvature, and (4) warpage from contact lens wear.[19] Whatever the explanation, the nature of the relationship between the topographic pattern and the astigmatic refractive error is difficult to determine. It has been suggested that an asymmetric bow-tie pattern may represent a forme fruste of keratoconus in some cases. We found no evidence of keratoconus in any of our subjects and do not think that this pattern is a reliable indicator of early keratoconus.

There was a 7.1% prevalence of irregular keratographs in our study. It seems unlikely that these eyes, which had normal spectacle-corrected visual acuity and normal-appearing corneas by slit-lamp microscopy, actually had such irregular topography. Possible explanations include tear film abnormalities, improper focusing of the keratoscope, or eccentric fixation. Significantly, eyes with an irregular pattern were consistently irregular on all four the keratoraphs taken.

Although the patterns identified in our classification system were distinctive, the divisions between groups were arbitrary. Variation in corneal topography probably forms a continuum, ranging from spherical to toroidal (Fig. 6.11). As pointed out by Dingeldein and Klyce,[19] the idea of separating the corneal surface into simple surface zones (central, spherical, paracentral, etc) probably has no anatomical correlate because the shape of normal corneas is so highly variable. Reassuringly, all of the cornea in this study exhibited peripheral flattening and nearly all exhibited radial asymmetry, confirming previous descriptions of the cornea as having a prolate, radially asymmetric, aspheric shape.

Because of the variability in corneal topographic patterns among individuals, developing a clinically meaningful classification

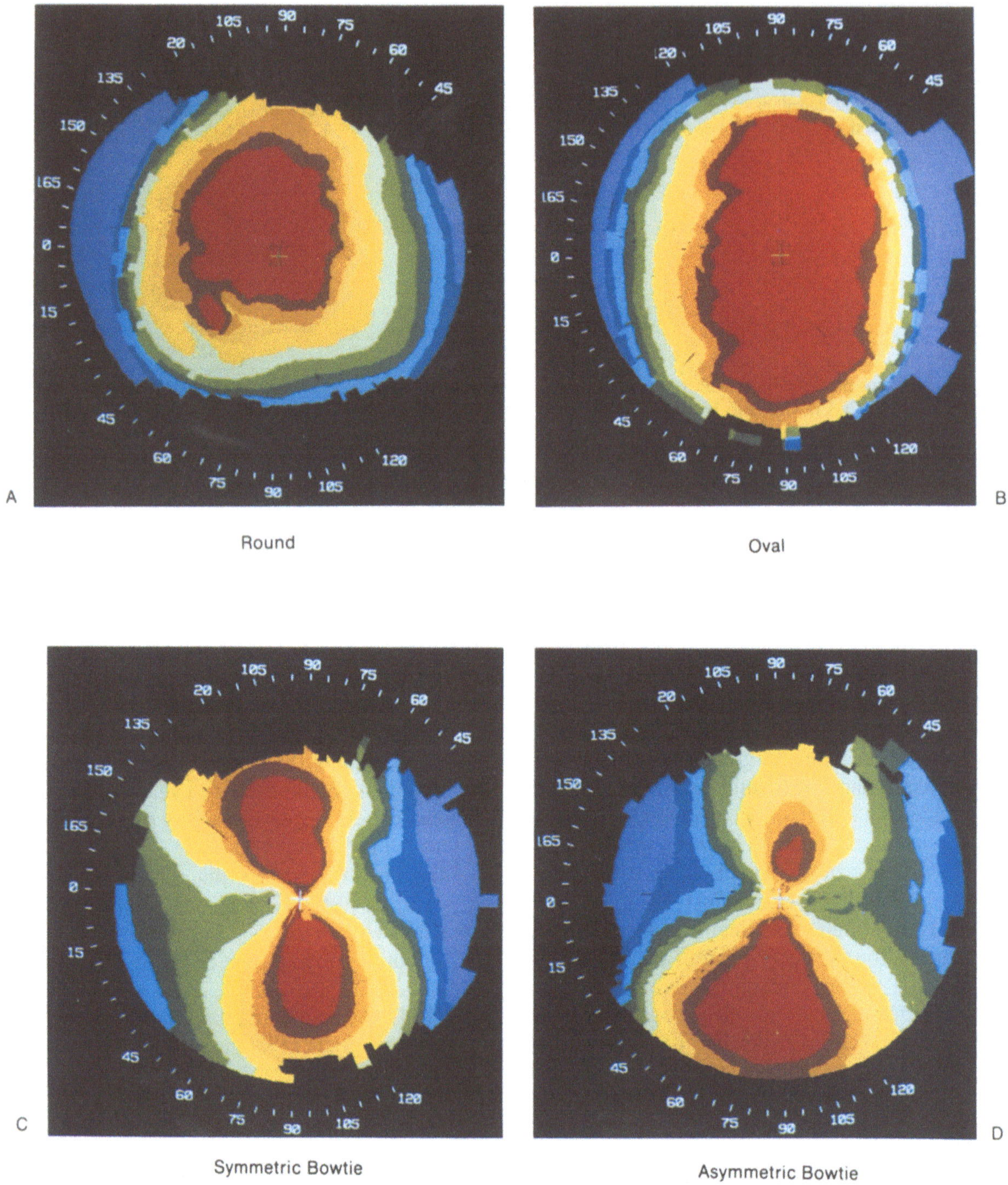

FIGURE 6.10. Five qualitative patterns of normal corneal topography based on computer-assisted videokeratography using the normalized scale. (A) round; (B) oval; (C) symmetric bow-tie; (D) asymmetric bow-tie; (E) irregular; (F) indicates the normalized scale the range of dioptric power (represented by each color) varies among eyes, depending on the amount of corneal asphericity. (From Bogan SJ, Waring GO, Ibrahim O, Drews C, Curtis L. Classification of normal corneal topography based on computer-assisted videokeratography. (With permission of *Arch Ophthalmol*. 1990;108:945–949. © 1990 American Medical Association.)

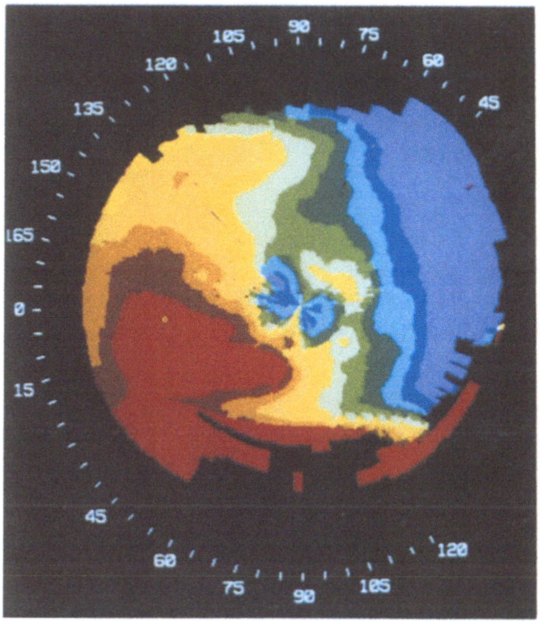

E

Irregular

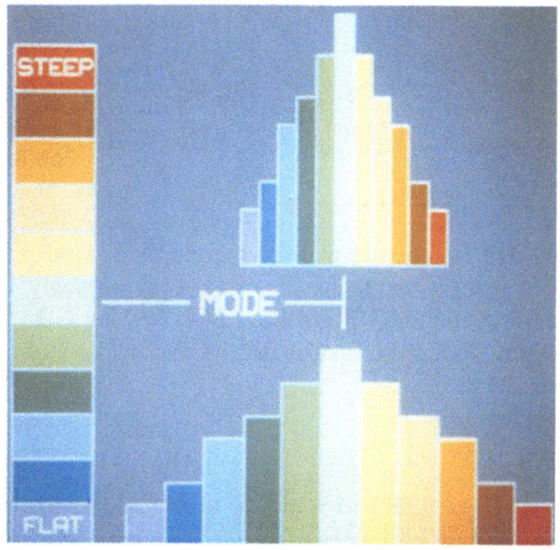

F

FIGURE 6.10 (E, F)

system is a challenge. Contributing to this is the problem of identifying which topographic characteristics are optically or visually important. As techniques for evaluating corneal topography have become more sophisticated, so too have the clinical applications. Our classification scheme is a simple qualitative description of patterns seen on color-coded maps and is intended as a preliminary step in the process of quantitatively characterizing and classifying corneal topography.

Corneal Topography After Radial Keratotomy

We used computer-assisted videokeratography (Computed Anatomy Corneal Modeling

TABLE 6.4. Relationship between the keratometric and refractive astigmatism and the videokeratographic pattern in 216 normal eyes.*

Videokeratographic pattern**	Keratometric astigmatism (D)		Refractive astigmatism (D)	
	(mean±SD)	%≥1.00 D	(mean±SD)	%≥1.00 D
Round	0.47 ± 0.34	10%	0.28 ± 0.39	8%
Oval	0.57 ± 0.30	20%	0.26 ± 0.41	7%
Symmetric bow-tie	1.40 ± 0.98	73%	1.00 ± 1.20	43%
Asymmetric bow-tie	0.89 ± 0.70	41%	0.47 ± 0.78	19%
Irregular	0.64 ± 0.53	27%	0.53 ± 0.51	27%

*One eye per subject.

**Normalized scale, Computed Anatomy Corneal Modeling System.

From Bogan SJ, Waring GO, Ibrahim O, Drews CD, Curtis L. Classification of normal corneal topography based on computer-assisted videokeratography. With permission of *Arch Ophthalmol* 1990;108:945–949. © 1990 American Medical Association.

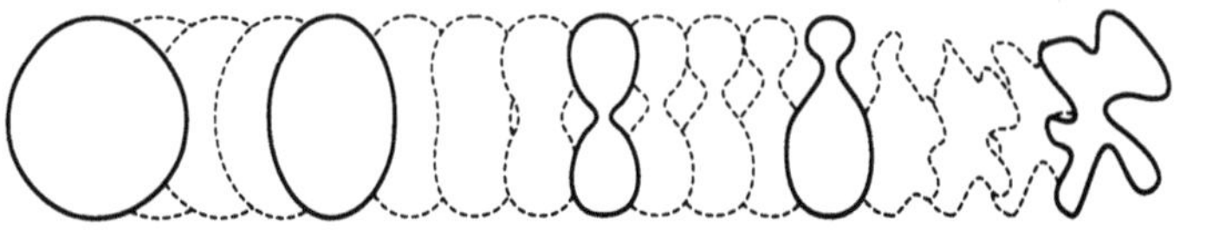

FIGURE 6.11. The five patterns recognized in color-coded topographic maps of normal eyes probably form a continuum. (From Bogan SJ, Waring GO, Ibrahim O, Drews C, Curtis L. Classification of normal corneal topography based on computer-assisted videokeratography. (With permission of *Arch Opthalmol.* 1990; 108:945–949. © 1990 American Medical Association.)

System), normalized scale, to compare the topography of 32 corneas from 23 subjects after radial keratotomy to the topography of 47 normal corneas from 47 subjects, matched for age and preoperative keratometric and refractive power.[21] Three ophthalmologists independently classified color-coded videokeratographs, based on the qualitative pattern of dioptric power distribution and the cross section of the shape.

Qualitative Descriptors

Topographic Pattern

The term "pattern" referred to the distribution of dioptric powers seen on color-coded topographic maps. Patterns included round, oval, symmetric bow-tie, asymmetric bow-tie, irregular, and polygonal (Fig. 6.12). One pattern that was seen after radial keratotomy, that was not seen in normal corneas, was a polygonal pattern. Criteria for identifying this pattern were that the color zones chosen for classification were roughly concentric, but instead of being round or oval, had two or more angles (≤ 135°) and three or more nearly straight lines. Polygonal patterns including squares, hexagons, and octagons appeared in 59% of radial keratotomy corneas.

Corneal Shape

Shape referred to the contour of a cross-sectional profile of the cornea. The corneas in the study fell into one of three configurations:[7] (1) prolate or positive shape factor, (2) oblate or a negative shape factor, (3) mixed prolate/oblate where the cornea had a prolate shape in one area and an oblate shape in another (Fig. 6.12). All normal corneas demonstrated a cross section that was steeper centrally than peripherally (prolate); 70% of corneas after radial keratotomy had a shape that was flatter centrally than peripherally (oblate). Normal corneas showed a smooth decrease in power of 1.9 ± 0.5 D (mean ± SD); corneas with radial keratotomy showed an increase in power of 2.8 ± 2.2 D from the center out to a radius of approximately 4.6 mm with a sharp inflection zone ("paracentral knee") at 2.7 ± 0.1 mm from the center.

Quantitative Descriptors

Asphericity

We represented the corneal asphericity by a curve that depicted the difference in dioptric power between ring 1 and each successive ring out to approximately ring 27. These differences were recorded for each eye in the 0°, 90°, 180°, and 270° semimeridians, and the values for all the eyes in each group at each ring, along each of the four cardinal semimeridians were averaged. Since the difference values were calculated by subtracting the dioptric power of ring 1 from the power of the more peripheral ring, a positive number represented steepening, while a negative number represented flattening.

We chose to report corneal power in diopters (D) rather than radius of curvature (mm) and to report distance from the center in millimeters rather in ring numbers. We thought that dioptric power was more clinically relevant than radius of curvature. In Figures 6.13 and 6.14 the distance of each data point from the center was calculated by averaging the distance of each ring from the center for all eyes along each of the cardinal semimeridians. However, the distance of each ring from the center of ring 1 may vary among semimeridians and among eyes. The standard deviation of these distances ranges from 0.02 mm centrally to 0.26 mm peripherally.

Rate of Change in Dioptric Power

The rate of change in dioptric power was calculated at each ring along the 0°, 90°, 180°, and 270° semimeridians in the following manner. From the dioptric power of each ring, we subtracted the dioptric power of the adjacent more central ring and divided the number by the distance in millimeters between the two rings. Average rate of change was calculated in each cardinal semimeridian by averaging the rates of change at that position for all corneas in each group.

Topography of the Entrance Pupil

We measured maximum range in dioptric power over a 4-mm area of cornea that was centered on the center of the entrance pupil, as determined on a frozen video image of the constricted pupil. Of course, not all pupils were 4 mm in diameter, but this approach allowed us to estimate the topograpahy of the corneas over the entire pupil.

Quantitative Corneal Topography After Radial Keratotomy

In this study, corneal asphericity after radial keratotomy was significantly greater than that of normal eyes (Fig. 6.13 and 6.14). Normal eyes demonstrated a relatively constant rate of change in dioptric power from the center to the periphery, but after radial keratotomy there was an increased rate of change in dioptric power between 2.6 and 3.3 mm from the center. Other authors have postulated the existence of this inflection zone (''paracentral knee''),[22] but its location has not been previously documented. The location of the inflection zone in the study agrees well with computer simulation of change in corneal shape after radial keratotomy, reported by Hanna and colleagues,[23] which predicted the flattening and posterior displacement of the central 6 mm diameter of the cornea and steepening and anterior displacement of the peripheral cornea between 6 and 11 mm in diameter.[23] The postulate of overall flattening of the cornea after radial keratotomy by other investigators[24] is untenable, based on the computer simulation model[23] and on our data from videokeratography. Analysis of the eight eyes for which we had pre- and postoperative videokeratographs also showed a trend toward peripheral steepening of the cornea after radial keratotomy.

The concept of the ''multifocal cornea'' has been used to explain good visual acuity despite residual refractive error in some patients after radial keratotomy.[24, 25] However, the cause of the multifocal effect has not been determined. Is it simply that the cornea has a greater range of power after radial keratotomy, or is it a certain pattern of power distribution required? We found that the cornea after radial keratotomy had a greater range in dioptric power from the center to the periphery than normal eyes. More important, the range of powers seen in the cornea over the standard 4 mm entrance pupil was nearly twice as great after radial keratotomy (3.8 ± 2.40) as in normal eyes (2.0 ± 0.5 D), indicating the potential for a multifocal lens effect.

Because the inflection point (''paracentral knee'') is located outside the entrance pupil (Figs. 6.13 and 6.14), it is unlikely that the increased asphericity caused by the inflection point accounts for the increased range of good visual acuity seen in some patients after radial keratotomy.[26] More likely, it is change in the topography over the entrance pupil (within the clear zone) that accounts for this finding. As Applegate and Gansel have observed, it is the location and size of the entrance pupil that is important when considering the optical function of the cornea after radial keratotomy.[27]

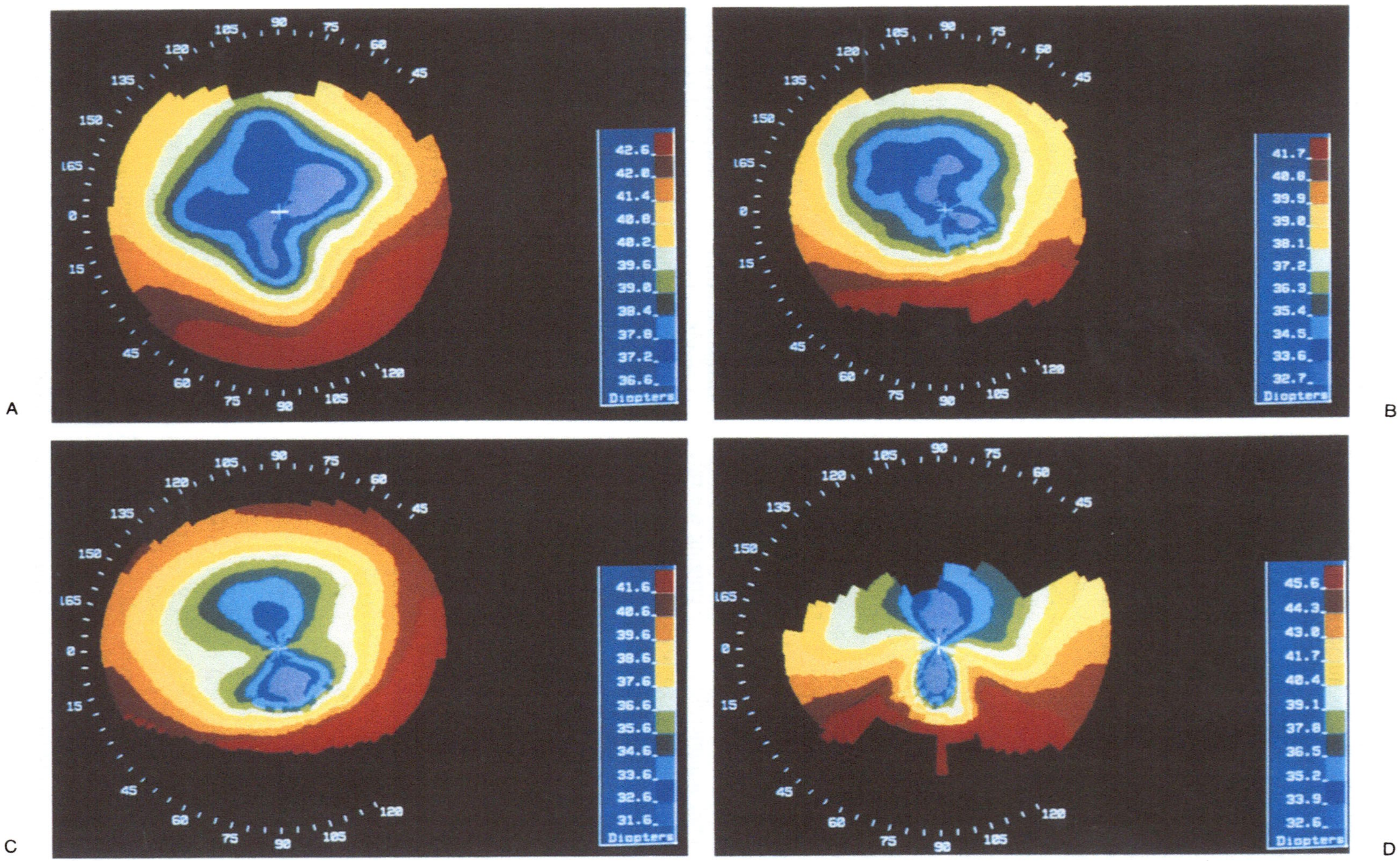
A
42.6
42.0
41.4
40.8
40.2
39.6
39.0
38.4
37.8
37.2
36.6
Diopters
B
41.7
40.8
39.9
39.0
38.1
37.2
36.3
35.4
34.5
33.6
32.7
Diopters
C
41.6
40.6
39.6
38.6
37.6
36.6
35.6
34.6
33.6
32.6
31.6
Diopters
D
45.6
44.3
43.0
41.7
40.4
39.1
37.8
36.5
35.2
33.9
32.6
Diopters

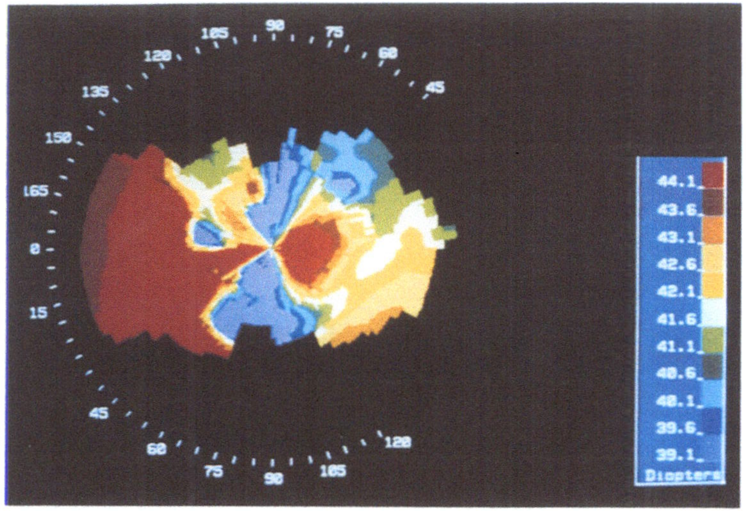

E

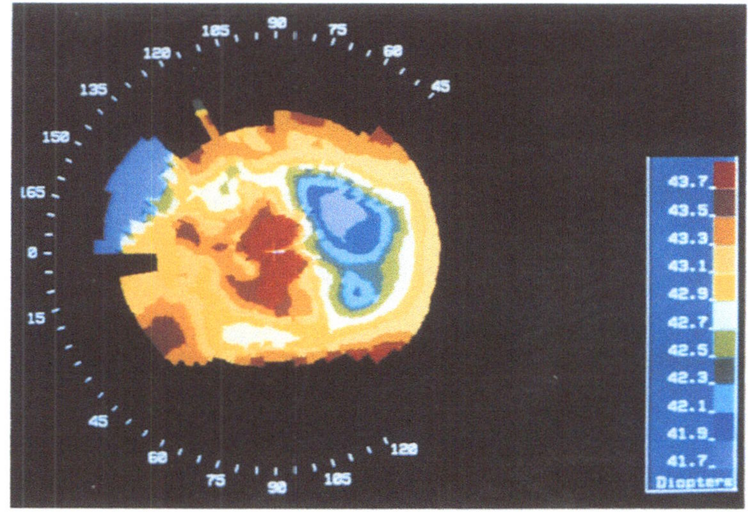

F

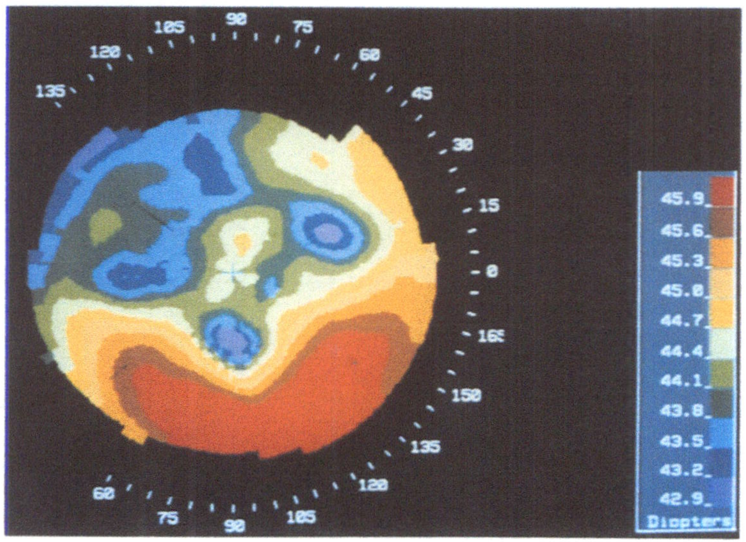

G

FIGURE 6.12. Videokeratographs showing seven patterns of power distribution in 32 corneas after radial keratotomy. The polygonal pattern was not seen in normal eyes. (A) Polygonal pattern, oblate shape. (B) Round pattern, oblate shape. (C) Symmetric bow-tie pattern, oblate shape. (D) Asymmetric bow-tie pattern, oblate shape. (E) Bow-tie pattern, mixed prolate/oblate shape. (F) Polygonal pattern, oblate shape. Steep/flat/steep ("nipple") configuration. (G) Irregular pattern, irregular shape (From Bogan SJ, Maloney RK, Drews CD, Waring GO. Computer-assisted videokeratography of corneal topography after radial keratotomy. (With permission of *Arch Ophthalmol*, June 1991; 109:834–841. © 1990 American Medical Association.)

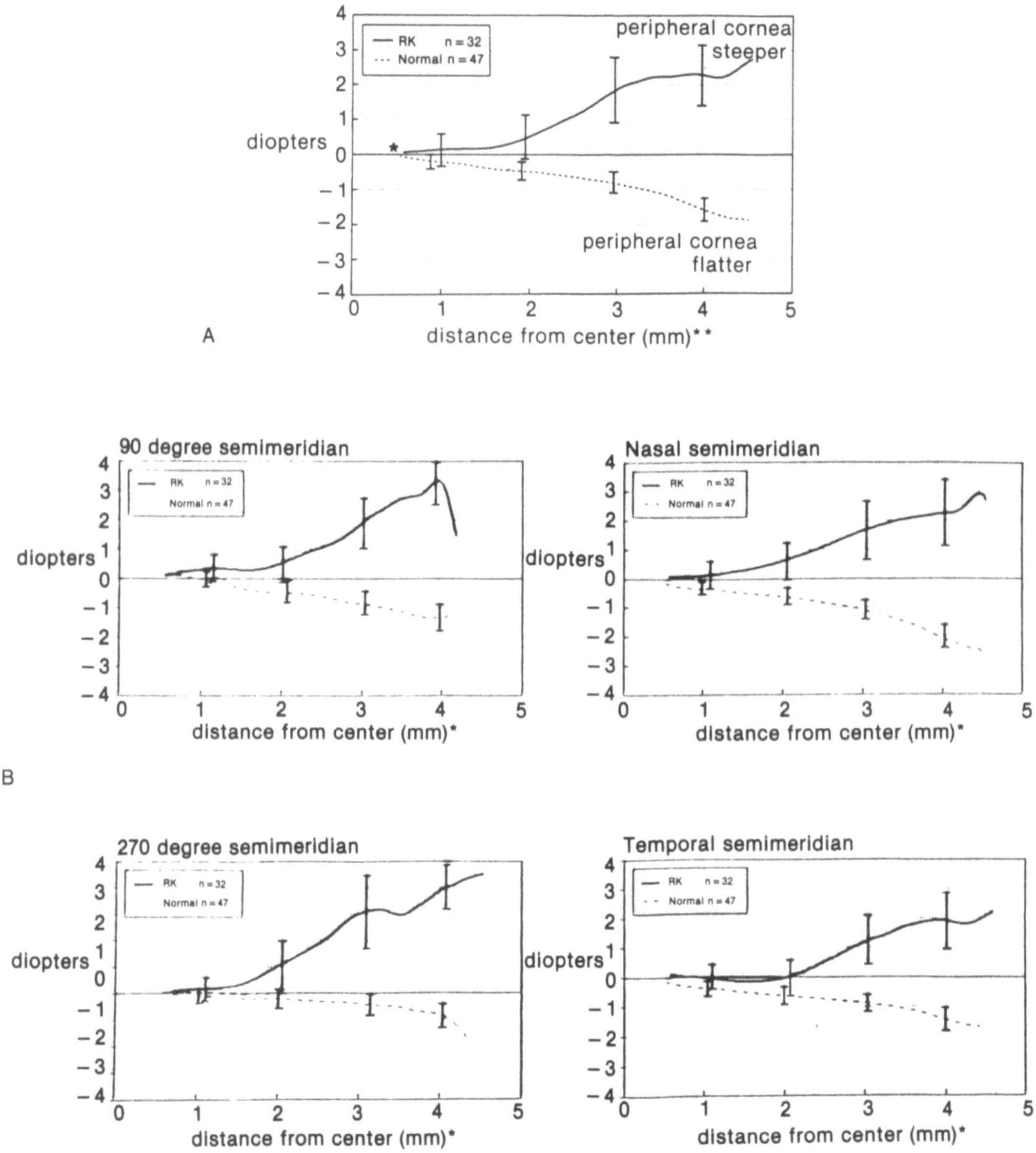

FIGURE 6.13. Corneal asphericity represented by a plot of the difference in dioptric power between rings 1 and rings 2 through 27 in normal corneas and corneas after radial keratotomy. (A) Average of values of 0°, 90°, 180°, 270° semimeridians combined. The curves demonstrate that after radial keratotomy the cornea is more aspheric and has more variable rate of change in dioptric power than normal corneas. (B) 0°, 90°, 180°, 270° semimeridians individually. Shows that asymmetry and asphericity among semimeridians is greater after radial keratotomy than in normal eyes. (From Bogan SJ, Maloney RK, Drews CD, Waring GO. Computer-assisted corneal topography after radial keratotomy. (With permission of *Arch Ophthalmol* June 1991; 109:834–841. © 1991 American Medical Association.)

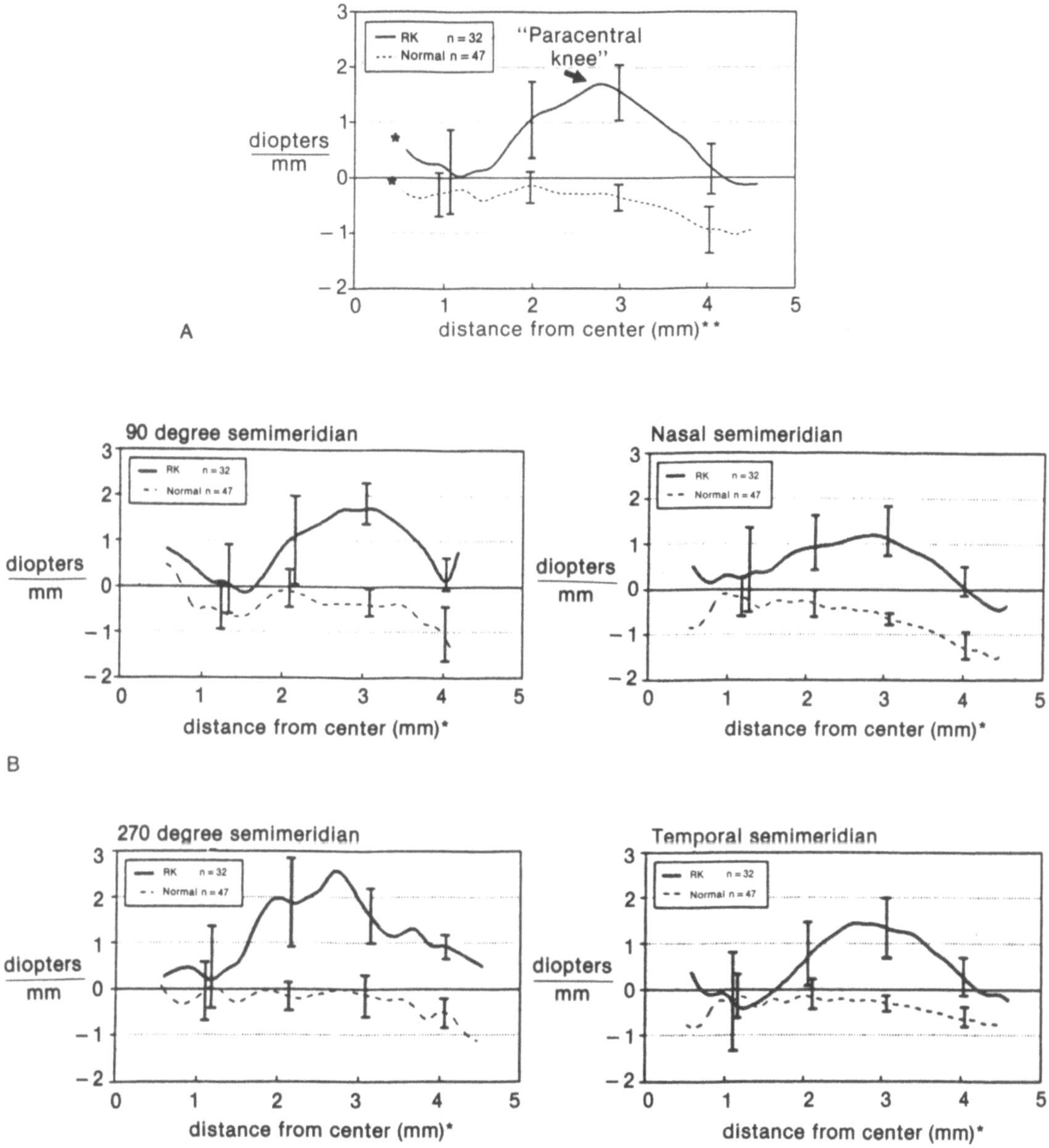

FIGURE 6.14. Rate of change in corneal dioptric power between ring 1 and rings 2 through 27. (A) Average of 0°, 90°, 180°, 270° semimeridians combined. The curves demonstrate a sharp inflection zone ("paracentral knee") after radial keratotomy located on a mean of 2.7 ± 0.1 mm from the center. (B) 0°, 90°, 180°, 270° semimeridians individually. The curves show asymmetry in the rate of change in corneal power along semimeridians, with a "paracentral knee." (From Bogan SJ, Maloney RK, Drews CD, Waring GO. Computer-assisted videokeratography of corneal topography after radial keratotomy.) (With permission of *Arch Ophthalmol.* June 1991: 834–841. © 1991 American Medical Association.)

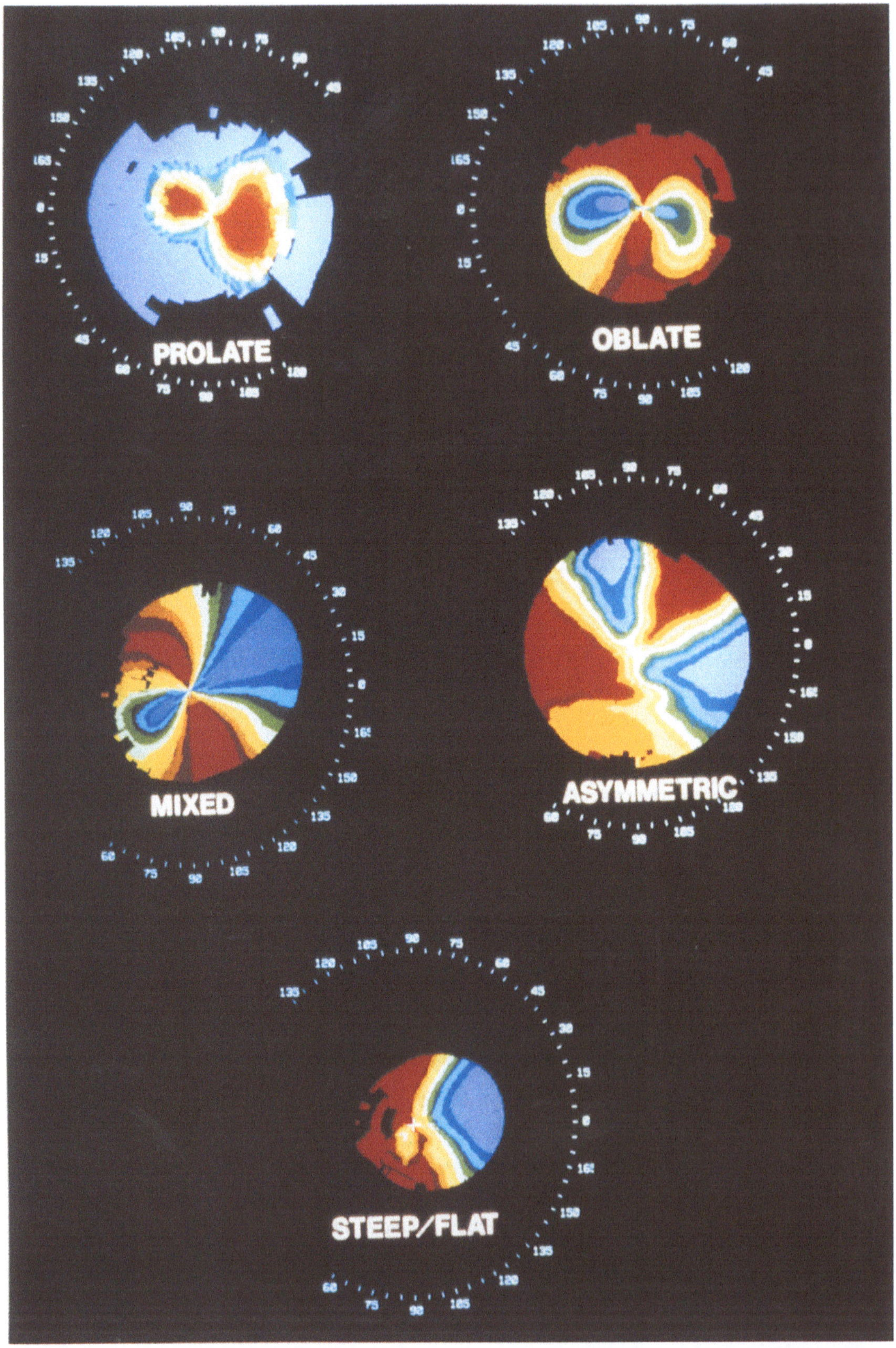

A B C D E

Further work correlating the range and pattern of power distribution over the entrance pupil with visual acuity and the optical quality of the corneal surface remains to be done.

Corneal Topography After Penetrating Keratoplasty

We classify qualitatively the topography of 45 corneas with clear penetrating keratoplasty and all sutures removed, observing five patterns[28] (Fig. 6.15).

1. Prolate (14, 31%). The cornea had regular astigmatism featured as a symmetric, red bow-tie pattern. Along the semimeridians of the bow-tie, color gradations showed steep central regions that became flatter toward the periphery.
2. Oblate (14, 31%). The cornea had regular astigmatism featured as a symmetric, blue bow-tie pattern. Along the semimeridians of the bowtie, color gradations showed flat central regions that became steeper toward the periphery.
3. Mixed prolate and oblate (8, 17.8%). The cornea had regular astigmatism with at least one of the four principal semimeridians depicted as a half red bow-tie, as seen in the prolate pattern and another principal semimeridian, depicted as a half blue bow-tie as seen in the oblate pattern. The half bow-ties were approximately 90° or 180° from one another.
4. Asymmetric (3, 8.7%). The principal semimeridians could be depicted by any of the previous patterns (red or blue, partial or complete bow-ties), but the two steep semimeridians were not aligned along a single meridian.
5. Steep/flat (6, 13.5%). The cornea was steeper on one side and became progressively flatter toward the other side.

The majority of corneas (approximately 90% comprising the prolate, oblate, mixed and asymmetric groups) had a large amount of astigmatism with a mean of approximately 5 D. Therefore, most of these corneas demonstrated a bow-tie configuration on the videokeratograph. In contrast, the steep/flat pattern had a statistically significantly lower amount of astigmatism (of approximately 3 D) and did not show the bow-tie pattern.

To provide a quantitative analysis of corneal topography after penetrating keratoplasty, Tripoli and colleagues[28] developed a method of quantitative analysis (Corneal Pattern Analysis Method CPAM) which measured the change in corneal power along each semimeridian, computing the average curvature and the slope of the line along each semimeridian. The quantitative analysis of each cornea was correlated with the five qualitative patterns mentioned above. For example, a prolate cornea would have a high central dioptric power and a lower peripheral dioptric power to produce a best fit line with the negative slope. An oblate cornea would have lower central dioptric power values in the center and higher values in the periphery, to produce semimeridians with a positive slope. The magnitude and sine of the slope measured the degree to which a cornea was prolate or oblate. The power distribution in different meridians would be bimodal because there were steep and flat semimeridians as a result of the astigmatism. Of the 41 corneas available for analysis, 25 were placed in the same pattern category by both the qualitative estimate of the ophthalmologists and the quantitative measurements of the CPAM. This was a statistically significant correlation ($P <$ 0.001, Kappa Statistic). Analysis of the reasons for disagreement among the remaining corneas indicated that the normal eyes scale may have been reason for disagreement, and such analyses and classifications may be better carried out using an absolute scale with 1.00 D steps. Qualitative algorithms may also be able

◁

FIGURE 6.15. Qualitative patterns of corneal topography after penetrating keratoplasty (sutures removed) based on computer-assisted videokeratography using the normalized scale: (A) Prolate. (B) Oblate. (C) Mixed prolate and oblate. (D) Asymmetric. and (E) steep/flat.

to distinguish keratographs in which the flat and steep semimeridians are not oriented orthogonally to each other.

The Future of Videokeratography

Computer-assisted videokeratography has greatly improved the ability of the clinician and researcher to understand the complexities of corneal shape and optical function. However, there are many topics and areas that still need refinement. Improved centering and focusing systems for the instruments will make them easier to use and more replicable. Algorithms based on aspheric optics will allow more accurate depiction of the aspheric cornea. The presentation of an outline of the location of the pupil will help identify the optically most important part of the cornea for each individual patient. The development of mathematical descriptors that can characterize the overall shape of the cornea (in a weighted manner to be more optically relevant) will improve the qualitative classifications presented in this chapter. Measurements of the entire corneal surface, from center to limbus, will be necessary for studies of the influence of corneal shape on the outcome of refractive surgery; that is, the information is important in deciding if topography is a predictive factor to be used to modify refractive surgical techniques for an individual eye. Topographic information will be more meaningful when combined with ray tracing algorithms to better determine the overall optical effect of the cornea on ocular refraction.

References

1. Waring GO. Making sense of keratospeak II: proposed conventional terminology for corneal topography. *Refract. Corneal Surg.* 1989; 5: 362–367.
2. Dabezies OH, Halladay JT. Measurement of corneal curvature: Keratometer (ophthalmometer). In: Dabezies OH, ed. *Contact Lenses: The CLAO Guide to Basic Science and Clinical Practice.* Orlando, FL: Grune and Stratton, 1984; pp 17.1–17.27.
3. Stone J. Keratometry. In: Ruben M, ed. *Contact Lens Practice: Visual, Therapeutic and Prosthetic.* Baltimore, Williams and Wilkins, 1975; pp 104–129.
4. Burk LL, Waring GO, Radjee B, et al. The effect of selective suture removal on astigmatism after penetrating keratoplasty. *Ophthalmic Surg.* 1988; 19:849–854.
5. Maguire LJ, Singer DE, Klyce SD. Graphic presentation of computer-analyzed keratoscope photographs. *Arch Ophthalmol.* 1987; 105:223–230.
6. Dingeldein SA, Klyce SD, Wilson SE. Quantitative descriptors of corneal shape derived from computer-assisted analysis of photokeratographs. *Refract Corneal Surg.* 1989; 5:372–378.
7. Rowsey JJ, Waring GO, Monlux RD, et al. Corneal topography as a refractive change predictor in PERK radial keratotomy. *Ophthalmic Surg.*, in press.
8. Miller D, Carter J. A proposed new division of corneal functions. In: Cavanagh HD, ed. *The Cornea. Transactions of the World Congress on the Cornea III.* New York: Raven Press, 1988; pp 155–158.
9. Ruben M. *Contact Lens Practice.* Baltimore; Williams and Wilkins, 1975; p 97.
10. Rowsey JJ, Schanzlin DJ. Corneal topography. In: Dabezies OH, Cavanagh HD, Farris RD, eds. *Contact Lenses: The CLAO Guide to Basic Science and Clinical Practice.* 2nd ed. Boston; Little, Brown , 1989; pp 1–16.
11. Hannush SB, Crawford SL, Waring GO, et al. Accuracy and precision of keratometry, photokeratoscopy, and corneal modeling on calibrated steel balls. *Arch Ophthalmol.* 1989; 107:1235–1239.
12. Hannush SB, Crawford SL, Waring GO, et al. Reproducibility of normal corneal power measurements with a keratometer, photokeratoscope, and video imaging system. *Arch Ophthalmol.* 1990; 108:539–544.
13. Clark BAJ. Mean topography of normal corneas. *Aust J Optom.* 1974; 57:107–114.
14. Knoll HA. Corneal contours in the general population as revealed by the photokeratoscope. *Am J Optom.* 1961; 38:389–397.
15. Clark BAJ. Topography of some individual corneas. *Aust J Optom.* 1974; 57:65–69.
16. Mandell RB, St Helen R. Position and curvature of the corneal apex. *Am J Optom.* 1969; 46: 25–29.
17. Clark BAJ. Variations in corneal topography. *Aust J Optom.* 1973; 56:399–413.

18. Kiely PM, Smith G, Carney LG. The mean shape of the human cornea. *Optom Acta*. 1982; 29:1027–1040.
19. Dingeldein SA, Klyce SD. The topography of normal corneas. *Arch Ophthalmol*. 1989; 107:512–518.
20. Bogan SJ, Waring GO, Ibrahim O, et al. Classification of normal corneal topography based on computer-assisted videokeratography. *Arch Ophthalmol*. 1990; 108:945–949.
21. Bogan SJ, Maloney RK, Drews CD, et al. Computer-assisted videokeratography of corneal topography after radial keratotomy. *Arch Ophthalmol*. 1990; 108.
22. Rowsey JJ, Waring GO, Monlux R, et al. Prospective evaluation of radial keratotomy (PERK) study. Photokeratoscope corneal topography. *Ophthalmology*. 1988; 95:322–334.
23. Hanna KD, Jouve FE, Waring GO. Preliminary computer simulation of the effects of radial keratotomy. *Arch Ophthalmol*. 1989; 107:911–918.
24. McDonnell PJ, Garbus J. Corneal topographic changes after radial keratotomy. *Ophthalmology*. 1989; 96:45–49.
25. Maguire LJ, Bourne WM. A multifocal lens effect as a complication of radial keratotomy. *Refract Corneal Surg*. 1989; 5:394–399.
26. Santos VR, Waring GO, Lynn MJ, et al. Relationship between refractive error and visual acuity in the prospective evaluation of radial keratotomy (PERK) study. *Arch Ophthalmol*. 1987; 105:86–92.
27. Applegate A. Gansel KA. The importance of pupil size in optical quality measurements following radial keratotomy. *Refract Corneal Surg*. 1990; 6:47–54.
28. Tripoli NK, Ibrahim OS, Coggins JM, et al. Quantitative and qualitative topography classification of clear penetrating keratoplasties. *Invest Ophthalmol Vis Sci*. 1990; 30 (suppl): 480.

7
Corneal Topography in the Diagnosis and Management of Keratoconus

Patrick J. Caroline and Craig W. Norman

Early reference to keratoconus was made by Mauchart (1748) and Taylor (1766), but the condition was first adequately described and distinguished from other corneal ectasias by Nottingham in 1854.[1] At that time, the treatment of keratoconus consisted of cauterization of the conical area with silver nitrate and the instillation of miotics accompanied by a pressure dressing.[2] In the early months of 1888, a French ophthalmologist, Eugene Kalt, began work on a crude glass shell designed to "compress the steep conical apex thereby correcting the condition." This was the first known application of a contact lens for the correction of keratoconus.[2, 3]

Since 1888, a wide variety of contact lens designs and fitting techniques have been promoted for keratoconus, most enjoying limited success.[4–8] Only in recent years have practitioners been able to adequately manage the condition with contact lenses. A number of technological advances made this possible, the most prominent being the development of modern photokeratoscopy techniques. Photokeratoscopy enabled clinicians to better understand keratoconus and also have allowed contact lens manufacturers to design more appropriate lens configurations for this complex condition.

To better understand modern contact lens fitting techniques for keratoconus, it is absolutely necessary to comprehend the corneal topography changes that occur in both the early and advanced forms of the disorder.

Corneal Topography in Keratoconus

Although the etiology of keratoconus remains somewhat unclear, the topographical changes have been well documented. It was Dekking (1920), and later Amsler (1932), who provided the first descriptions of these changes based on early photokeratoscopy findings.[9–11] The system introduced by Amsler classified keratoconus into four stages[12]:

Stage 1: Oblique astigmatism with inequality of the keratoscopy mires
Stage 2: Intensification of the above signs
Stage 3: Pronounced conical shape with corneal thinning but no opacities
Stage 4: Opacities at the apex

More recently, A. E. Reynolds (personal communication, 1985), L. Bronstein (personal communication, 1988) and Rowsey[13] have further described the geometry of the keratoconus eye based on photographs obtained using the Corneascope (Kera Inc., Santa Clara, CA) photokeratoscopy instrument. Tomlinson and Schwartz,[14] Townsley,[15] and Wesley[16] have also contributed to our understanding of the corneal topography in keratoconus through the use of the Photo Electric Keratometer. Recent advances in computer-based analysis of keratoscopy images (described elsewhere in this book) have enabled even greater understanding of the topographic patterns characteristic of the early as well as late stages of keratoconus.[17]

These modern photokeratoscopy techniques have demonstrated that in early keratoconus there is characteristically a pear-shaped pull of the central keratoscopy rings with steepening initially occurring inferiorly, usually in the temporal quadrant (Fig. 7.1). In this early stage, the superior cornea (above the midline) remains relatively unaffected and thus "normal" in curvature, similar to a nonkeratoconic eye (Fig. 7.2.)[18] This combination of topographic findings—pear-shaped inferotemporal steepening plus normal curvature of the superior half of the cornea—is sufficiently pathognomonic to allow photokeratoscopy to be the primary diagnosis tool for early keratoconus. Additionally, the normal superior corneal topography becomes the most important consideration in fitting contact lenses for early keratoconus, because the "normal" portion of the cornea, not the steeper conical area, determines the lens design and fitting technique.

As previously noted, the earliest keratoscopic change noted in keratoconus is a paracentral steepening most commonly located in the inferotemporal quadrant. As the condition progresses, the steepening spreads nasally to include the inferior (6 o'clock) and inferonasal cornea. In advanced forms of the condition, rotational steepening occurs at and above the midline along a path that eventually includes the temporal, superotemporal, and superior (12 o'clock) cornea (Fig. 7.3). The superonasal quadrant of the cornea is always the last to be affected, and thus an "island" of normal corneal topography often remains in this area even in the most advanced stages of the condition (Fig. 7.4) (L. Bronstein, personal communication, 1985, and Ref. 13). Additionally, it should be mentioned that, even in the advanced forms of keratoconus, the superior 3 to 4 mm of the cornea remains relatively "normal" in curvature. Although there are exceptions to these patterns of corneal changes in keratoconus, the vast majority of eyes have been noted to follow this "spiral" progression. Many of these changes obviously occur well beyond the area evaluated by the keratometer. The keratoscope, and now its photo- and video-based progeny, is absolutely essential to document the complex topographic changes in keratoconus. Furthermore, as will be discussed below, modern contact lens management of this condition depends almost entirely upon adequate documentation of these topographic abnormalities.

Corneal Topography in Advanced Keratoconus

Throughout the years, authors have described keratoconus as a noninflammatory steepening of the central cornea resulting from stromal thinning. Although few will argue with this definition, it is clear today that the diagnosis of advanced keratoconus is one that encompasses an entire spectrum of *diversely shaped* ectatic conditions. The only common topographical finding present in these corneas is central or paracentral corneal steepening. Beyond the central 5 mm, structural changes take place in the area of the midperipheral and peripheral cornea creating shapes that have been classified as either "nipple," "oval,"[20] or "globus" (Fig. 7.5).[19] In addition to determining classification, the peripheral corneal changes in keratoconus will have a profound effect on the choice of contact lens design and the fitting technique; in the most advanced cases, they also may affect the degree of postkeratoplasty astigmatism.

For contact lens fitting purposes, we have devised a specific fitting philosophy for each of the three corneal shapes found in advanced keratoconus. This system is based not on central corneal curvature, but primarily on the status of the peripheral corneal topography as determined by photokeratoscopy.

Nipple-Shaped Topography

The nipple form of keratoconus characteristically consists of a small central ectasia less than 5 mm in diameter.[21] The most striking feature of the nipple contour is the nearly 360° of "normal" cornea that surrounds the base of the cone (Fig. 7.6). The topography of the nip-

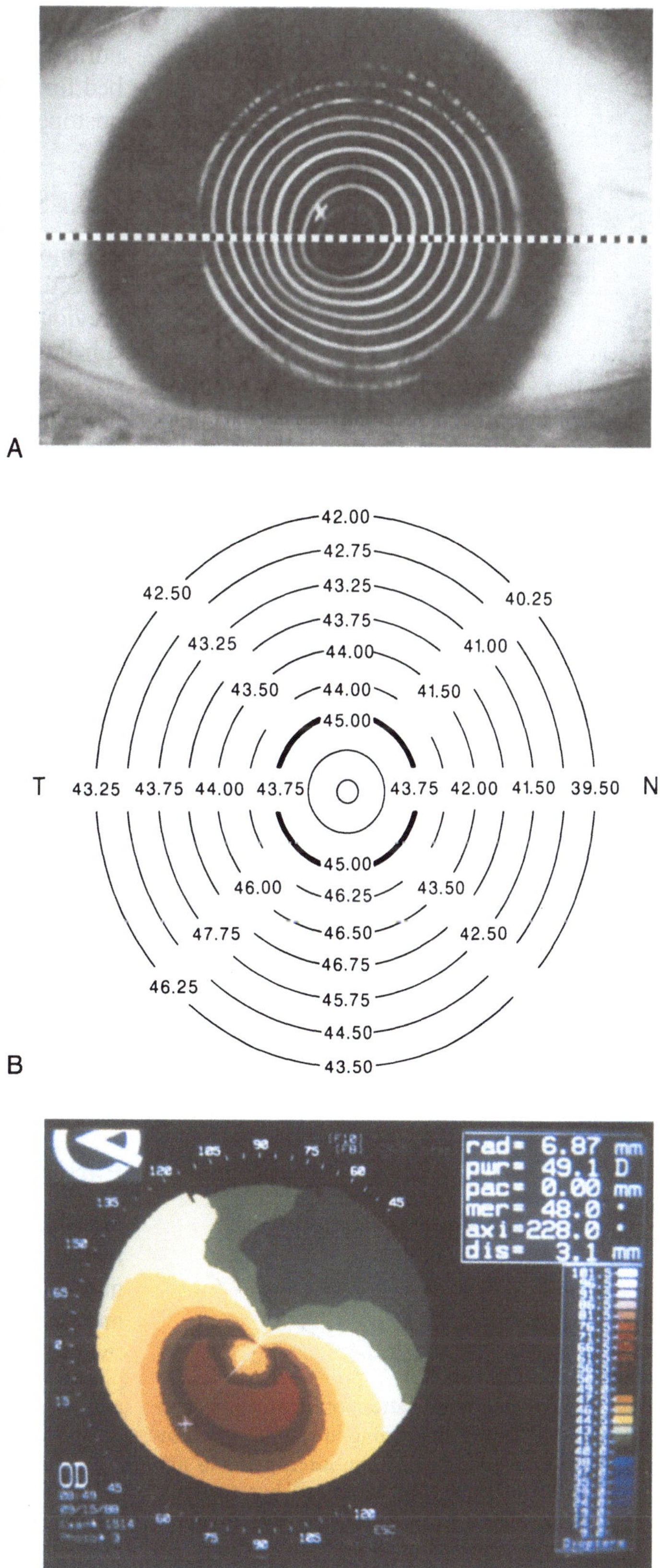

FIGURE 7.1. (A) Photokeratoscopy of early keratoconus. Note the pear-shaped pulling of the central keratoscopy reflex and the relatively normal cornea above the midline. (B) Topographical analysis of Figure 7.1a. (C) Computer-based color-coded mapping more clearly illustrates the power distribution commonly noted in early keratoconus.

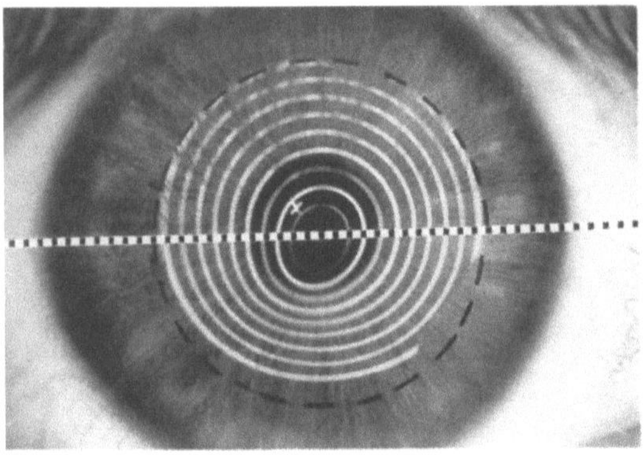

FIGURE 7.2. Photokeratoscopy of early keratoconus. The black broken lines illustrate a sphere that aligns the normal superior cornea and falls far beyond the ninth ring inferiorly.

ple form of keratoconus has tremendous implications for its management. The rapid change in curvature from the steep center to the more normal midperipheral cornea creates numerous fitting obstacles that will be discussed later in this chapter. Although difficult to fit with contact lenses, the nipple-shaped topography may be ideally suited for keratoplastic surgery. The small-diameter central location of the cone permits complete removal of the ectasia within the area of trephination. The 360° of relatively normal recipient cornea creates an optimum bed for wound closure and helps to minimize postoperative corneal astigmatism.

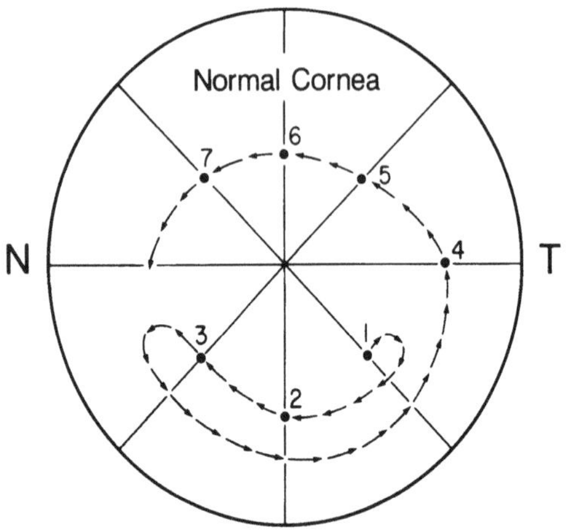

FIGURE 7.3. Quadrantal pattern of keratoconus progression with initial steepening in the inferior temporal quadrant followed by the inferior (6:00) and inferonasal quadrants. In advanced keratoconus, the cornea, above to midline, becomes involved with the superior nasal quadrant, the last to be affected.

Oval-Shaped Topography

The most common corneal shape found in advanced keratoconus is the oval topography. As previously discussed, the nipple-shaped cone is hallmarked by nearly 360° of normal peripheral topography. In the oval form of keratoconus, the topography below the midline will exhibit varying degrees of corneal steepening. An "island" of more normal corneal topography remains above the midline of the cornea and is the single characteristic feature of the oval cone. (Fig. 7.7).

Globus-Shaped Topography

The "globus" form of keratoconus is the largest, involving nearly three quarters of the corneal surface. Because of its size, most or all of the keratoscope rings will be encompassed in the area of the cone (Fig. 7.8). Unlike the nipple and oval forms of keratoconus, the "globus" cone has no "islands" of normal cornea present in the typical photokeratograph.

Corneal Topography and Contact Lens Fitting

Early Keratoconus

In fitting early keratoconus, the central keratometry ("K") readings are of little value and may be misleading. Instead, knowledge of the more normal superior midperipheral cornea (which lies beyond the area measured by the keratometer) becomes the single most important fitting consideration.[22] In Figure 7.9, a computerized color-coded photokeratograph "map" illustrating a patient having early keratoconus with inferior temporal steepening is presented. The central cornea dioptric power is 54.4 D (Fig. 7.9A), while the dioptric power

FIGURE 7.4. (A) Photokeratoscopy of advanced keratoconus with an island of "normal" cornea in the superior nasal quadrant. (B) Topographical analysis of (A).

A

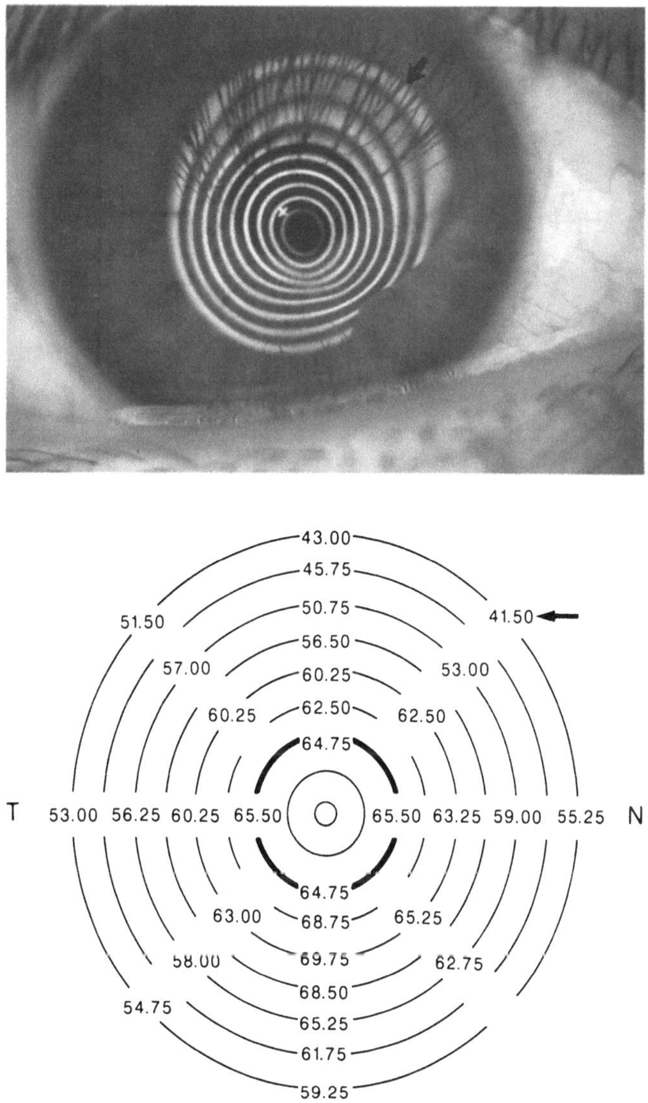

B

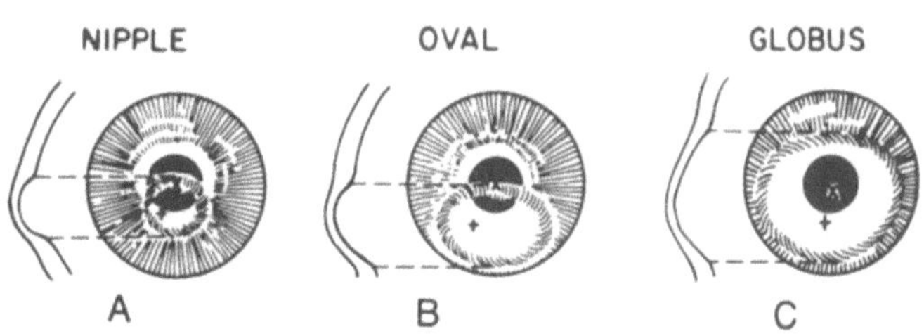

FIGURE 7.5. Size, shape, and location of the three forms of advanced keratoconus: (A) nipple, (B) oval, and (C) globus.

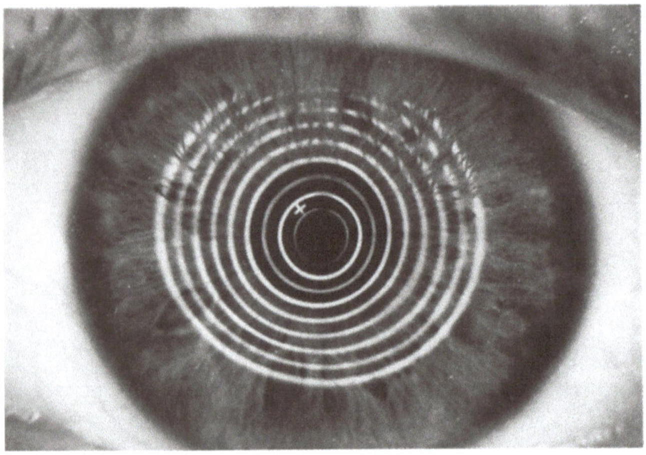

A

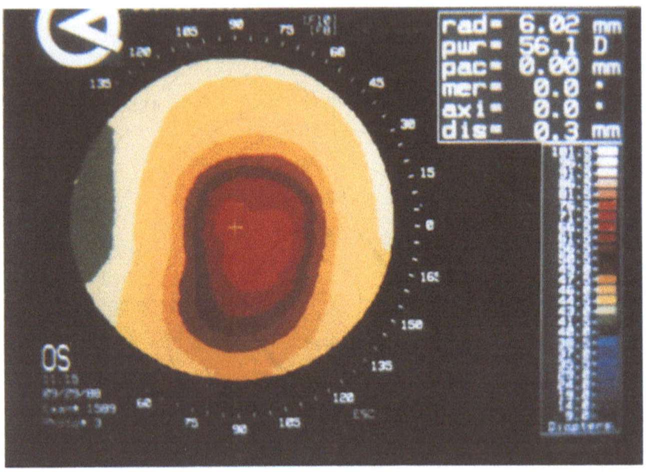

B

FIGURE 7.6. (A) Photokeratoscopy of nipple-type keratoconus. Note to near 360° of normal cornea that surrounds the steep central ectasia. (B) Color-coded mapping of (A) more clearly demonstrates the power distribution in nipple keratoconus.

3.1 mm superior to the center is approximately 10 D flatter, 44.7 D (Fig. 7.9B).

Figure 7.10 illustrates the role of the superior paracentral cornea in fitting early keratoconus. Topographical analysis of Figure 7.10A reveals: a central K reading (third ring) of 46.25 D/49.75 D, inferior meridianal steepening to 51.25 D and superionasal meridianal flattening to 41.00 D. If a contact lens is fitted on "K" (46.25 D) or steeper than "K," the lens will be forced downward due to impingement of the steep curve on the more normal superior cornea. This would prevent the lens from freely traversing along the vertical meridian with each blink (Fig. 7.11). In this situation, the misleading information of the central "K" reading could lead to an excessively steep fitting relationship.

Figure 7.12 illustrates a more advanced form of keratoconus, with central "K" readings of 48.75 D/53.75 D and the inferior corneal steepening to 56.25 D. The flattest point, 41.50 D, remains at the area of the ninth ring in the superonasal quadrant. If a contact lens is fit on "K" (48.75 D), the lens will again be excessively steep in relation to the superior cornea resulting in an inferiorly-fixed lens position and subsequent corneal compression by the contact lens edge (Fig. 7.13). In photokeratoscopy, this compression is best noted by broken keratoscopy lines, as well as by broadening and flattening of the reflected rings. Initially, patients may be comfortable with the steeply fitted lenses; however, with time, there generally is an increased lens awareness and a decreased wearing time. Therefore, it is impor-

FIGURE 7.7. (A) Photokeratoscopy of oval-type keratoconus. Note the "island" of normal cornea above to midline and the loss of normal cornea temporally (9:00). (B) Color-coded mapping of (A).

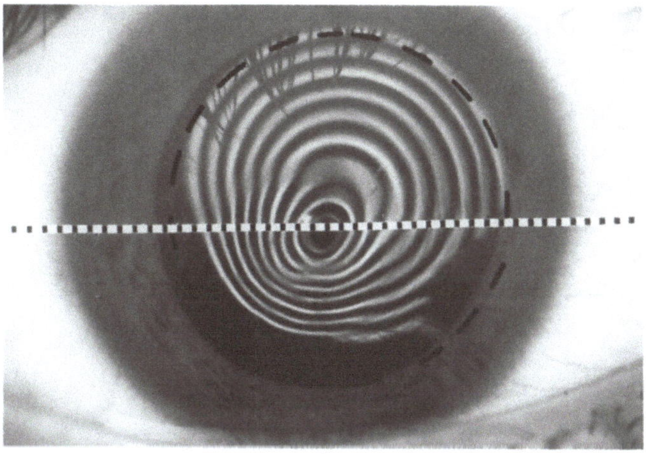

A

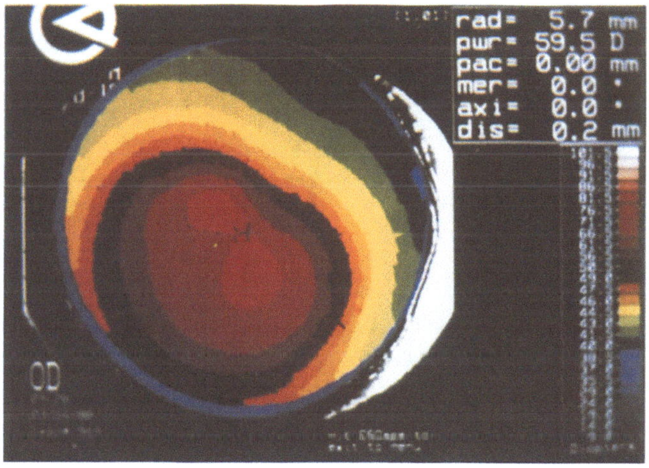

B

tant to select a lens design that is flat enough so that there will be no superior corneal compression, and only slight, "feather" touch (Fig. 7.14). Any attempt to align or vault the *apex* of the cone will result in a fixed lens inferiorly and a tight-fitting relationship superiorly. This is not only true in fitting early keratoconus, but equally critical in all stages of the condition.

In keratoconus, the superior cornea dramatically flattens beyond the steeper conical apex, limiting the effective use of spherical lens designs. An aspheric design can often provide greater lens alignment across the more peripheral cornea. Whether a spheric or aspheric lens design is used, the same fitting criteria must be maintained.

The following is our step-by-step approach to fitting early keratoconus based on photokeratoscopy or diagnostic lens findings.

1. Diagnostic lens fitting begins by performing photokeratoscopy and obtaining a dioptric topographical analysis of the corneal shape (Fig. 7.15A).
2. The steeper central cornea (Fig. 7.15B) and the flatter superior cornea (ninth ring or approximately 3 mm above the visual center of the cornea) (Fig. 7.15C) regions are identified for reference.
3. A diagnostic lens with a base curve *equal* to the dioptric power at the superior (12:00 meridian) ninth ring (or 3.0 mm above the visual center) is placed on the eye and its position and relationship to the cornea are

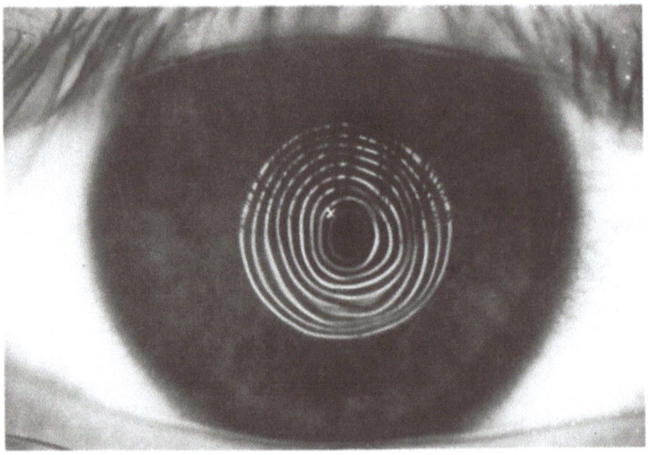

A

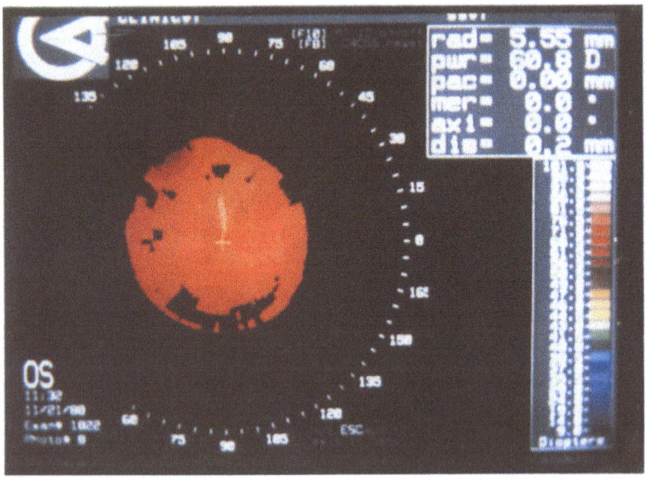

B

FIGURE 7.8. (A) Photokeratoscopy of the globus form of keratoconus. Note that all nine rings of the keratoscopy image are encompassed into the area of the cone. (B) Color-coded mapping of (A).

evaluated. In diagnostic fitting, the superior lens/cornea relationship should be evaluated to determine when alignment occurs. This is best accomplished by pushing the lens up to the superior limbus and evaluating the fitting relationship with fluorescein (Fig. 7.15D).

In its normal resting position, the lens should lie slightly high on the cornea and near, but not beyond, the superior limbus. In this position, the upper lid controls the orientation and movement of the contact lens as though the lens itself were attached to the upper lid. If the diagnostic lens lies low over the apex of the cone, this generally indicates that the lens is too steep or its posterior optical zone is too large. The steeper the lens is in relationship to the cornea, the more limited will be the upward excursion of the lens following each blink.[23]

The optical zone of the diagnostic lens should drape across the central portion of the cornea, creating 2 mm to 4 mm of feather apical touch. It is important that the lens curvature be equivalent to, or slightly *flatter* than, the "normal" superior cornea. The lower lens edge should lift away from the cornea due to the inferior corneal steepening. Intermittent bubbles or frothing may thus be noted inferiorly. This is not only acceptable but essential to ensure both adequate superior alignment and vertical

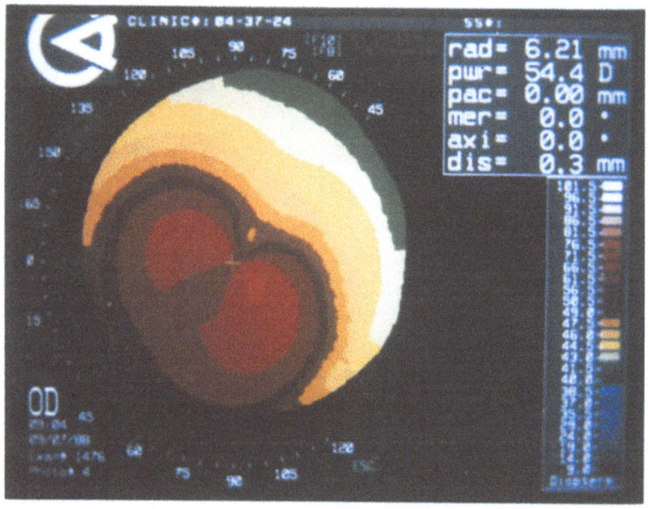

A

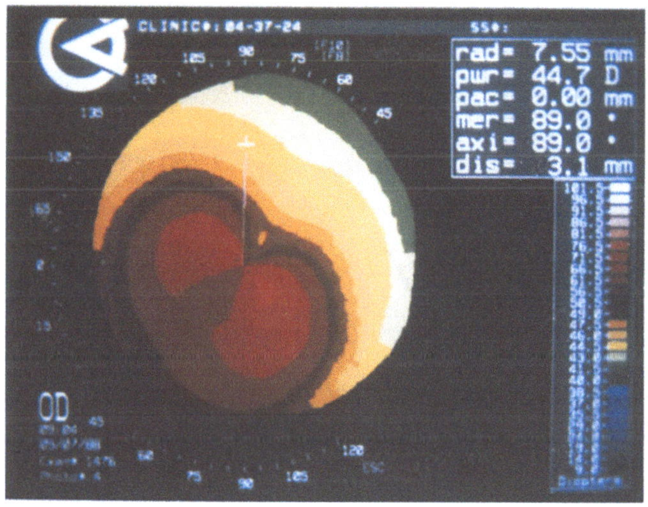

B

FIGURE 7.9. (A) Color-coded mapping of early keratoconus with central power readings of 54.4 D. (B) Illustrates the same photograph as (9). The corneal power 3.1 mm superior to the geometric center has flattened to 44.7 D.

lens movement with the blink. Any attempt to decrease the inferior edge lift (i.e., steepening the base or peripheral curves), will result in a tight lens/cornea relationship superiorly. Furthermore, with a steep fitting relationship, the lens edge may cause further mechanical distortion of the cornea and exacerbate the condition.

4. Lens size is best determined by measuring the horizontal visible iris diameter (V.I.D.) and ordering a lens 2.3 mm smaller; for example V.I.D. 11.5 mm, lens diameter 9.2 mm.
5. Having achieved the desired fit, an overrefraction is used to determine the final contact lens power.

Fitting Advanced Keratoconus

Because of the varying peripheral corneal topographies found in advanced keratoconus, no one lens design or fitting philosophy will consistently result in optimal fit. For this reason, a variety of different fitting approaches must be employed, each based solely on the status of the peripheral corneal topography. The following describes our fitting approach for advanced keratoconus, based on the photokeratoscopic

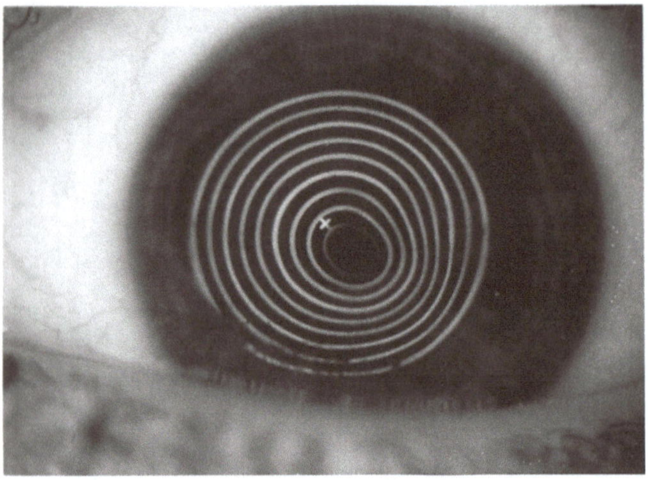

A

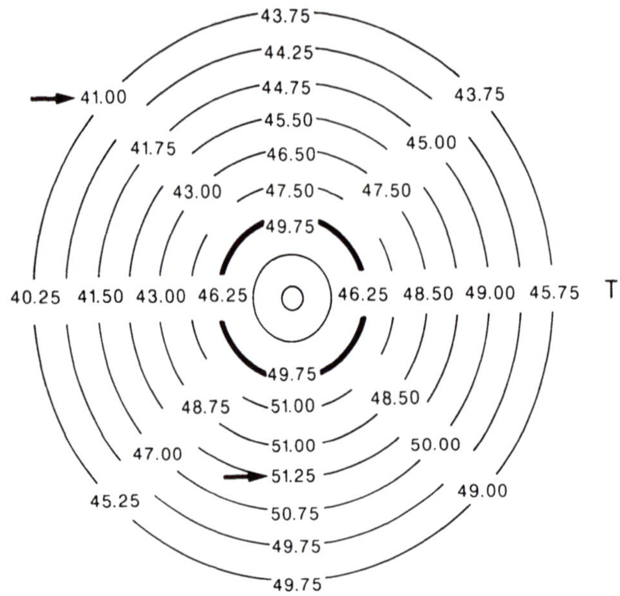

B

FIGURE 7.10. (A) Photokeratoscopy and (B) topographical analysis of early keratoconus with central K readings 46.25/49.75 and inferior 6:00 steepening to 51.25. The flattest area lies in the superior nasal quadrant 41.00.

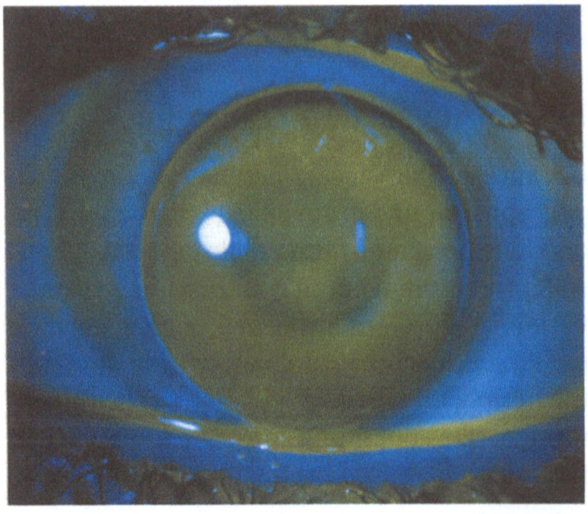

FIGURE 7.11. Illustrates an "O.K." fit, 46.25 D. Note the superior impingement on the more normal superior cornea. At that point to lens is 3.00 to 5.00 D steeper than the superior cornea. This fitting relationship forces the lens downward and prevents the lens from freely transversing the vertical meridian with the blink.

FIGURE 7.12. (A) Photokeratoscopy and (B) topographical analysis of advanced keratoconus, with central K readings 48.75/53.75 and inferior corneal steepening to 56.25. The flattest area remains in the superior nasal quadrant 41.50.

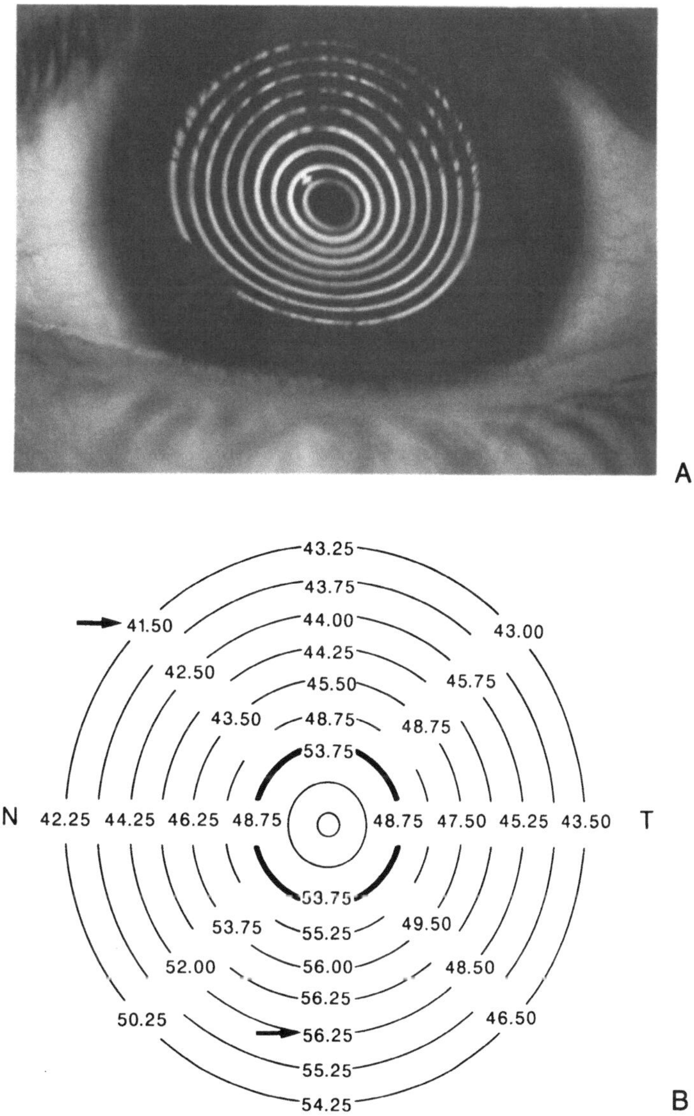

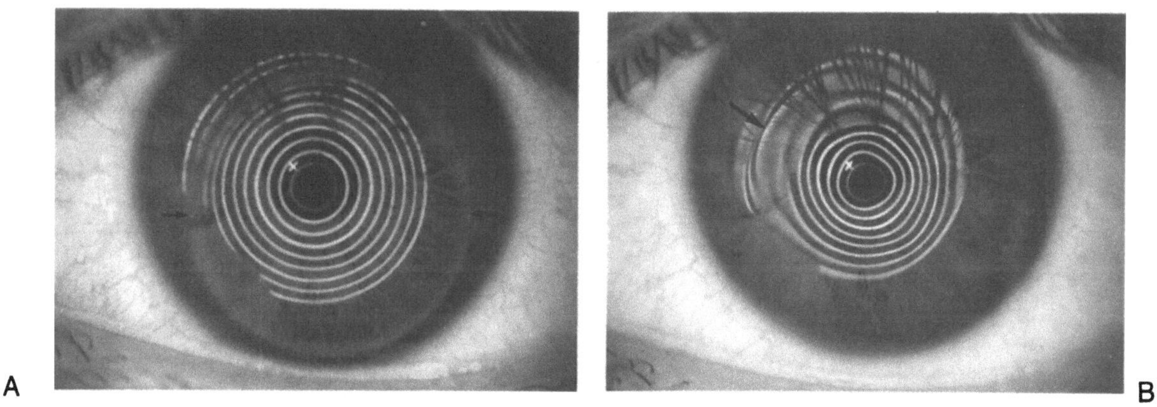

FIGURE 7.13. (A) Photokeratoscopy over the top of a contact lens fitted on "K." Note the inferior temporal fixed lens position. (B) Photokeratoscopy following lens removal. Note the compression ring present in the superior nasal quadrant.

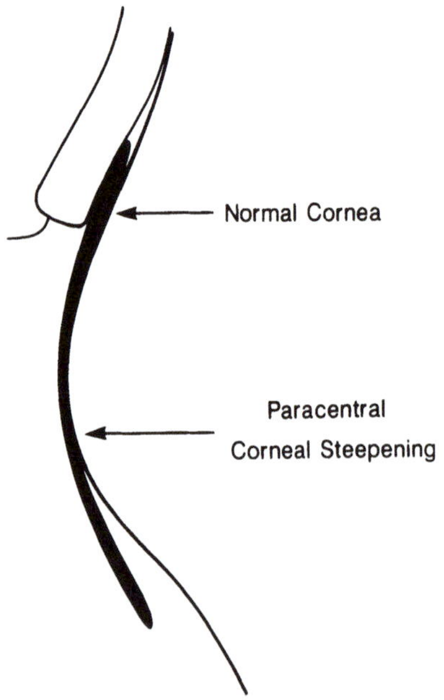

A

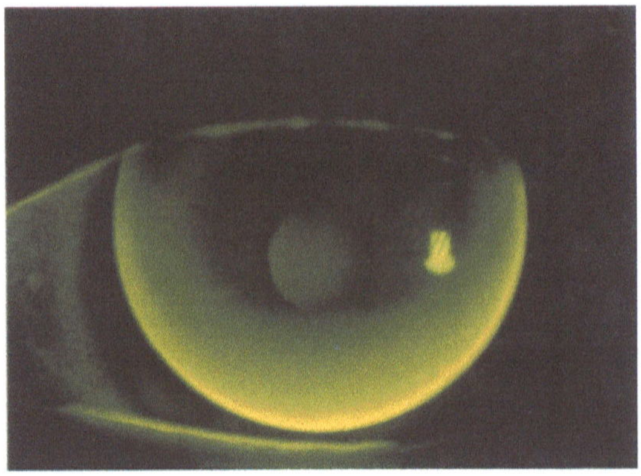

B

FIGURE 7.14. (A) A sectional view of the superior alignment fitting philosophy in early keratoconus. Note the inferior lens clearance secondary to the steeper paracentral cornea. Any attempt to bring the inferior edge into closer apposition to the cornea will result in superior impingement. (B) The anticipated fluorescein pattern of a well-aligned lens in early keratoconus.

classification of peripheral corneal topographies (as either nipple, oval, or globus).

Fitting the Nipple Cone

The nipple-shaped topography creates numerous fitting obstacles because of the rapid change in corneal shape from center to midperiphery. As previously discussed, the nipple cone (Fig. 7.16) consists of central ectasia measuring 5 mm or less surrounded by 360° of essentially normal cornea.

The superior alignment fitting philosophy previously described in early keratoconus is often successful in the early stages of the nipple-shaped topography. However, as the central ectasia progresses, the superior alignment fit creates greater localized apical bear-

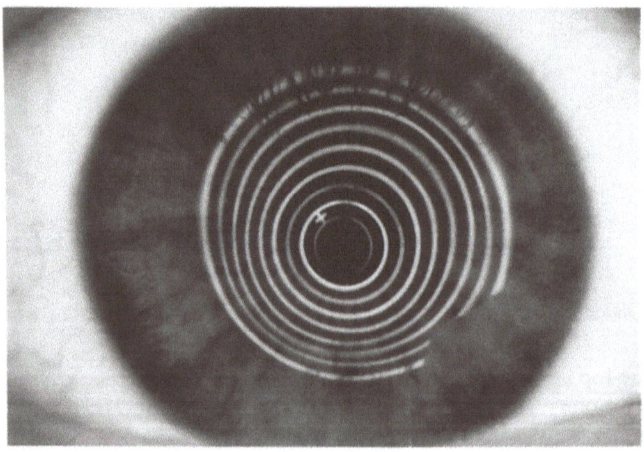

A

FIGURE 7.15. (A) Photokeratoscopy of early keratoconus with inferior temporal steepening and relatively normal superior cornea topography. (B) Color-coded mapping with a central diopteric power of 50.2 D. (C) Approximately 3.0 mm above the central cornea, the diopteric power drops to 42.3 D. (D) The fluorescein pattern of a superior alignment lens fitted on the cornea described in Figures 7.15a–c.

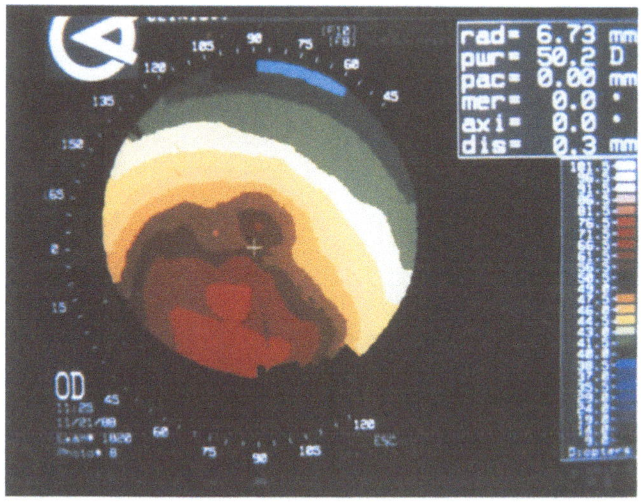
rad= 6.73 mm
pwr= 50.2 D
pac= 0.00 mm
mer= 0.0 °
axi= 0.0 °
dis= 0.3 mm
OD
Diopters

B

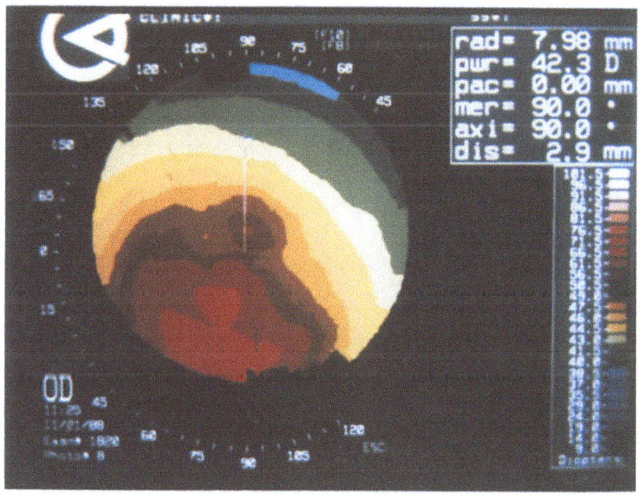
rad= 7.98 mm
pwr= 42.3 D
pac= 0.00 mm
mer= 90.0 °
axi= 90.0 °
dis= 2.9 mm
OD
Diopters

C

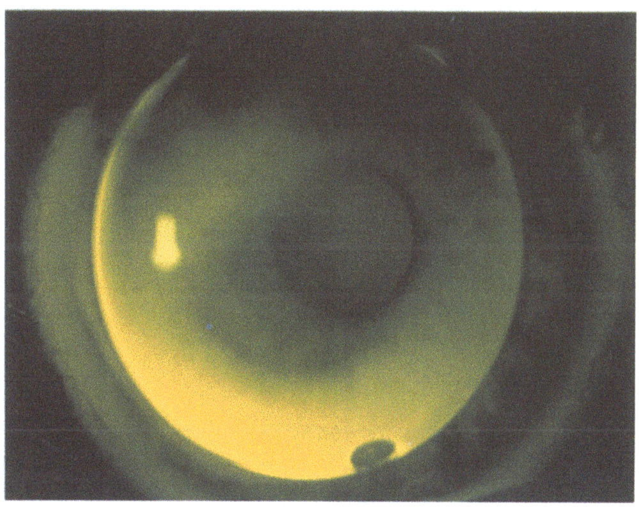

D

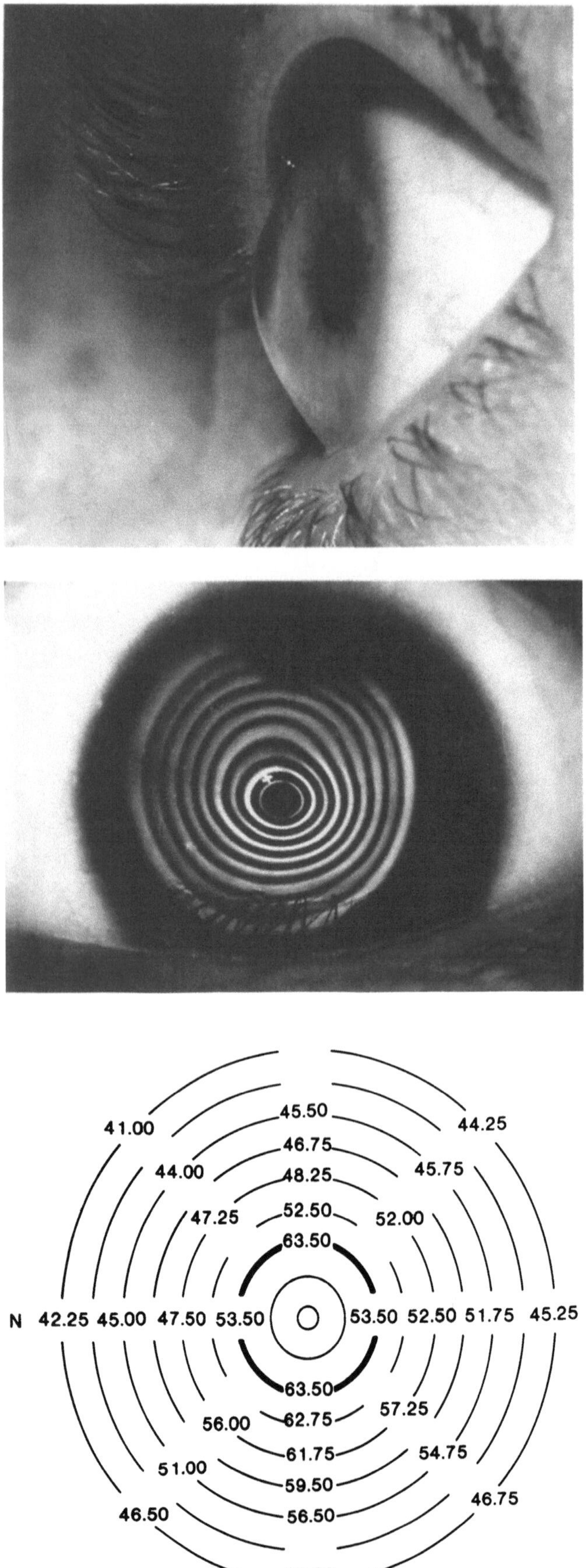

FIGURE 7.16. (A) An advanced nipple cone in profile. Note the steep central ectasia and the 360° of normal peripheral cornea. (B) Photokeratoscopy and (C) topographical analysis of nipple-shaped keratoconus.

ing. This can lead to excessive lens rocking and instability, resulting in symptoms of lens awareness.

Our clinical experience has shown that the advanced nipple topography responds more favorably to a contour fitting technique. This is best accomplished with lens designs that incorporate a small diameter (8.1 mm or less) and a small optical zone (eg, 5.5 mm). Our spherical design of choice is the McGuire nipple cone design, which incorporates a small, 5.5-mm posterior optical zone and four wide and flat peripheral curves to contour the flatter, more normal midperipheral cornea. The posterior optical zone must be large enough to encompass the steep ectatic portion of the cornea and the lens periphery flat enough to avoid impingement of the midperipheral cornea (Fig. 6.17). Again, photokeratoscopy is essentially part of this fitting technique.

Fitting the Oval Cone

As discussed earlier, the oval cone (Fig. 7.18) is hallmarked by inferior steepening with varying degrees of normal corneal topography superiorly. In fitting the oval-shaped cone, careful attention must be directed to the status of the superior and horizontal (along the 180° meridian) corneal topography. A superior alignment technique, similar to that used in early keratoconus, can be considered only if the superior topography and the horizontal topography are relatively normal. In this situation, the normal cornea at 9:00, 12:00, and 3:00 provides a sufficient base by which to support the superior alignment fitting lens.

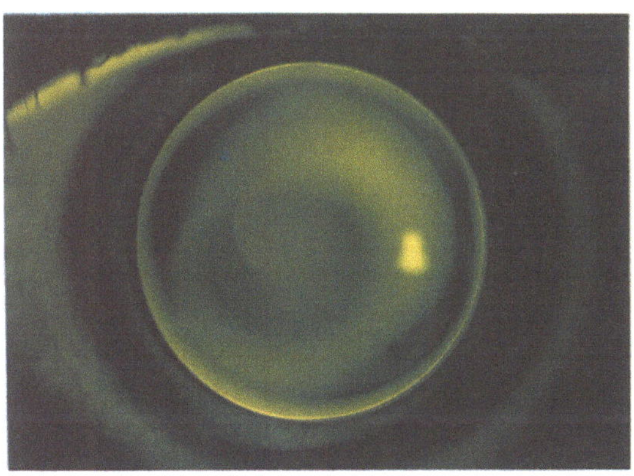

FIGURE 7.17. Fluorescein pattern of a contour fitting McGuire cone lens for nipple keratoconus. Note the 2 to 3 mm of central feather touch surrounded by 360° of fluorescein pooling. This clearly illustrates how quickly the cornea topography changes from center to midperiphery.

As the oval cone progresses, the normal corneal topography in the temporal horizontal meridian is lost. The superior alignment fitting philosophy is less likely to provide an adequate fit due to a lack of horizontal fulcrum (contact point) temporally (Fig. 7.19). This loss of normal cornea temporally is followed by involvement of the superior cornea, resulting in the last "island" of normal cornea being in the superonasal quadrant.

At this point, a contour fitting philosophy is again required to provide adequate lens stability (Fig. 7.20). In our experience, this is best accomplished with the spherical McGuire oval cone lens design, or with an aspheric lens design having adequate peripheral eccentricity to provide the needed clearance and lens stability. Again, mastery of photokeratoscopy is a prerequisite to successful contact lens fitting in advanced keratoconus.

Fitting the Globus Cone

The globus form of keratoconus signifies a nearly total involvement of the cornea by the disease process. As discussed earlier, in nipple keratoconus the ectatic central cornea is surrounded by 360° of normal cornea. In the oval form, 180° or less of normal cornea remains above the midline of the cornea. Keratoscopically, in the globus form, all of the rings of the image are reflected in the steepened area. In this advanced stage, the only "normal" unaffected portion of the cornea is in the superior paralimbal area (Fig. 7.21A, B).

Because of the size and the extensive involvement of the peripheral cornea, contact lens fitting for globus conus requires large lens diameters and steeper base curves. Our lens of choice is the McGuire globus cone design, which utilizes a larger 9.1 mm diameter and a 6.5 mm optical zone for lens stability. Again, it is important to adjust the base curve of the lens

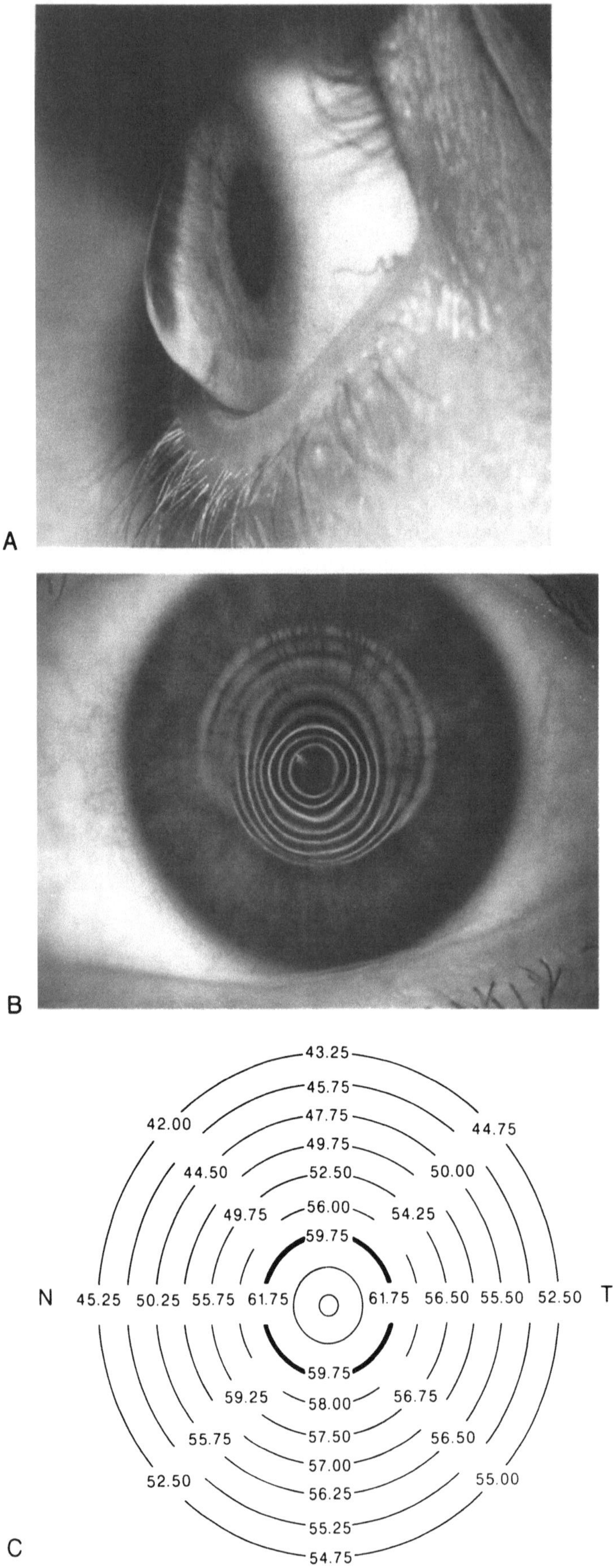

FIGURE 7.18. (A) Profile view of an oval cone with normal superior corneal topography and paracentral steepening below the midline. (B) Photokeratoscopy and (C) topographical analysis of oval-shaped keratoconus. Note the relatively normal superior topography and the inferior, below-the-midline steepening.

A

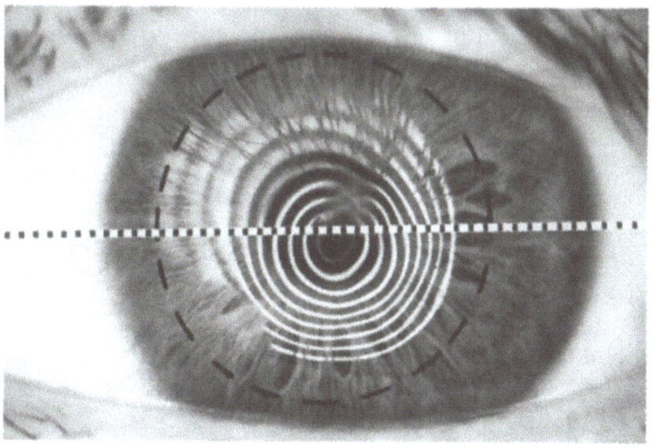

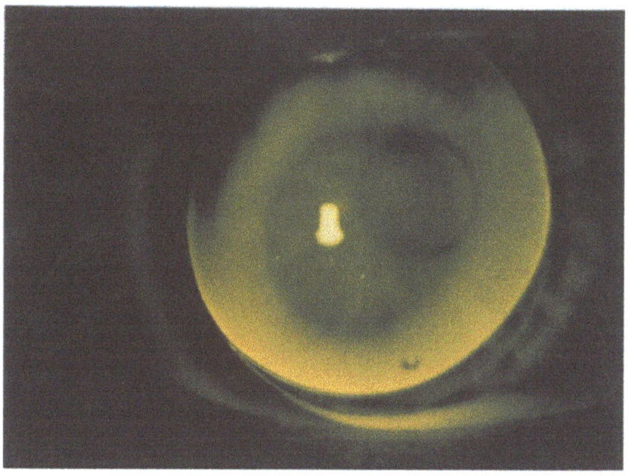

B

FIGURE 7.19. (A) A more advanced oval cone with loss of normal cornea contour temporally along the horizontal meridian. An "island" of normal cornea remains in the superior nasal quadrant. (B) Demonstrates a superior alignment lens fitted to the cornea in (A). Note the loss of fulcrum (contact) temporally and the slight bearing nasally along the more normal corneal topography.

to allow 3 to 4 mm of feather apical touch, in order to avoid excessive impingement of the peripheral cornea.

Refraction over the Trial Lens

Overrefraction is an integral part of the diagnostic fitting. It may be important to overrefract using large- diopter steps (0.50 D or even 1.00 D), as keratoconus patients find it difficult to distinguish small changes in power due to the high degree of myopia and irregular astigmatism. It is not uncommon for keratoconus patients wearing rigid contact lenses to manifest moderate to high amounts of residual astigmatism. This can be easily evaluated by placing a ±0.50 cross-cylinder at 90°, 180°, 45°, and 135° and asking the patient if there is any subjective improvement in visual acuity. Correcting the residual astigmatism is best accomplished with glasses, which often improves visual acuity three to four lines. Front surface toric rigid lens designs have been successfully fitted in keratoconus patients resistant to wearing spectacles over their contact lenses.

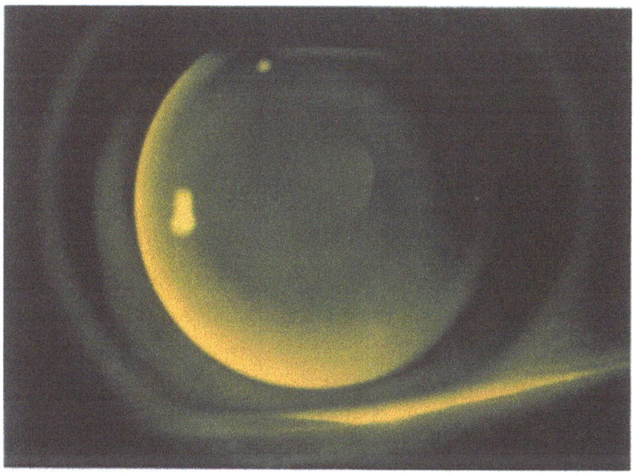

FIGURE 7.20. An oval cone design—McGuire lens on a cornea with an island of normal contour superior nasal (upper right). The base curve must be steep enough to maintain lens stability along the horizontal meridian, yet flat enough to avoid excessive peripheral impingement in the superior nasal quadrant.

All lenses should be ordered in a rigid gas permeable (RGP) material to avoid epithelial hypoxia and corneal erosions during the long wearing schedule of the keratoconus patient. All lenses must be manufactured under the strictest controls possible. Not only must the laboratory be capable of manufacturing one perfect lens for the patient, but they must also be able to duplicate that lens should the patient need a replacement. Every aspect of the lens design (base curve, optical zone, diameter, edge, etc.) plays an integral role in the overall success of the patient. Therefore, the practitioner should evaluate the lens prior to dis-

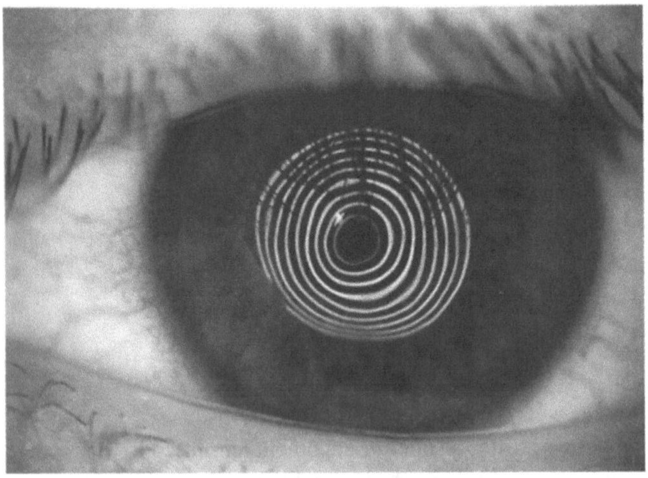

A

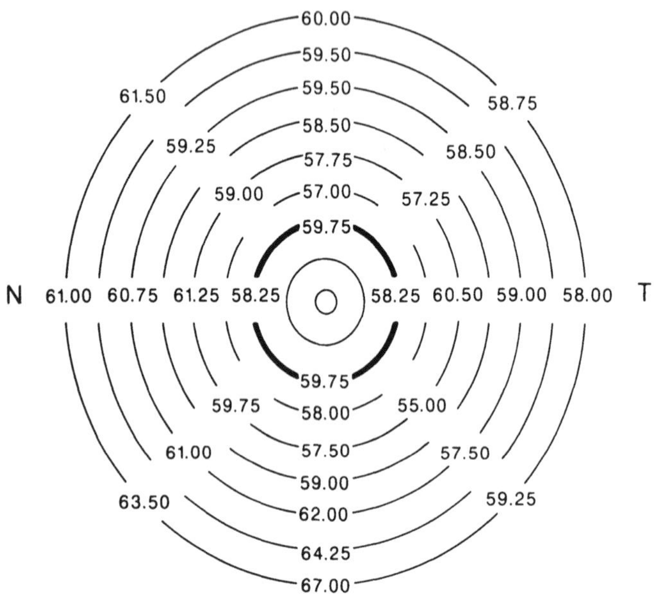

B

FIGURE 7.21. (A) Photokeratoscopy and (B) topographical analysis of globus-shaped keratoconus.

pensing and communicate any design concerns to the manufacturer.

Summary

No other group of patients has benefited more from contact lenses than has those with keratoconus. Unfortunately, the contact lens fitting process can be a frustrating experience for both patient and practitioner. To better manage the condition, practitioners may want to re-evaluate the concept that keratoconus always requires steep lens designs. This begins by avoiding the misleading information provided by central keratometry readings, and instead, designing the lens from the information obtained by sophisticated photokeratoscopic assessment of the topography of the midperipheral and peripheral cornea.

For many practitioners, the use of flatter fitting philosophies will be a major departure from their traditional approach to managing the keratoconus patient. To fit the keratoconus patient successfully requires a complete rethinking of the corneal topography; it must be recognized that the disease affects the cornea far beyond the range of the keratometer.

Therefore regardless of the fitting technique used, it will be important for the contact lens practitioner to envision a three-dimensional picture of the corneal shape during the fitting process so that steep fitting relationships (which will eventually lead to superior corneal compression, increased lens awareness, and decreased wearing time) may be avoided.[22] It is anticipated that as new and more accurate computer algorithms are developed for the quantitative assessment of corneal topography, our ability to successfully fit even advanced stages of keratoconus will be greatly enhanced.

References

1. Duke-Elder S. *Cornea and Sclera. Part II. System of Ophthalmology: Diseases of the Outer Eye*. Vol. 3. St Louis: CV Mosby, 1965; pp 964–976.
2. Heitz R. *History of Contact Lenses: The CLAO Guide to Basic Science and Clinical Practice, Part I*. Orlando, FL., Grune and Stratton, 1984; pp. 1–19.
3. Panas P. Presentation of instruments and apparatus. *Bull Acad Med Services*. March 20, 1988;3(19):400–401.
4. Moss HI. The contour principle in corneal contact lens prescribing for keratoconus. *J Am Optom Assoc*. March 1959; 570–572.
5. Girard LJ, Soper J, Sampson W. Corneal contact lens. St Louis: CV Mosby, 1970; 297.
6. Chiquair Arias V: A new technique of fitting contact lenses on keratoconus. *Contacto*. 1959;3(12):393–415.
7. Korb D. Recent developments in fitting contact lenses for keratoconus. *J Am Optom Assoc*. 1984;55(3):172–174.
8. Caroline P, Doughman D, McGuire J, et al. Report on a new contact lens design for keratoconus. *Contact Intraocular Lens Med J*. 1978;4(3):69–73.
9. Dekking H. Zur Photographic der Hornhauto ber Flache. *Klin Mbl Augenheilk*. 1929;82:640–647.
10. Amsler M. Ueber Photo Keratoskopie. *Bericht Heidelberg*. 1930;48:202–209.
11. Amsler M. Le Keratocone Fruste. *Bull Mem Soc Fr. d' Opht*. 1937;50:100.
12. Amsler M. Quelques Donnees du Probleme du Keratocone. *Bull Soc Belge Ophth*. 1961; 129:331–354.
13. Rowsey J, Reynolds AE, Brown R, et al. Corneal topography corneascope. *Arch Ophthalmol*. June 1981,99:1093–1100.
14. Tomlinson A, Schwartz C. Position of the corneal apex in keratoconus. *Am J Optom Physiolog Optics*. January 1980;11(4):72–81.
15. Townsley M. New equipment and method for determining the contour of the human cornea. *Contacto*. 1967;11(4):72–81.
16. Wesley N. Practical application and new concepts with the photo-electronic keratoscope. *Contacto*. 1969;13:32–43.
17. Maguire L, Bourne W. Corneal topography of early keratoconus. *Am J Ophthalmol*. August 1989; 108:107–112.
18. Rowsey J. Topographical analysis of the cornea. *Int Ophthalmol Clin*. 1983;23(4):1–32.
19. Caroline P, Doughman D, McGuire J, et al. A new contact lens design for keratoconus. *Contact Lens J*. June/August 1978;12(1):69–71.
20. Buxton J. Therapeutic use of contact lenses in keratoconus. *Ophthalmic Dig*. January 1975;29.
21. Rich G. The geometry of keratoconus: alternative approaches to fitting. *Rev Optom*. April 15, 1979;116(4):88–91.
22. Bronstein L. Formcom Keratoconus Fitting Manual. Phoenix: Bronstein Laboratories.
23. International Diagnostic Instruments. Corneascope/Comparator Operations Manual. Ed. III, Tulsa, July 1980.

8
Corneal Topography Following Traumatic Lacerations

Timothy T. McMahon

Ocular trauma is a common phenomenon and is the leading cause of vision loss in young adults.[1, 2] Its prevalence encompasses both sexes, and all races and ages; young males, however, are the group most commonly affected. Injuries to the cornea represent a significant percentage (57 to 63%) of all ocular injuries.[3, 4] The high prevalence of these injuries is most likely related to the prominent anatomical exposure of the cornea to projectiles and other sources of trauma.

With the advent of antimicrobial agents, the operating microscope, improved suture materials, and better microsurgical techniques, a higher percentage of cases of corneal and other ocular trauma are being treated successfully, with preservation of not only the globe but also vision.

With these advancements, an understanding of surface topography takes on much more importance. Corneal topographic considerations must now be included in the treatment of ocular trauma from the moment an individual presents with a corneal laceration to the final vision rehabilitation phases.

Wounds to the cornea result in three significant visual or optical effects: scar formation producing opacities within the cornea and possibly within the line of sight, regular astigmatism, and irregular astigmatism. Of these three, irregular astigmatism, which is produced by variable tractional forces on the corneal surface, is frequently the most important factor leading to visual loss.

This chapter reviews topographic aspects of corneal injuries that should be considered. These include the type of trauma; the location, shape, and size of wounds; tissue loss; wound closure; wound healing factors; and management considerations of healed lacerations.

Type of Laceration

Corneal lacerations can be clinically classified into two significantly different categories: penetrating corneal injuries and perforating corneal injuries.

Penetrating corneal injuries constitute those insults that involve the corneal stroma but do not pass through the cornea to the inner structures of the eye. Penetrating corneal injuries may be simple punctures or lacerations and, at times, may involve tissue loss. Distinguishing between perforating and penetrating injuries is important.

With penetrating corneal injuries, endophthalmitis and retained intraocular foreign bodies are not of concern. Loss of intraocular contents does not occur with penetrating injuries, even though significant shock-wave induced injury to intraocular structures may have occurred. Additionally, if any surgical intervention is necessary, only the anterior surface of the cornea will require surgical reapposition. If the posterior aspect of the stroma is reasonably intact, good apposition of the wound is quite possible, thus minimizing any associated irregular astigmatism. Although penetrating injuries are likely to be less severe than are perforating injuries, they can demonstrate comparable effects on corneal topography and visual acuity.

In perforating corneal injuries, the source of the trauma passes through all the layers of the cornea into, or through, the eye. If the object involved passes within the eye but not through the globe, the injury is termed a penetrating ocular injury with corneal perforation. If the insulting object passes through both the cornea and the globe, the injury is referred to as both a perforating corneal and perforating ocular injury or, more commonly, as a double perforating injury.

Wound apposition is more difficult following perforating injuries. Loss of corneal tissue is more common than in penetrating corneal injuries. Incarceration of iris within the wound can also complicate the picture, contributing to broad, vascularized, elevated scar formation and to surface irregularity.

Wound Location

The location of the wound plays an extremely important role in the visual outcome of a corneal injury. In the assessment of a wound and the associated topographic influences from the scar, it is helpful to divide the cornea into three zones: central, peripheral, and limbal-scleral (Fig. 8.1).

The central zone constitutes the central 3 mm of the cornea centered about the line of sight. Lacerations to this area are likely to demonstrate visual deficits from the opacity of the scar as well as from corneal irregularity. The visual impact of the scar is directly related to its surface area and its proximity to the center of the line of sight. Thin scars can pass directly over the visual axis and have only mild influences on visual acuity (Fig. 8.2). On the other hand, dense thick scars that blanket much of the pupillary space, not surprisingly, may have a profound effect on vision (Fig. 8.3). In addition to the visual blockade effect from an opacity in the central zone, topographic effects from surface irregularities may contribute significantly to visual loss (Fig. 8.4). Scattering of light and diffraction effects may be important in wounds to this region, but their impact compared to astigmatism and opacification is not well understood.

The peripheral zone is the area extending 3 mm out from the border of the central zone in all directions (Fig. 8.5). Wounds to this area are likely to result in a loss of spectacle-corrected visual acuity through effects on corneal topography only. This may be in the form of induced regular astigmatism as well as irregular astigmatism. In this area, unless there are major alterations to the architecture of the iris and shape of the pupil, the resultant corneal opacity from the wound plays little or no role in visual loss. Conversely, the topographic effects of peripheral wounds are frequently profound and account for most of the visual loss.

Mild disturbances in surface topography can have a major visual impact. For example, the patient in Figure 8.6 suffered a partial-

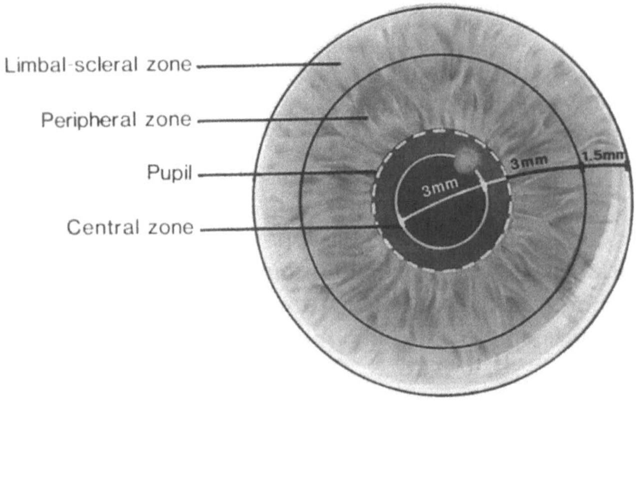

FIGURE 8.1. Diagram representing the three zones of topographic importance following corneal trauma. The central zone encompasses the central 3 mm of the cornea. The peripheral zone is the 3 mm surrounding the central zone. The limbal-scleral zone extends outward from the peripheral zone by about 1.5 mm.

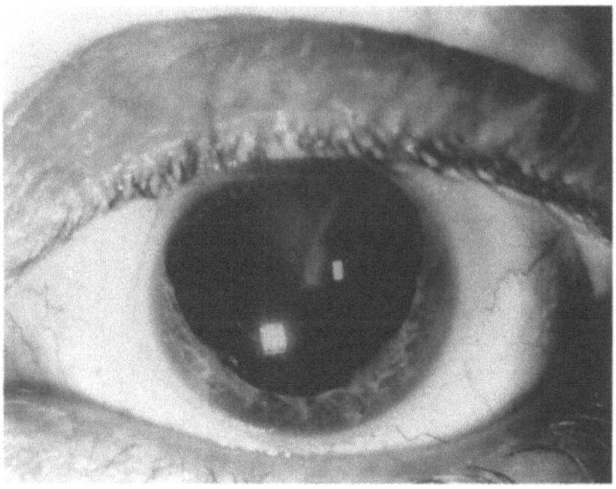

FIGURE 8.2. A thin scar remains in the central and peripheral zones of a patient following a perforating corneal laceration caused by a piece of aluminum.

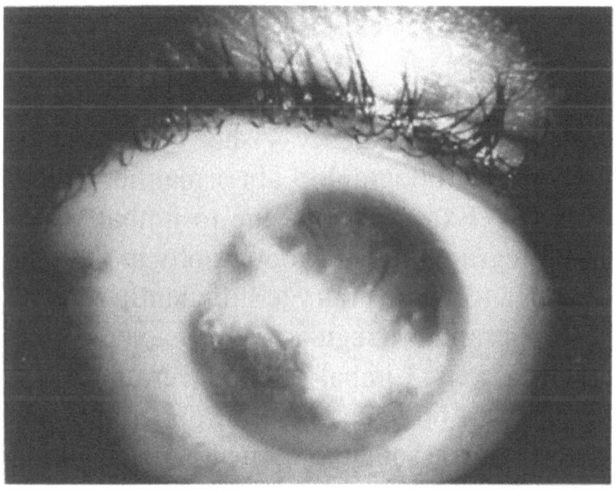

FIGURE 8.3. A massive corneal scar completely occluding the pupillary space remains in a patient who suffered blunt trauma.

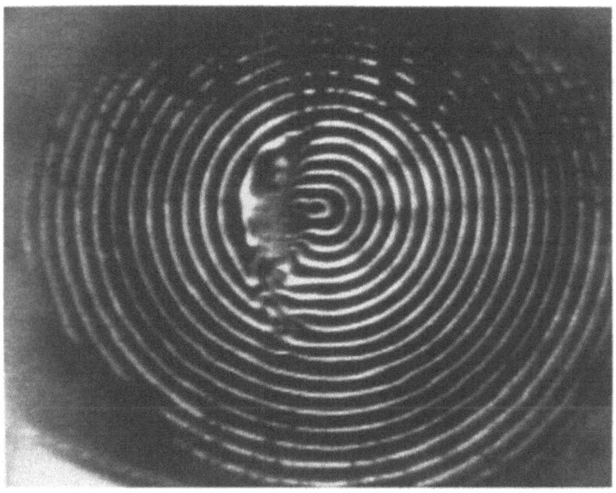

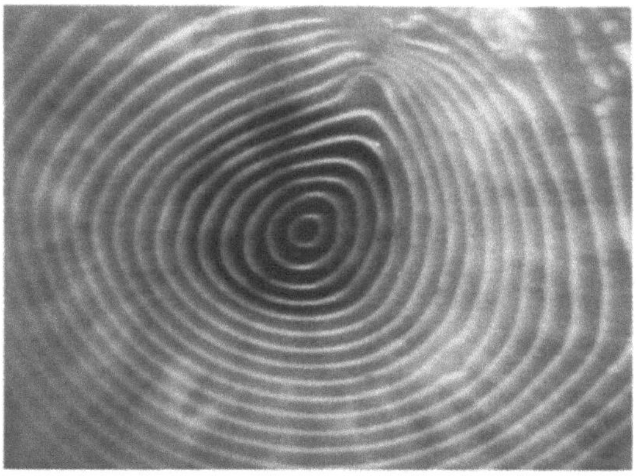

FIGURE 8.5. A superior nasal perforating corneal laceration has healed, leaving a superotemporal to inferonasal oriented scar in the peripheral zone. No scarring invades the visual space. A dragging of the rings toward the superior nasal quadrant can be seen resulting in both regular, against-the-rule astigmatism and irregular astigmatism. There is compaction of the rings immediately adjacent to the scar representing a steep area.

thickness (70% depth) corneal laceration to his left eye that was not repaired. The wound healed leaving a thin, mildly tortuous avascular scar located in the peripheral zone. No limbal involvement was present and minimal elevation of the scar was noted. Photokeratoscopy demonstrated only a subtle irregularity to the rings in the area of the scar (Fig. 8.7). Without the examiner's knowledge that a corneal defect was present, the area of irregularity seen on analysis of the rings would likely have been overlooked. The patient's best spectacle-corrected visual acuity was 20/50. His vision with a rigid gas permeable corneal contact lens was 20/15 and with a soft contact lens was 20/20.

Unlike central and peripheral corneal injuries, limbal and scleral wounds need to be

FIGURE 8.4. Photokeratoscopy picture demonstrating surface irregularities that can be found with thin healed lacerations. The superior-inferior oriented laceration has distinct alterations to the ring pattern over the scar. Additionally, flattening along the horizontal meridian toward the center of the cornea is evident.

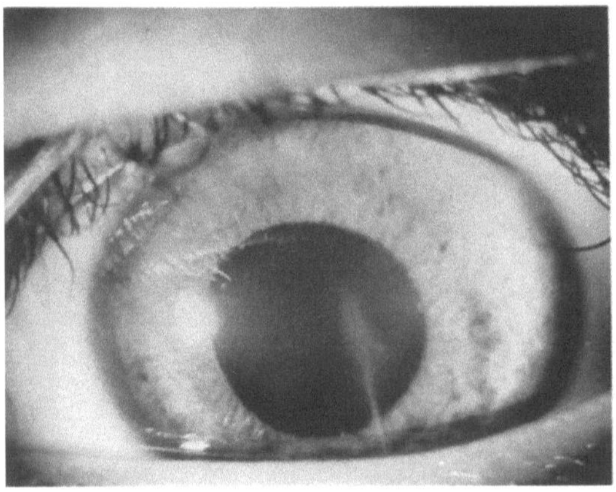

FIGURE 8.6. In a patient who suffered a penetrating corneal laceration involving the central and peripheral zones, the wound healed without sutures being placed. The scar demonstrates virtually no elevation and is quite thin and linear.

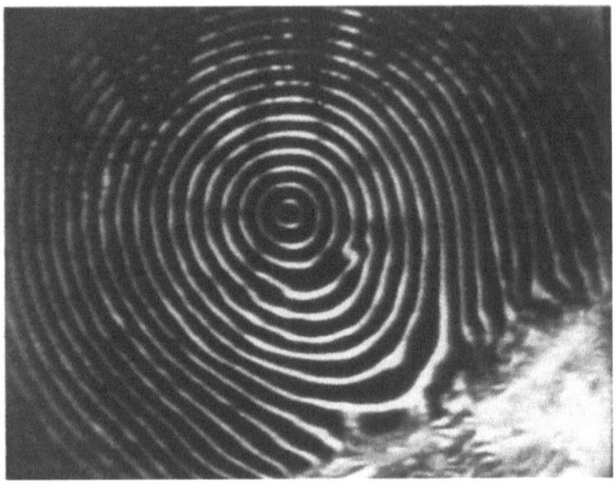

FIGURE 8.9. Photokeratoscopy image of the cornea shown in Figure 8.8, demonstrating marked topographic irregularity over the scar. Flattening from the scar to the central cornea is also evident.

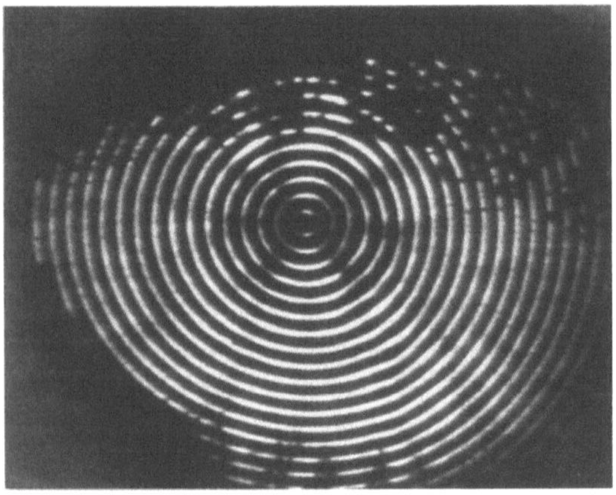

FIGURE 8.7. Photokeratoscopy of the cornea shown in Figure 8.6, demonstrating only a subtle irregularity to the rings.

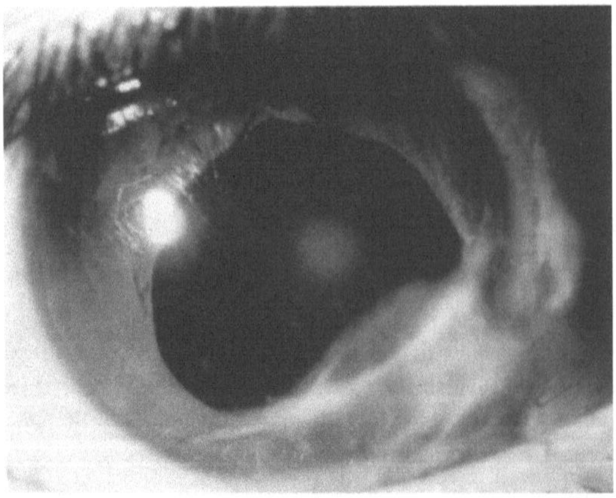

rather severe for a visual effect to be present. These wounds influence visual optics exclusively from topographic abnormalities (Figs. 8.8–8.10). Extensive damage to limbal structural integrity will alter topography in the limbal area and, if the injury is sufficiently severe, the topographic irregularity may extend into the visual axis. Limbal-scleral lacerations that are likely to influence central topography are those having associated tissue loss or resulting in massive elevated scar formation. Additionally, those lacerations in which sutures are tied very tight may affect central topography.

Wound Size

The topographic importance of wound size is closely related to the location of the wound. In general, longer wounds exhibit a greater area of topographic influence than do shorter lacer-

FIGURE 8.8. Perforating corneal laceration located in the limbal-scleral zone. Note the Y-shaped broad scar that resulted from blunt trauma.

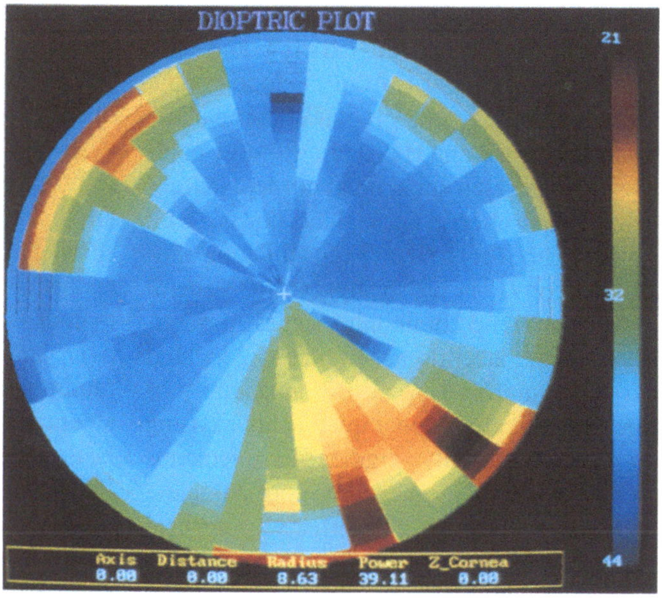

FIGURE 8.10. Visioptic EH270 dioptric plot derived from the photokeratoscopy image in Figure 8.9 showing marked flattening from the center of the cornea toward the scar site. The color-coded bar to the right of the plot indicates the range in diopters found in the plot. Flat curvatures are shown as warmer (red) colors and steeper curvatures are located toward the blue end of the spectrum.

ations. Also, the closer the wound is to the line of sight, the greater the effect of wound length on vision. Snell[5] reported that in patients who had perforating lacerations greater than 4 mm in length, only 14 to 26% achieved a visual acuity of 20/40 or better; conversely, in those who had lacerations less than 4 mm, approximately 50% obtained 20/40 or better acuity. Eagling,[3] in her series of isolated injuries to the cornea and sclera, noted that if the laceration was less than one third of the corneal diameter, a low incidence of corneal astigmatism resulted. With wounds involving one third of the corneal diameter or less, the maximum astigmatism found was 4.00 diopters (D); however, three fourths of the cases had cylinders less than 2.25 D. In wounds greater than one third of the corneal diameter in length, a wide range of postrepair astigmatism was found, but all the cases in the series with greater than 4.00 D of astigmatism had lacerations greater than one third of the corneal diameter. Eagling also found that complete transverse (limbus-to-limbus) lacerations resulted in no more astigmatism than did injuries that involved one third to two thirds of the corneal diameter. My experience would seem to contradict this finding (unpublished data).

Other important features of wound size are the width, and the thickness or elevation of the resultant scar. The horizontal width of the scar is less important, except in the central zone, where the opacity of the scar can play a significant role in vision loss.

Wound Shape

The importance of wound shape with regard to post repair topography is not well defined. Eagling[3] observed that the shape of the laceration did not have a significant effect on astigmatism. Her experience may represent the case for lacerations that have good wound closure and no tissue loss. In cases where the wound is not well apposed during suturing and where tissue has been lost, high levels of astigmatism resulting from substantial corneal flattening over the wound area can be expected.[6, 7]

Tissue Loss and Wound Closure

Rowsey[8] has enumerated 10 caveats in refractive surgery that can generally be applied to the primary management of traumatic lacerations leading to some control of postrepair corneal topography (Table 8.1). Caveats 1, 4, and 9 are of significant concern from a topographic standpoint in the primary repair of corneal lacerations. Rowsey and Hays[7] and Rowsey et al[9] have demonstrated substantial corneal flattening over experimental corneal incisions as well as over sutured corneal incisions utilizing photokeratoscopy. They also suggest that general corneal flattening commonly occurs, particularly in longer lacerations and in those located near the visual axis. With the availability of more sophisticated topographic analysis using computer analyzed, digitized, videokeratoscopy (CADVK) systems, a more complete picture of the topographic effects of corneal lacerations can be seen.[10–15]

The Corneal Modeling System manufactured by Computed Anatomy (New York) and the Visioptic EH-270 Corneal Topographer designed by El Hage (Houston) are two of the CADVK instruments presently available. These devices have several advantages over standard photokeratoscopy instruments in the evaluation of the traumatized cornea, including more keratoscopy rings (enabling better appreciation of the peripheral cornea) as well as quantitative analysis providing dioptric power information for a very large percentage of the cornea.

As an example, photokeratoscopy of the right eye in the patient in Fig. 8.11 demonstrates an inverted teardrop pattern representing apparent flattening and inducement of an against-the-rule corneal astigmatism plus cylinder axis 180 centrally. Inferiorly, both over and immediately adjacent to the scar, minimal ring separation is noted, representing steepening of the cornea. In Figure 8.12 a Corneal Modeling System topographic map for the same patient demonstrates substantial steepening over the healed scar as well as in the immediately adjacent area. Flattening occurs relatively rapidly away from the injury site in lateral and superior directions. This pattern is not consistent with Rowsey's caveat of flattening over a sutured wound (Table 8.1, caveat 4).

The patient in Figure 8.13 suffered a traumatic V-shaped corneal perforation that encompassed the central zone. The angle of the V was greater than 100° and was closed using small interrupted sutures. Following removal

TABLE 8.1. Ten caveats in refractive surgery as applied to the management of traumatic corneal lacerations.

1. The normal cornea flattens over a vertical incision.
2. Radial corneal incisions flatten the adjacent cornea and the cornea 90°.
3. The corneal flattening effect of radial incisions increases as incisions approach the visual axis.
4. The cornea flattens directly over any sutured incision.
5. The cornea flattens adjacent to loose limbal sutures and flattens 180° away and steepens 90° away.
6. The cornea steepens adjacent to tight limbal sutures and steepens 180° away and flattens 90° away.
7. The cornea flattens over wedge resections or tucks.
8. The cornea steepens anterior to wedge resections or tucks.
9. Tissue removal produces corneal flattening over the site of tissue removal, whether traumatic or surgically induced.
10. Full-thickness corneal limbal tissue addition produces corneal steepening over the site of the tissue addition and flattens the adjacent cornea.

From Rowsey JJ. Ten caveats in refractive surgery. *Ophthalmology*. 1983;90:148–155.

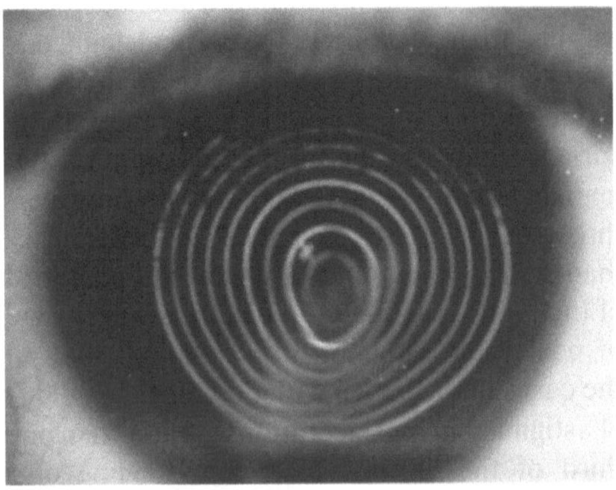

FIGURE 8.11. Photokeratoscopy image of a cornea with an inferior corneal laceration. An inverted teardrop pattern is evident suggesting a flattening of the vertical meridian in the central cornea. Inferiorly, over the scar and immediately adjacent to the scar a compaction of the rings can be seen, representing steepening in this area.

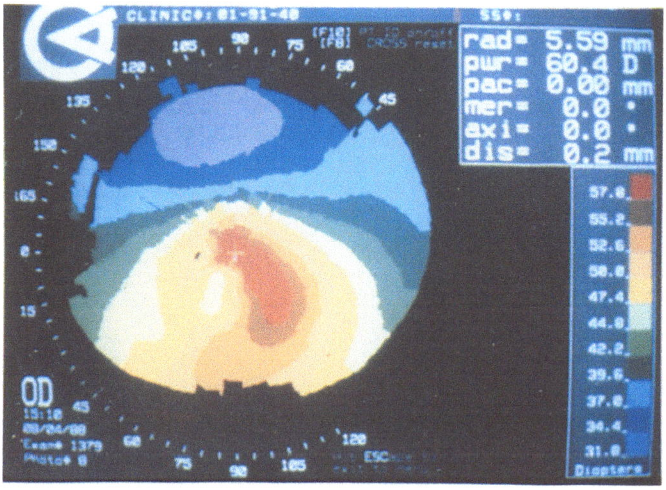

FIGURE 8.12. Corneal map produced by the Corneal Modeling System of the patient in Figure 8.11, demonstrating steepening at the site of the scar and in the immediate area.

of the sutures, regular and irregular astigmatism remained, reducing spectacle acuity to 20/70. A rigid contact lens corrected acuity to 20/30. Photokeratoscopy of this eye demonstrates flattening of the cornea central to the wound and steepening immediately adjacent to it (Fig. 8.14). The Visioptic EH270 dioptric plot derived from the photokeratoscopy image quantitatively demonstrates this phenomenon (Fig. 8.15).

Wound Healing Factors

Wound healing, particularly stromal wound healing, plays an important part in postrepair corneal topography. Approximately 12 hrs after a corneal laceration, the fibroblastic phase begins. The beginning of this phase is apparently associated with successful epithelial wound healing and represents the point in time at which stromal keratocytes take on fibroblast-like characteristics and produce type III collagen and scariform glycosaminogly-

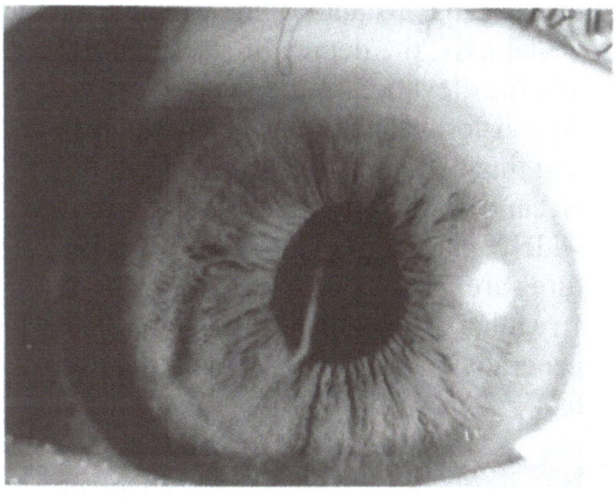

FIGURE 8.13. Angulated or V-shaped perforating corneal laceration involving the central zone. This wound was well closed at suturing and did not demonstrate any tissue loss. Visual acuity with spectacles was 20/70 and with a contact lens was 20/30.

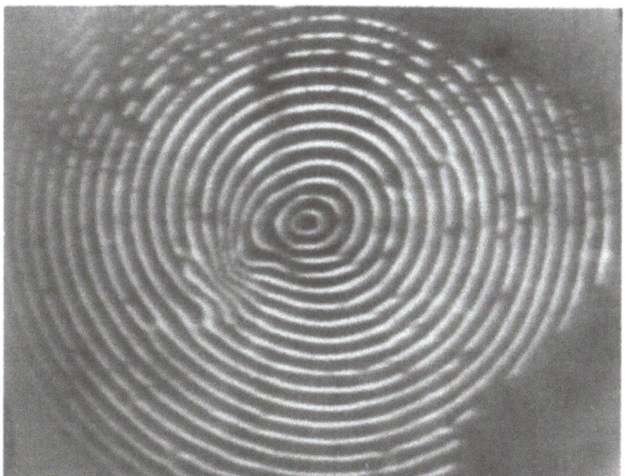

FIGURE 8.14. Photokeratoscopy image of the patient in Figure 8.13, showing the flattest central corneal meridian to be oriented toward the scar. Adjacent to the scar is an area of steepening.

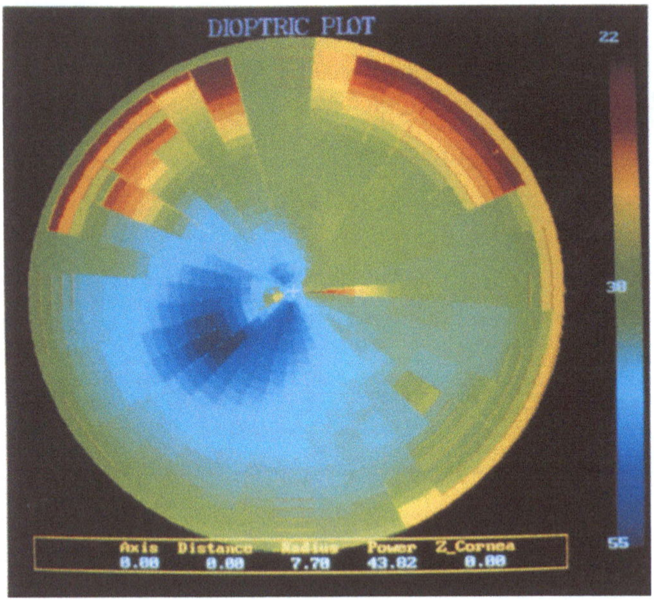

FIGURE 8.15. Visioptic EH270 dioptric plot made from the keratoscopy image found in Figure 8.14, quantitatively showing the flattening in the central cornea toward the scar and the steepening about the scar site.

cans.[16] One week after the injury, alignment of the type III stromal collagen to the normal type I collagen of the stroma begins to take place and then the scar contracts. This contraction appears to be of substantial importance in the topography of the scar and the area immediately adjacent to it. The two cases shown in Figures 8.11–8.15 demonstrate what appears to be a manifestation of stromal contraction at the wound site.

Topographic Considerations in the Management of Healed Lacerations

The corneal topography of the healed eye following penetrating and perforating corneal lacerations demonstrates some general characteristics that can be useful in visual rehabilitation of the patient. These six general topographic features are as follows:

1. The topography along the laceration scar generally demonstrates flattening, although this may be localized to the most anterior aspect of the scar only (Fig. 8.16). At times, steepening of the healed wound site can be found (Fig. 8.12).
2. The corneal surface immediately adjacent to the scar is steep if there is elevation of the scar or significant contracture of the scar (Figs. 8.13 and 8.14).
3. For lacerations not crossing the apex of the cornea, central flattening usually occurs, with the flattest meridian pointed toward the scar the majority of the time (Figs. 8.9 and 8.10).
4. The amplitude of the topographic effect on the central cornea is related to the length of the scar, the distance of the wound from the visual axis, the degree of scar contracture, and the elevation of the scar.
5. Apical corneal flattening can be substantial, and this flattening will be enhanced if there is central corneal tissue loss or if large, widely placed interrupted or running sutures are used.
6. Irregular astigmatism is common and will generally be the major visually limiting effect.

In the presence of irregular astigmatism extending into the visual axis, maximum visual acuity can be obtained only by masking the astigmatism, altering the visual axis or by eliminating the irregular astigmatism.

Masking of corneal astigmatism is accom-

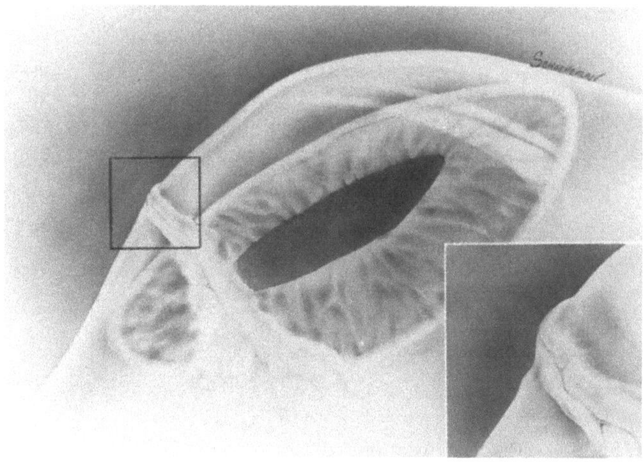

FIGURE 8.16. Graphic representation of the steepening found adjacent to many healed lacerations. Elevated scar tissue may have a steep or, more commonly, a flat anterior surface. Tractional forces or tissue loss produces the flattening found extending from the scar to the central cornea.

plished with the use of either rigid or, less frequently, soft contact lenses. Rigid contact lens fitting has been demonstrated to be an effective treatment option in the visual rehabilitation of patients with corneal lacerations.[17] Contact lenses create a new optical surface in front of the injured cornea. Tears fill in the area between the lens and the cornea, optically eliminating surface irregurities.

Eliminating irregular corneal astigmatism following repair of a traumatic corneal laceration is presently limited to selective suture placement and removal, penetrating keratoplasty, or rotating the affected area out of the line of sight by using a rotated autograft.[18] Photoablative refractive surgery may, in the future, provide an alternative to these choices. By sculpting the affected surface using the excimer laser, the corneal surface may be sufficiently smoothed to effectively eliminate irregular astigmatism.

Penetrating corneal surgery, whether an autologous or homologous transplant, is limited to cases in which visual rehabilitation using glasses or contact lenses has failed, and where sufficient clinical evidence of visual potential exists.

References

1. Roper-Hall MJ. The treatment of ocular injuries. *Trans Ophthalmol Soc UK.* 1959;79:57–92.
2. *Vision Problems in the U.S.A.: A Statistical Analysis.* New York: National Society to Prevent Blindness, Occupation Research Department, 1980.
3. Eagling EM. Perforating injuries of the eye. *Br J Ophthalmol.* 1976;60:732–736.
4. Adhikary HP, Taylor P, Fitzmaurice DJ. Prognosis of perforating eye injury. *Br J Ophthalmol.* 1976;60:737–739.
5. Snell AD: Perforating ocular injuries. *Am J Ophthalmol.* 1945;28:263–281.
6. Eisner G. *Eye Surgery: An Introduction to Operative Techniques.* New York: Springer-Verlag, 1980.
7. Rowsey JJ, Hays JC. Refractive reconstruction for acute eye injuries. *Ophthalmic Surg.* 1984;15:569–574.
8. Rowsey JJ. Ten caveats in keratorefractive surgery. *Ophthalmology.* 1983;90:148–155.
9. Rowsey JJ, Reynolds AE, Brown R. Corneal topography. Corneascope. *Arch Ophthalmol.* 1981;99:1093–1100.
10. El Hage SG. Differential equations for the use of the diffused ring keratoscope. *Am J Optom Arch Acad Optom.* 1972;49:436–442.
11. Klyce SD. Computer-assisted corneal topography: High resolution graphical presentation and analysis of keratoscopy. *Invest Ophthalmol Vis Sci.* 1984;25:1426–1435.
12. Maquire LJ, Singer DE, Klyce DS. Graphic presentation of computer analyzed keratoscopic photokeratographs. *Arch Ophthalmol.* 1987; 105:223–230.
13. Klyce SD, Wilson SE. Methods of analysis of corneal topography. *Refractive Corneal Surg.* 1989;5:368–371.

14. El Hage SG. A computerized corneal topographer for use in refractive surgery. *Refractive Corneal Surg*. 1989;5:418–424.
15. Wang J, Rice DA, Klyce SD. A new reconstruction algorithm for improvement of corneal topographical analysis. *Refractive Corneal Surg*. 1989;5:379–387.
16. Yanoff M, Fine BS. *Ocular Pathology: A Text and Atlas*. Philadelphia: Harper & Row, 1982.
17. Smiddy WE, Hamburg TR, Kracher GP, et al. Contact lenses for visual rehabilitation after corneal laceration repair. *Ophthalmology*. 1989;96:293–297.
18. Bourne WM, Brubaker RF. A method of ipsilateral rotational autokeratoplasty. *Ophthalmology*. 1978;85:1312–1316.

9
Radial Keratotomy and Corneal Topography

Joseph F. Fleming

Considering the little understanding we have of radial keratotomy, it is suprising that the operation has been successful. Currently, predictability remains an area of concern.[1] The level of predictability is reasonable enough that the surgery continues to be done in considerable numbers. Most would agree, however, that radial keratotomy would be more successful if it were possible to predict the refractive outcome with greater precision.

Efforts have been made to refine predictability.[2] Realistically, no significant strides have been made since improvement of basic instrumentation reduced the chance of erroneous corneal thickness measurements and blade settings.

Most surgeons take into account certain variables in planning radial keratotomy. These may include preoperative myopia and age.[2,3] More controversial preoperative factors include sex, intraocular pressure, central corneal curvature, corneal thickness, and corneal diameter. Certain intraoperative factors such as optical zone size, number of incisions, and incision depth are accepted determinants of outcome.[2,3] A less certain intraoperative factor used by some surgeons is incision redeepening.[4,5] Postoperative interventions are important. Steroids appear to influence outcome, especially in women.[6] Some surgeons use ocular hypotensive agents in hopes of modifying surgical outcome.[7]

Corneal topography is one area that holds promise in the realm of radial keratotomy predictability. The optical effect seen with radial keratotomy is attributable to change on the anterior corneal surface. We will discuss some new concepts regarding the mechanism of corneal change with radial keratotomy.

Preoperative Corneal Topography

Asphericity

The aspheric shape of the anterior corneal surface is well recognized.[8] Theoretically, individual corneal curvature falls on a continuum ranging from positive aspheric shape (steeper centrally, flatter peripherally) to negative aspheric shape (flatter centrally, steeper peripherally). As visualized in Fig. 9.1, a spherical shape where the radius of curvature is the same, centrally and peripherally, lies in the middle of the continuum. Most human corneas fall toward the end of the spectrum representing positive asphericity.[9,10] The gradual peripheral flattening associated with positive asphericity compensates for the image defocusing noted with sperical refracting surfaces (spherical aberration).[11] Some human corneas may have a virtually spherical shape, whereas a negative aspheric contour is not generally recognized in the preoperative cornea.[12] One may relate the type of aspheric curvature to the two major curves of an ellipse.[10] The positive aspheric shape is a prolate curve and the negative aspheric shape is an oblate curve.

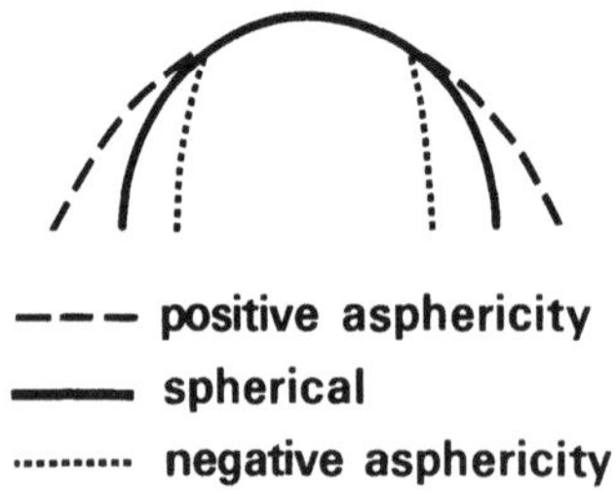

FIGURE 9.1. Range of corneal curvature.

Determinants of Central to Peripheral Corneal Contour

Three anatomic determinants are associated with central to peripheral corneal contour. These are corneal diameter, corneal sagittal height, and central corneal curvature (Fig. 9.2). We will consider how these three factors interact. Corneas with the same central curvature may have markedly different shapes. Figure 9.2, for example, shows three different corneas with the same average keratometry readings. Despite the same central curve, one is spherical, one is negatively aspheric, and one is positively aspheric. Sagittal height being constant in these three examples, it is the variation in diameter that accounts for the differences in contour. Using the spherical cornea as a reference, we can see that a smaller diameter pushes the shape toward negative asphericity while the larger diameter allows positive asphericity. Figure 9.3 emphasizes the effect of sagittal height on corneal contour. With the central curve and diameter constant, a small sagittal height favors positive asphericity while large sagittal height allows negative asphericity.

Postoperative Corneal Topography

Corneal Flattening

Single radial incisions flatten the cornea. Rowsey[13] has indicated that the adjacent cornea (same meridian) is flattened, while the cornea in a meridian 90° away is flattened to a lesser degree.

Symmetrically placed multiple radial incisions flatten virtually all of the cornea.[14] There is a misconception that true peripheral steepening occurs with radial keratotomy. In fact, radial keratotomy flattens all of the cornea, and only relative peripheral steepening occurs. This is true because the diffuse flattening observed is greater centrally than peripherally. In general, the postoperative corneal contour must be considered negatively aspheric.

In that diffuse (central and peripheral) corneal flattening occurs with radial keratotomy, we should recognize radial keratotomy as a tissue addition procedure. Flattening of the entire anterior corneal surface implies tissue addition because a net increase in corneal surface area must occur.

Optical Effect of Negative Asphericity

In most cases, radial keratotomy causes relative peripheral corneal steepening and a negatively aspheric shape (Fig. 9.1).[14] This results in significant optical consequences.

The positive asphericity of the normal cornea is meant to compensate for spherical aberration.[11] A spherical cornea (or lens) brings

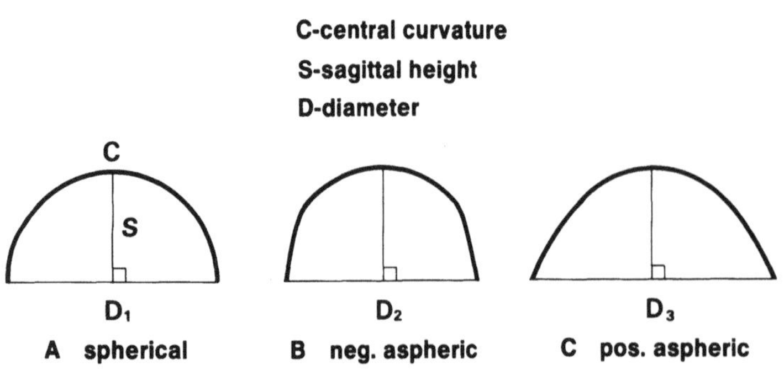

FIGURE 9.2. Variance in corneal diameter is a determinant of corneal contour.

FIGURE 9.3. Variance in corneal sagittal height is a determinant of corneal contour.

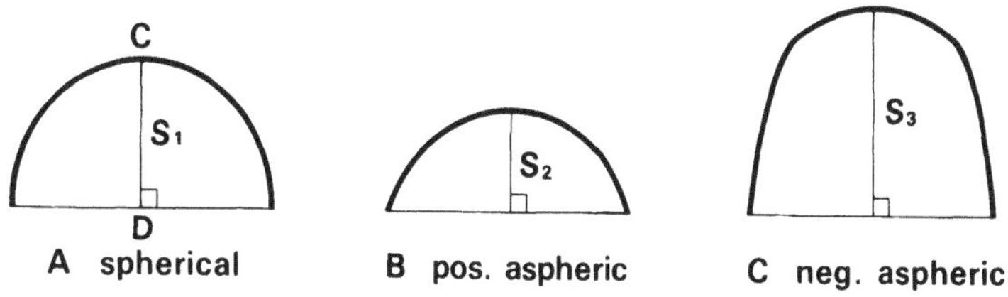

peripheral light rays to focus in front of more central rays (Fig. 9.4). This is important at night, when pupillary dilation allows entrance of more peripheral rays and the image defocusing results in "night myopia." The post-radial keratotomy negative corneal asphericity actually accentuates this problem by inducing more positive spherical aberration.[14] The relative peripheral steepening increases the amount of defocusing by bringing peripheral rays to focus more anteriorly. We know that only some of those radial keratotomy patients with subjective complaints of diurnal visual fluctuation have measurable change in refraction or keratometry throughout the day.[15] It may be that post-radial keratotomy negative asphericity is a factor contributing to subjective diurnal fluctuation.

There is new evidence to suggest that negative asphericity after surgery also has some positive visual consequences. Holliday et al (16) observe that radial keratotomy patients displaying a myopic shift when refracted before, then after, dilation see better without correction than matched normals. The tendency of these patients to become more myopic with dilation is attributed to positive spherical aberration, a condition induced by negative asphericity. In this situation, the dilated pupil allows entrance of peripheral light rays that traverse a gradually steepening cornea. These rays focus more anteriorly than paraxial rays. This shifts the circle of least confusion anteriorly and minus power must be added to the refraction. One would expect some night visual dysfunction to result. However, the condition may impart some significant visual advantage in better illumination (undilated state). When compared to normal eyes at the same refractive error, these radial keratotomy patients showed significantly better undilated and uncorrected Snellen acuity. The authors speculate that the negative aspheric cornea has a multifocal optical property causing increased depth of field. This results in better uncorrected vision when the pupil is small.

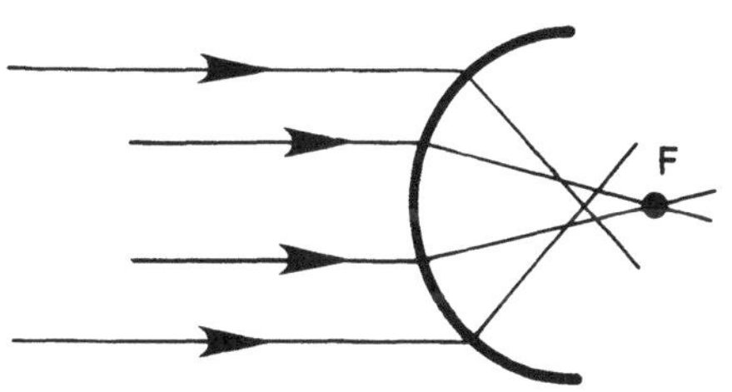

FIGURE 9.4. Image defocusing results from spherical aberration.

I have recently correlated measurements of negative asphericity in radial keratotomy patients with their uncorrected, undilated visual acuities (unpublished data). For optical zones less than 4.0 mm, greater postoperative negative asphericity is associated with better uncorrected vision. In patient subgroups with the same optical zone size and same postoperative spherical equivalent, greater negative asphericity imparted significantly better undilated, uncorrected Snellen acuity. For optical zones of 4.0 mm and greater, the opposite was true. Subgroups with the same optical zone size and same postoperative spherical equivalent demonstrated a significant relationship between greater negative asphericity and lesser undilated, uncorrected vision. One may speculate as to the difference between those with optical zones less than 4.0 mm and those with optical zones equal to or greater than that level. Patients with smaller optical zones achieve greater central flattening and more postoperative negative asphericity than patients with larger optical zones.[12] A large degree of negative asphericity may be required to obtain a visually meaningful increase in depth of field; that is, a desirable multifocal effect may require a threshold level of negative asphericity. Only patients with optical zones small enough to produce this threshold obtain uncorrected vision better than expected for their postoperative spherical equivalent. In patients with larger optical zones and less negative asphericity, the minimal multifocal effect may be overshadowed by the image defocus caused by the negative aspheric surface. Larger optical zone patients thus get no benefit and some deficit if they tend toward a larger degree of negative asphericity.

The shape of the cornea after radial keratotomy plays a role in the quality of vision after surgery. Negative corneal asphericity has the advantage of producing better than expected uncorrected vision in some patients while probably creating difficulty with night vision in others.

Visual Axis Orientation in Radial Keratotomy

Most surgeons orient the optical zone on the visual axis in radial keratotomy. Likewise, with corneascopy the rings may be oriented on the visual axis. In that most individuals have a positive angle κ, the visual axis usually lies about 1mm nasal to the geometric center of the cornea. The nasalmost radial incisions, therefore, pass through different portions of the corneal curvature than the temporalmost incisions (Fig. 9.5). In fact, with a 3.0 mm optical zone, the temporalmost incision is relatively close to the geometric center. A glance at the scan of a preoperative photo (Fig. 9.6) will show that the midperipheral rings encompass an area of greater curvature temporally than they do nasally, since the photokeratograph scanned was taken with visual axis orientation.

Effect of Radial Keratotomy as Observed by the Corneascope

The Corneoscope photograph reveals a dramatic picture of the topographical change that occurs with radial keratotomy. Let's arbitrarily select ring 4 of the Corneoscope. Figure 9.6 shows a pre-radial keratotomy and a post-radial keratotomy photograph. Ring 4 on the postoperative photo has a greater circumference than that on the preoperative photo. This represents corneal flattening. We will examine this change in greater detail.

To better understand the corneoscopic shift that occurs with radial keratotomy, we will create a Corneoscope radial keratotomy model (Fig. 9.7). Corneoscopy is, in reality, a two-dimensional representation of three-dimensional phenomena. In corneoscopy we deal with hemichords, as represented by R_1 and R_2 in Fig. 9.7. The hemichord of a given Corneoscope ring is actually the radius of that ring, and it may be easily measured on the photograph with a ruler. The hemichord for a given ring will vary from photo to photo. After all, we use change in ring circumference to qualitatively identify flattening and steepening. The digital scanner actually measures hemichords in various meridians in assigning curvature measurements to the Corneoscope ring.[17] If the hemichord length for a given ring varies from photo to photo, one would wonder what

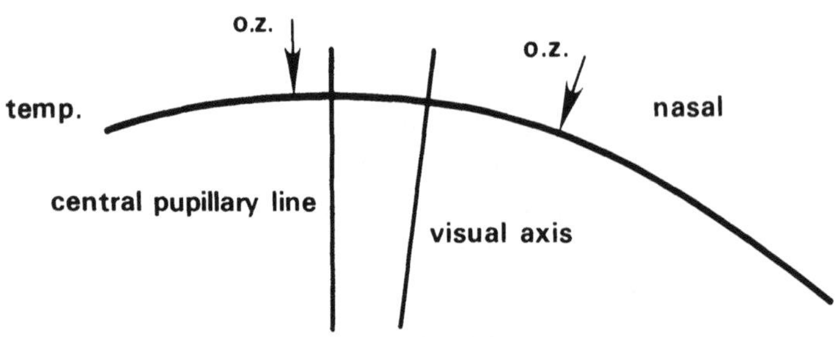

FIGURE 9.5. Orientation of the optical zone mark on the visual axis causes nasal decentering of the optical zone.

is constant in corneoscopy. The constant parameter for each ring is sagittal depth; the sagittal depth from one photo to the next should be consistent for a given ring. Rings 1 through 12 represent progressively increasing, theoretically fixed sagittal depths. Thus sagittal depth, S, for the Corneoscope ring represented in Fig. 9.7 is the same preoperatively and postoperatively. However, the hemichord, R, varies. The flatter postoperative cornea exhibits a hemichord R_2 greater than R_1 of the preoperative cornea. Following suit, the circumference ($2\pi R$) of the noted ring is larger postoperatively. In this fashion, corneoscopy represents corneal flattening with radial keratotomy by expansion of ring circumference.

The corneoscope gives us an indirect view of the corneal surface. On one end of the horizontal instrument axis of the device is mounted a camera. On the other end is positioned the patient's cornea such that the visual axis is aligned with the instrument axis. The corneoscope faceplate contains the object locus, the collection of lighted concentric rings. Each point source of light on the object rings releases a ray of light that reflects from the corneal surface and courses toward the camera film. This ray is distinguished by the fact that the normal to the corneal reflection point bisects the incident and reflected arm of the ray. Once the ray is reflected from the corneal surface, it crosses the instrument axis at the center of the camera lens and is finally imaged on the film. The two-dimensional film image, however, is not of the rings as they are actually reflected from the cornea. In fact, the cornea acts as a convex mirror creating a virtual image. The corneoscope photograph as we observe it contains the virtual image, which is located spatially several millimeters posterior to the corneal surface.[18]

The ideal method of understanding corneal change with radial keratotomy would involve the observation of an actual ring of corneal tissue. We can make such an observation mentally (as will be done later in this chapter), but we do not have a clinical method of actual observation currently. The Corneoscope gives us a practical clinical method of approximating this observation. Corneoscope rings do not represent actual rings of corneal tissue; that is, the changes seen in the two-dimensional Corneoscope ring after radial keratotomy surgery are not the same as would be observed with an actual ring of corneal tissue. However, the similarities between the two are sufficient enough to make corneoscopy a clinically useful method of understanding corneal change with radial keratotomy.

Radial Keratotomy Theories

Ligament Theory

Fyodorov[19] explained the corneal change observed after radial keratotomy as being due to dissection of the circular ligament of the cornea. He proposed the idea that anterior radial incisions would lead to dissection of the peripheral circular collagen fibers. The resultant weakening of this ligament would allow marked reduction of the mechanical stability of the corneal periphery. Peripheral bulging of the cornea would allow peripheral steepening and central flattening.

To date, there has been no convincing histologic evidence of a peripheral corneal ligament. In addition, true peripheral corneal steepening has not been observed after radial keratotomy.[14] However, this theory did correctly attribute the refractive change observed after radial keratotomy to central corneal flattening.

Wound Gape Model

The principal goal of this chapter is the introduction of the wound gape theory as proposed by A.E. Reynolds (personal communication, 1986). The realization that radial keratotomy results in diffuse (central and peripheral) corneal flattening indicates that radial keratotomy is a tissue-addition procedure; radial keratotomy allows an increase in the total amount of tissue constituting the cornea, with a net increase in anterior corneal surface. The radial incisions gape and gradually fill in with fibroblasts and epithelium. Binder and colleagues[20] suggest that this early stage of wound healing

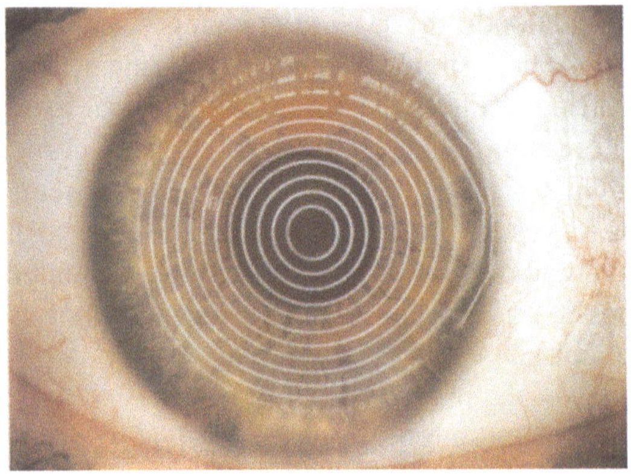

A

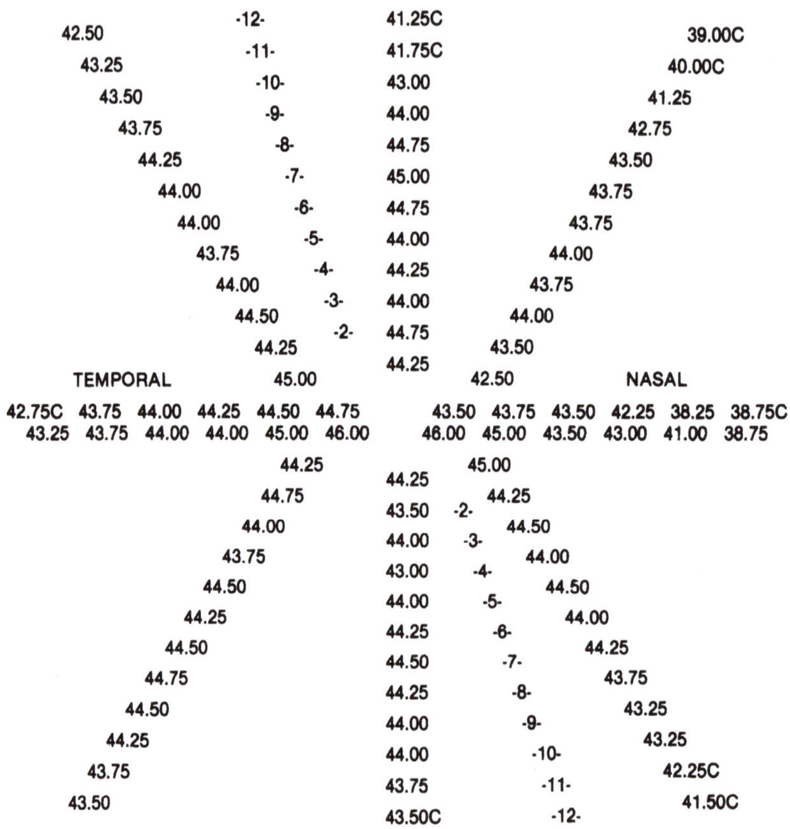

B

FIGURE 9.6. (A) Preoperative photokeratograph. (B) Postoperative (radial keratotomy) photokeratograph. (C) Digital scan (diopters) of preoperative photokeratograph from (A). (D) Digital scan (diopters) of postoperative photokeratograph from (B).

eventually progresses to complete wound healing, documented as early as 66 months after surgery.

A multiplicity of factors may contribute to the degree of wound gape and resultant degree of corneal flattening in any one case. We may, in a given case, estimate the degree of gape using preoperative and postoperative photokeratographs. If we look at the case represented by the photographs in Fig. 9.6, the computer scanner can identify the hemichord length (R) for ring 4 of the preoperative photo

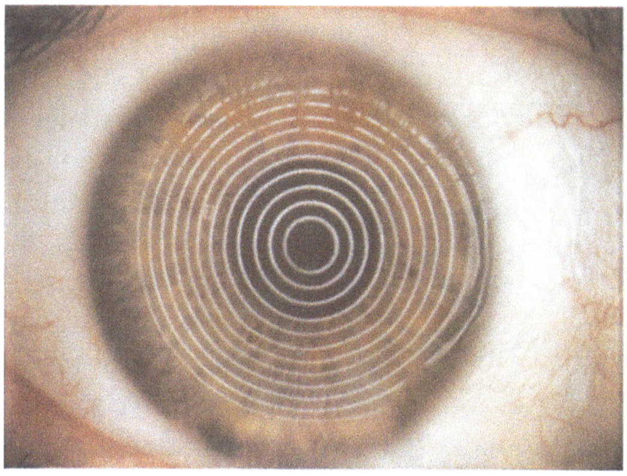

C

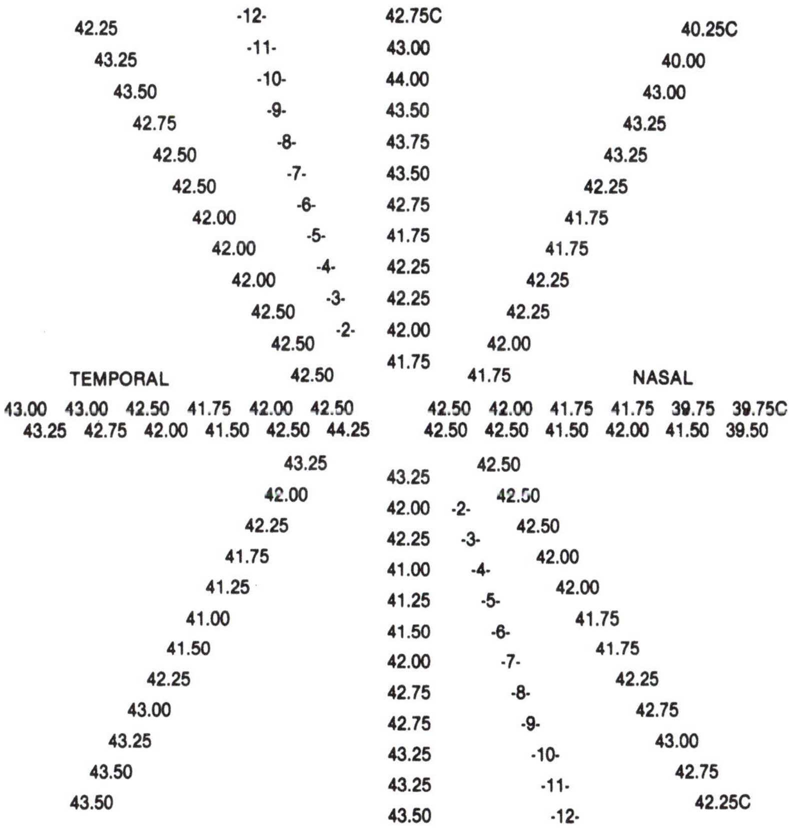

D

FIGURE 9.6. (C, D)

(Fig. 9.6). From this, we calculate the circumference of ring 4 as 11.56 mm. We perform the same procedure on the postoperative photo (Fig. 9.6B). The postoperative circumference of ring 4 is calculated as 12.25 mm. Therefore, the circumference of ring 4 has been increased by 0.69 mm as a result of radial keratotomy. If we divide this value by 8 (the number of incisions), we obtain an average per-incision gape fo 0.09 mm. This gape factor will vary depending upon which ring is chosen for the calculation. Remember, this method at best estimates

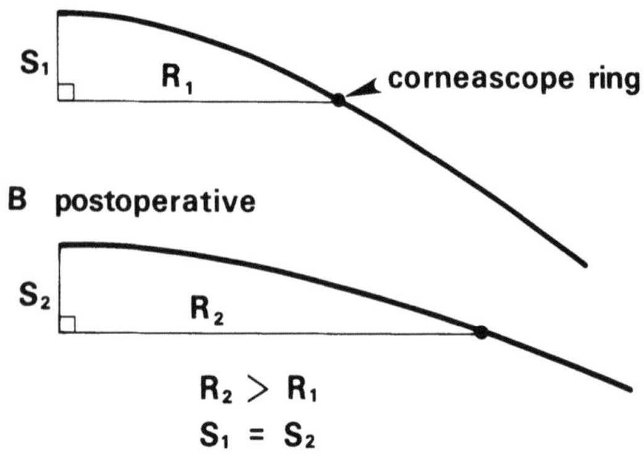

FIGURE 9.7. (A) Preoperative position of a Corneascope ring relative to the corneal surface. (B) The flattened postoperative corneal surface allows an increase in the radius (R) of the Corneascope ring.

the amount of gape, as the Corneascope ring does not truly represent an actual ring of corneal tissue.

The wound gape model theory offers a versatile model of the mechanism of radial keratotomy. It can account for variations in surgical effect previously related to preoperative, intraoperative, and postoperative factors. It may also explain some previously unrecognized predictors of surgical effect. We will consider the wound gape model in greater detail.

A Mental Radial Keratotomy Model

I previously discussed the fact that the Corneascope ring does not behave exactly like a ring of corneal tissue. We will, therefore, examine a mental radial keratotomy model to study the changes in a ring of corneal tissue that will result from the gaping of multiple radial incisions.

To gain understanding of the effect of wound gape, let us construct a mental radial keratotomy model. We will first observe a hypothetical ring of corneal tissue centered around the corneal apex (Fig. 9.8). We choose this ring to be large enough in diameter that a 3.0 mm optical zone radial keratotomy will allow all incisions to pass through our ring of tissue (Fig. 9.8). If we draw a straight line from the corneal apex to any point on our tissue ring, we can assign this line a length X_1 (Fig. 9.9). We now drop a line from the corneal apex perpendicular to the iris plane. We can identify on this line, a distance, S_1, representing the sagittal depth of our tissue ring. Next we perform radial keratotomy on this cornea. Figure 9.9 B represents the postoperative cornea. The incisions gape, and this increases the circumference of our tissue ring. In fact, our tissue ring is elevated (the cornea flattens). The postoperative sagittal depth, S_2, is less than the preoperative value, S_1. Because the corneal flattening results in an increase in the distance between the corneal apex and our ring, X_2 is greater than X_1. These changes occur due to an overall increase in midperipheral corneal surface area as a result of wound gape. In that corneal diameter remains constant, the increase in midperipheral surface area also allows central corneal flattening.

The graphics of this model may appear similar to those of the corneascope radial keratotomy model, but there are substantial differences.

Reynolds–Kilmer Corneal Model

The Reynolds-Kilmer model cornea (Fig. 9.10) is designed to exaggerate corneal surface characteristics. The model consists of a rubber

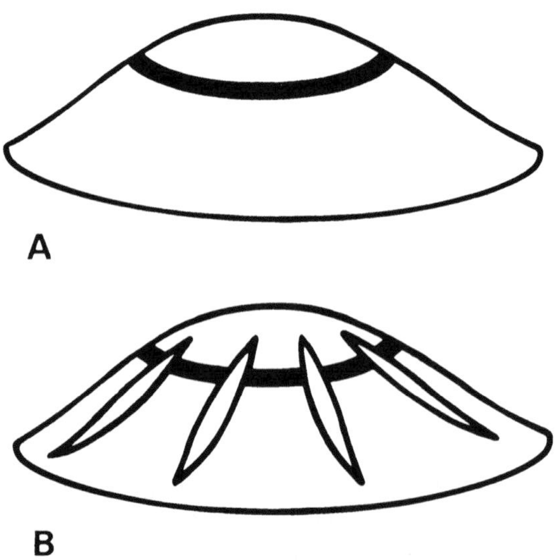

FIGURE 9.8. (A) A hypothetical ring of corneal tissue is chosen. (B) The radial incisions pass through this tissue ring.

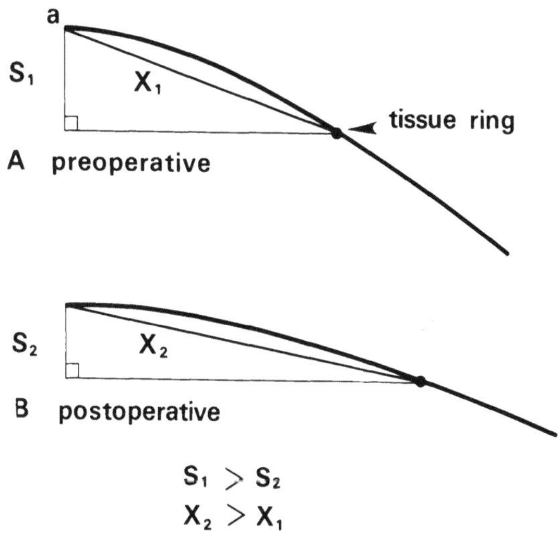

FIGURE 9.9. (A) The hypothetical tissue ring lies at a given chord length (X_1) and a given sagittal depth (S_1) from the corneal apex (a). (B) After radial keratotomy, the tissue ring on the newly flattened corneal surface is elevated such that sagittal depth (S_2) decreases and chord length (X_2) increases.

sheet placed over a wooden form. Incisions may be placed in the rubber surface of the model. Because of the large size of the model (12 cm in outside diameter), variations in degree of incision gape may be observed with the naked eye.

How Wound Gape Explains Radial Keratotomy Results

Much of the following information is based on the Reynolds–Kilmer model cornea (personal communication with A.E. Reynolds, O.D., 1986). In addition, estimates of wound gape based on measurement of Corneascope ring circumference support these conclusions.

Depth

Deeper incisions exhibit greater gape. This is consistent with the observation that deeper radial keratotomy incisions result in greater surgical effect.[2, 3] This also casts interesting light on the controversial concept of incision re-deepening.

Incision Length

Longer incisions show greater gape.

Number of Incisions

In comparing 4, 8, and 16 radial incisions, we find interesting results. The amount of gape per incision is greater with 4 than 8. However, the total gape (sum of incision gapes) is greater with 8 than with 4. The same relationship holds in comparing 8 and 16 incisions. This supports the observation that if 16 incisions achieve 100% of possible surgical effect, four incisions will achieve 70%, whereas 8 incisions will achieve 90%.[21]

Healing

This elusive factor is probably affected by such variables as age, sex, and postoperative steroid use. It is likely that variability in healing will result in greater or lesser final wound gape. It is common to see some regression in surgical effect during the first 30 days postoperatively.[22] This is likely due to a gradual decrease from the immediate postoperative gape level due to the initial healing stages. Steroids may retard this tendency.

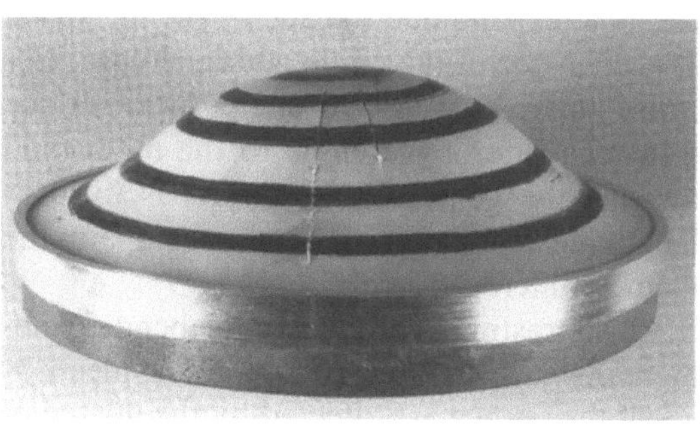

FIGURE 9.10. The rubber surface of the Reynolds–Kilmer model cornea allows placement of incisions at different locations to demonstrate variance in wound gape.

The Bending Moment Theory

Au and Rowsey[23] have proposed a mechanical model of the cornea that assumes certain tissue dynamics in response to surface incisions. The model encompasses many facets of the wound gape theory with the addition of interesting and simple mechanical concepts.

Bending moment theory considers central flattening seen with radial keratotomy as the indirect result of paracentral corneal flattening that occurs between adjacent radial incisions. Such paracentral flattening is explained by a change in stress within the corneal stroma precipitated by placement of radial incisions. The incisions create a negative bending moment, whereby mechanical stress is redistributed from the entire corneal thickness to the thin layer of unincised cornea at the incision base. The stress redistribution in the stroma between incisions causes stretching of posterior stromal layers and compression of anterior layers. The net effect of this negative bending moment is flattening of the cornea between incisions.

The bending moment theory further explains why paracentral flattening between incisions leads to central flattening. A key assumption is that an arc length on the corneal surface is fixed if not interrupted by an incision; the cornea is assumed to be inelastic such that an arc passing through the center of the cornea from one side to the other cannot be expanded by forces that deform the cornea. A circle is imagined on the corneal surface such that it will pass through the midpoint of any radial incisions placed with radial keratotomy. When incisions are made the circumference of the circle must expand due to gape of the incisions. The diameter of the circle must increase. Because an arc passing over the corneal surface from one side of the circle to the other (and through the center of the circle) is fixed in length, central flattening must accompany the diameter increase.

An interesting byproduct of the bending moment theory is the suggestion that the mechanics of the cornea are affected by the degree of peripheral asphericity. The model predicts that those with greater peripheral asphericity (those that flatten more in the periphery) will respond more to radial keratotomy.

Finite Element Theory

Several investigators[24, 25] have applied finite element theory in modeling corneal response to radial keratotomy. Finite element technique is an established engineering tool for studying the stress-strain behavior of a structure. The structure is theoretically constructed of a finite number of bricks (elements) connected to one another by nodes. By analyzing the response of each element to specific forces, the response of the entire structure is understood.

Vito, Shin, and McCarey[25] created a computer simulation of radial keratotomy incorporating the finite element technique. The model predicts that higher intraocular pressure, lesser corneal thickness, deeper incisions, and smaller optical zones will result in more corneal flattening with surgery. The authors noted that the model should be considered in qualitative agreement with clinical observations with radial keratotomy. They also pointed out the limitations of the model due to the assumptions required in applying the theory. For example, the study assumes the cornea to be homogeneous with all layers having the same toughness (isotropic). The cornea, of course, is composed of non-homogeneous layers, and these layers possess different mechanical properties (non-isotropic). The study also assumes the cornea to be spherical with symmetrical curvature about an axis. The cornea in reality is aspheric and rotationally asymmetric.[26]

Finite element modeling is a promising technique with potential applications in various refractive procedures. To bring this method to fruition, investigators must identify the value of Young's modulus for Bowman's and Descemet's membranes. Also, a rotationally asymmetric model with an aspheric contour is necessary.

The Predictive Role of Corneal Asphericity in Radial Keratotomy

Recognized predictors of radial keratotomy outcome include optical zone size, patient age, and incision depth. Multiple regression analyses in large radial keratotomy studies indicate that these three variables explain only 75 percent of variation in response to surgery.[2 3] This is concluded because multiple coefficients of determination (R^2) in these studies have not exceeded 0.75. It is reasonable to wonder if a corneal shape factor might account for a portion of the remaining 25 percent. Specifically, it is reasonable to ask if preoperative corneal asphericity is a predictor of radial keratotomy outcome.

I examined 81 cases of eight-incision radial keratotomy in 81 patients. Optical zone size ranged from 3.0 mm to 5.0 mm. Key preoperative measurements included corneoscopy and manifest refraction, and 3 month postoperative measurements included manifest refraction.

Preoperative photokeratographs were scanned with a digital analyzer. Ninety-six hemichord measurements were taken representing each of 12 rings in the 8 major semimeridians. These values were used to calculate an aspheric index, a quantitative measure of corneal asphericity.[26] The aspheric index technique is based upon the idea that asphericity represents a deviation from central corneal sphericity. A positive value indicates positive asphericity, while a negative value describes negative asphericity.

Regression analysis was used to examine the relationship between preoperative asphericity and 3 month change in refraction after radial keratotomy. Linear regression and second-order polynomial regression showed very low correlation between these two variables. However, third-order polynomial regression showed a large increase in the coefficient of correlation (R=0.41) with statistical significance at $p < 0.001$. The plot of this equation (Fig. 9.11) indicates that corneas with low preoperative asphericity respond less to radial keratotomy. Those corneas with high asphericity respond more to surgery. Within the midrange of preoperative aspheric index values, little effect from asphericity was observed.

Several comments are in order regarding these observations. Multiple regression analysis of the same data revealed preoperative asphericity as a statistically significant, but minor, predictor of radial keratotomy outcome.

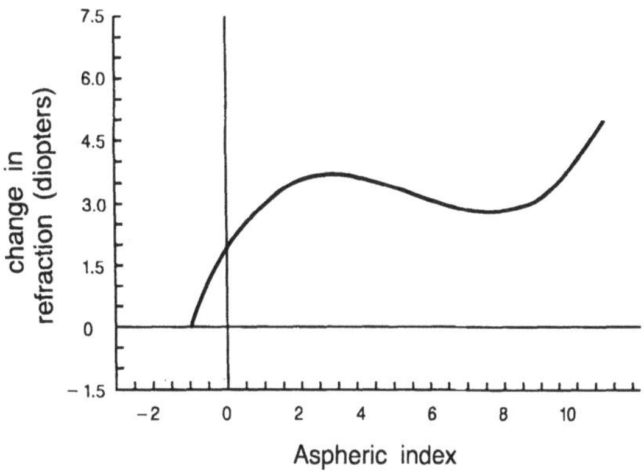

FIGURE 9.11. Plot of third-order regression equation describing relationship between preoperative aspheric index (x-axis) and 3 month change in refraction (Y-axis).

Addition of asphericity to a multiple variable predictor equation (along with recognized predictive variables such as optical zone size, age, and incision depth) resulted in only a 2 percent increase in the coefficient of multiple determination. Another feature of this patient series is the use of manifest refraction rather than cycloplegic refraction. This was done to avoid the artifactual change in refraction that can occur in dilation of eyes with negative asphericity.[16, 27] Also deserving comment is the level of the correlation coefficient of 0.41 for the third-order polynomial equation. This is not extraordinarily strong correlation, but it is consistent with that seen for other accepted radial keratotomy predictors. With an R value of 0.41, the coefficient of determination (R^2) is calculated as 0.16. This would suggest that preoperative asphericity explains 16 percent of the variation in response to radial keratotomy. By way of comparison, in the PERK study the R^2 value for age was 0.12 and for incision depth was 0.04.[3]

Conclusion

Knowledge of corneal topography is essential in understanding radial keratotomy. The wound gape theory may explain many of the topographical changes observed with radial keratotomy. Corneoscopy possesses some limitations in representing corneal topography. New instruments may allow us to better understand topographical shifts by permitting direct observation of change at any point on the anterior corneal surface. However, corneoscopy will remain a clinically useful, practical tool for the ophthalmologist who performs radial keratotomy.

References

1. Binder PS. Radial keratotomy in the United States. *Arch Ophthalmol.* 1987;105:37–39.
2. Sanders DR, Deitz MR, Gallagher D. Factors affecting predictibility of radial keratotomy. *Ophthalmology.* 1985;92:1237–1243.
3. Lynn MJ, Waring GO, Sperduto RD, et al. Factors affecting outcome and predictibility of radial keratotomy in the PERK study. *Arch Ophthalmol.* 1987;105:42–52.
4. Arrowsmith PN, Marks RG. How predictible is radial keratotomy? *Cataract.* 1986:7–14.
5. Waring GO. The changing status of radial keratotomy for myopia. Part II. *Refract Surg.* 1985;1:119–137.
6. Hays JC, Rowsey JJ, Balyeat HD. Effect of post-operative steroids on the refractive result of radial keratotomy. *Invest Ophthalmol Vis Sci.* 1985;26(suppl):150.
7. Sawelson H, Deitz MR, Arrowsmith PN. Postoperative care and complications. In: Arrowsmith PN, Deitz MR, Marks RG, et al, eds. *Radial Keratotomy.* Thorofare, NJ: Slack, 1984; pp. 91–100.
8. Ludlum H, Wittenbuerg S. Measurements of optical dioptric elements using photographic methods: II. Corneo-theoretical considerations. *Am J Optom.* 1966;42:249–267.
9. Clark BA. Mean topography of normal cornea. *Aust J Optom.* 1974;57:107–115.
10. Kiely PM, Smith G, Carney LG. The mean shape of the human cornea. *Optica Acta.* 1982;8:1027–1040.
11. Ogle KN. *Optics.* 2nd ed. Springfield, IL: Charles C Thomas, 1979.
12. Rowsey JJ, Balyeat HD, Monolux R, et al. Prospective evaluation of radial keratotomy: Photokeratoscope corneal topography. *Ophthalmology.* 1988;3:322–334.
13. Rowsey JJ. Topographical analysis of the cornea: ten caveats in keratorefractive surgery. In: Binder PS, ed. *Refractive Corneal Surgery: The Correction of Astigmatism.* Boston: Little, Brown, 1983: pp. 1–32.
14. Fleming JF. Corneal topography and radial keratotomy. *Refract Surg.* 1986;2:249–254.
15. Schanzlin DJ, Santos VR, Waring GO, et al. Diurnal change in refraction, corneal curvature, visual acuity, and intraocular pressure after radial keratotomy in the PERK study. *Ophthalmolgy.* 1986;98:167–175.
16. Holladay JT, Lynn MJ, Waring GO, et al. The relationship of visual acuity, refractive error, and pupil size after radial keratotomy. *Arch Ophthalmol.* 1991;109:70–76.
17. Rowsey JJ, Isaac M. Corneoscopy in keratorefractive surgery. *Cornea.* 1983;2:133–142.
18. Ludlum WM, Wittenberg S. Measurement of the ocular dioptric elements utilizing photographic method. Part II. Cornea-theoretical considerations. *Amer J Optom.* 1966;43:249–267.
19. Fyodorov SN, Durney VV. Operation of dosaged dissection of corneal circular ligament in cases of myopia of mild degree. *Ann Ophthalmol.* 1979;11:1885–1890.
20. Binder PS, Nayak SK, Deg JK, et al. An ultrastructural and histochemical study of long-term wound healing after radial keratotomy. *Am J Ophthalmol.* 1987;103:432–440.
21. Salz J, Lee JS, Jester JV, et al. Radial keratotomy in fresh human cadaver eyes. *Ophthalmology.* 1981;88:742–746.
22. Arrowsmith PN, Sanders DR, Marks RG. Visual, refractive, and keratometric results of radial keratotomy. *Arch Ophthalmol.* 1983; 101:873–881.
23. Au Y, Rowsey JJ. Bending moment modeling in radial keratotomy. In:Spaeth GS, ed. *Current Therapy in Refractive Surgery.* Philadelphia:BC Decker, 1989:47–53.
24. Bryant MR, Velinsky SA, Plesha ME, et al. Computer-aided surgical design in refractive keratotomy. *CLAO J.* 1987;13:238–242.
25. Vito RP, Shin TJ, McCarey BE. A mechanical model of the cornea: The effects of physiological and surgical factors on radial keratotomy surgery. *Refractive and Corneal Surgery.* 1989;5:82–88.
26. Kiely PM, Smith G, Carney LG. Meridional variations of corneal shape. *Am J Optom Physiol Opt.* 1984;10:619–626.
27. Fleming JF. Should refractive surgeons worry about corneal asphericity. *Refractive and Corneal Surgery* 1990;6:455–457.
28. Applegate RA, Gansel KA. The importance of pupil size in optical quality measurements following radial keratotomy. *Refractive and Corneal Surgery.* 1990;6:47–54.

10
The Corneascope-Comparator Method of Hard Contact Lens Fitting

Maureen K. Lundergan

The history of hard contact lens fitting has been a unique combination of art and science. One need only to look at the myriad of fitting techniques to realize that any single method has been unsatisfactory in the individual case. Variations in corneal shape, diameter, interpalpebral zone, refractive error, and tear film have traditionally meant spending considerable time fitting trial lenses, regardless of which fitting method is used.

The goal of every hard contact fitting procedure is to provide a comfortable fit and maximize visual acuity while minimizing the impact of the lens on normal corneal physiology. The cornea has a high rate of aerobic metabolism, nine tenths of which takes place in the epithelial layer.[1–5] The oxygen necessary to maintain normal corneal epithelial metabolism is obtained primarily by diffusion from the tear layer (Figs. 10.1 A,B). Without adequate tear exchange, the rate of anaerobic metabolism increases, resulting in increased levels of lactic acid and subsequent intracellular epithelial edema formation.

The key problem, then, is one of maximizing the exchange of tears beneath the lens with each blink. This is even more important in dry eye states. Oxygen-permeable lens materials provide some latitude in fitting but cannot replace adequate tear exchange.

Corneal Topography

The normal cornea is aspheric with a changing radius of curvature from the center to the periphery. Traditionally, the corneal contour has been divided into two zones.[6] The central zone has been described as relatively spherical with the radius of curvature averaging 7.9 mm (range 7.2 to 8.7 mm). The annular peripheral zone flattens progressively toward the limbus. This two-zone concept is now considered inadequate to describe the actual change in corneal contour from center to periphery. The entire cornea actually flattens as one moves away from the center, though the flattening occurs at a somewhat faster rate in the corneal periphery. The normal adult cornea measures approximately 12 mm in diameter. If the central 3 mm of the cornea, as measured by the keratometer, has a radius of curvature of 7.8 mm (43.25 diopters), it must flatten rapidly to maintain an average sagittal height of 2.4 mm and a diameter of 12 mm. Because the visual axis is usually slightly nasal to the geometric center of the cornea, giving a positive angle K, the keratograph gives slightly more information about the nasal cornea (Fig. 10.2). This also means that the cornea flattens more rapidly nasal to the visual axis than temporal to it.

A study was conducted in 1959 to determine the common characteristics among patients comfortably wearing hard contact lenses (written communication with A.E. Reynolds, O.D., January 1986). The study was designed to ascertain the relationship between the cor-

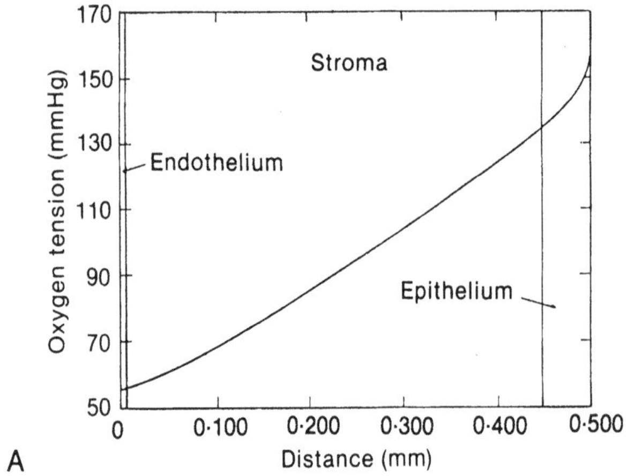

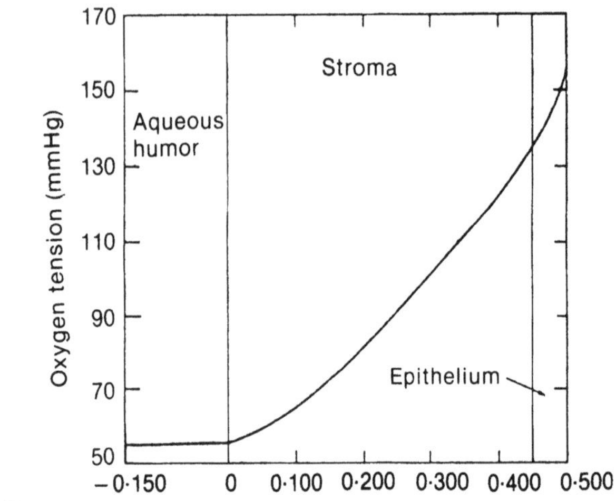

FIGURE 10.1. (A) Oxygen tension distribution in the in vivo cornea open to the area at the epithelial surface. (B) Oxygen tension in the in vivo cornea with a 0.150 mm stagnant layer of aqueous humor on the posterior surface and no endothelium. The epithelial surface is open to the air. (Fatt and Bieber: The steady-state distribution of oxygen and carbon dioxide in the in vivo cornea. I. The open eye in the air and the closed eye (A) and (B) from *Exp Eye Res.* 1968;7:109–112, with permission.

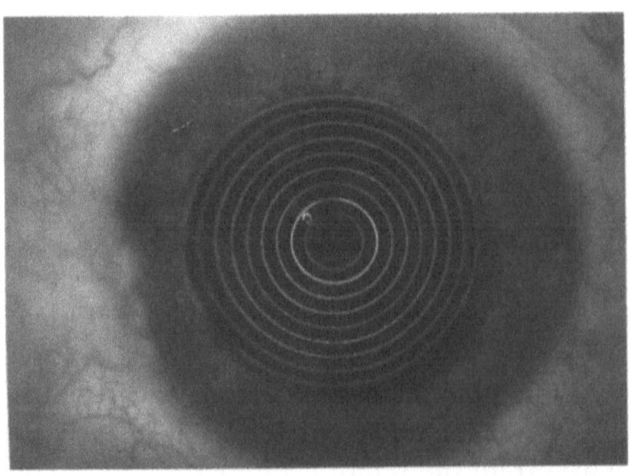

FIGURE 10.2. Positive angle K. Corneal rings decentered nasally, left eye.

neal contour and the spherical rigid lens. One hundred patients (10 patients were referred by each of 10 different doctors), who were all wearing their lenses in complete comfort, were studied. Some were fit on K, some steeper than K, some flatter than K, and various diameters were used. A mold of each patient's cornea was made; a pantograph was used to trace the mold in four meridians. These were then enlarged 10× and a corresponding model of each lens was made. In all cases, there was lens rocking in the vertical meridian with points of touch in the midline or above. The point of touch varied from the apex to the periphery, depending on whether the lens was fit on K, was steeper than K, or was flatter than K. The bevel and intermediate curve played very little role in the actual fit. However, the clearance between the optical zone margin and the cornea in the vertical meridian, which measured between 0.05 and 0.10 mm in most cases, proved to be an important variable: it provided a vertical rocking motion with each vertical lens excursion and therefore good tear exchange during each blink. The optical zone itself, in most cases, covered 40 to 43% of the corneal surface area. The Comparator was designed for use with the Corneascope keratograph to fit rigid lenses using these guidelines.[7]

Corneascope and Comparator in Contact Lens Fitting

The use of the Corneascope with the Comparator provides an efficient, accurate way of fitting hard lenses over a wide range of corneal contours (Fig. 10.3). It can also be used for soft contact lens fitting; however, this will not be discussed here. The Polaroid keratograph of the Corneascope image provides a permanent record of the virtual image of nine Placido rings projected onto the cornea.[8] The image is magnified 2.8×. Ring 9 encompasses approximately 40 to 50% of the total corneal surface area.[9] This area is inversely proportional to the corneal power; specifically, a cornea of 40 D has a chord length of 8.3 mm measured from the inside of ring 9, whereas a 50 D cornea has a chord length of 6.7 mm.[10]

The keratograph, then, is a contour map of the cornea. Since ring 3 corresponds to the central 3 mm measured by a standard keratometer, rings 4 through 9 give us information about the midperiphery of the cornea. This additional information is a key asset in contact lens fitting, since the optical zone of a rigid lens usually has a much larger diameter than the corneal surface as measured by the keratometer. This results in a steeper lens-to-cornea relationship, which can be altered by changing trial lenses after viewing the fluorescein pattern. Figure 10.4A demonstrates the typical keratographic appearance of contact lens compression. Rings 3 through 9 are broad and distorted due to compression by a tight-fitting lens. One hour after removing the lens, the corneal distortion is markedly improved, although irregularities in rings 6 through 9 persist (Fig. 10.4B). The information provided by the keratograph helps avoid this complication of fitting the normal cornea with a contact lens and is invaluable in fitting a cornea with irregular astigmatism due to keratoconus, or scarred or postsurgical corneas.

The Comparator takes the keratograph at a known magnification and compares it to theo-

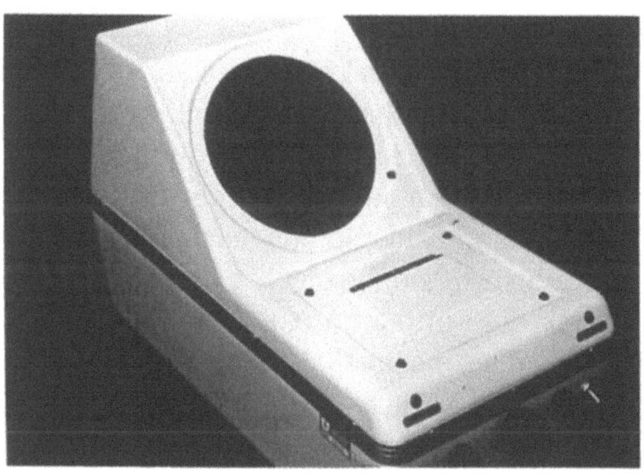

FIGURE 10.3. The Comparator.

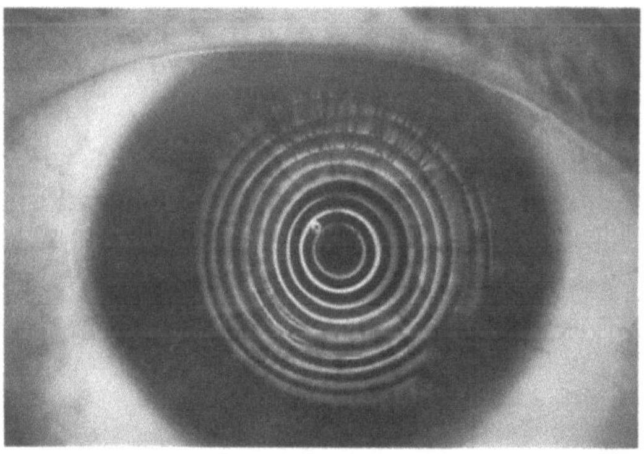

A

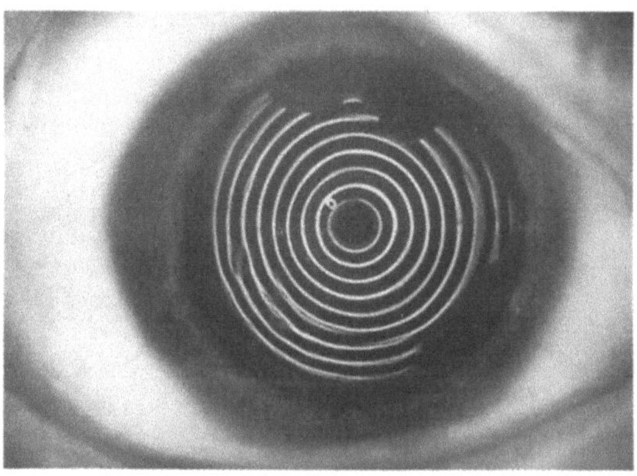

B

FIGURE 10.4. (A) Typical keratographic appearance of contact lens compression from a tight-fitting contact lens. (B) Same eye 1 hr after contact lens removal. Note marked improvement in corneal distortion.

retical spheres of known radii of curvature and chord length to approximate the radius at any of the nine rings.[8] Although it does not reveal the actual shape of the cornea, it does give us the curvature of the sphere that would pass through the apex and the point on the inside of a given ring (Fig. 10.5). The range of corneal radii that can be interpreted by the Comparator is 6.35 to 9.60 mm. The actual contour of the cornea in any given meridian is accurately represented only by an infinite number of spheres of differing radii of curvature.

The Comparator allows the contact lens fitter to choose that portion of the cornea he wishes to fit. It gives us the base curve and optical zone diameter necessary to provide peripheral support and adequate clearance in the vertical meridian for proper tear exchange. The Comparator simulates an infinite number of trial contact lenses, allowing the trial lens fitting to be performed before a lens is actually placed on the eye. The magnified image on the Comparator viewing screen shows the trial lens necessary to fit a given area of the cornea, and its points of bearing, points of clearance, and a simulated fluorescein staining pattern. Minor adjustments in the base curve of the lens can be made simply by changing the magnification of the keratograph on the screen, thus eliminating the need for placement of numerous trial lenses on the patient.

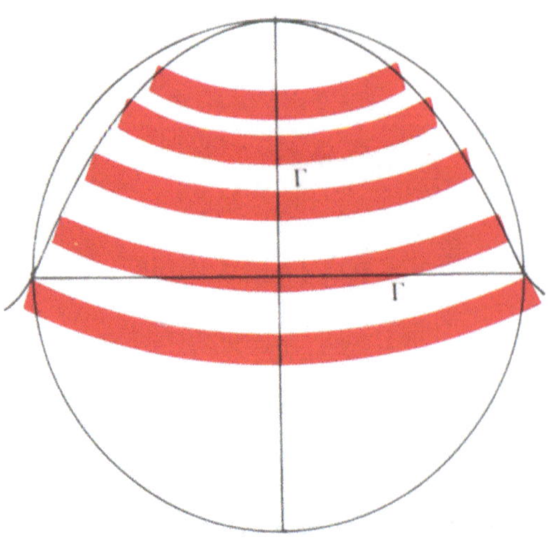

FIGURE 10.5. Comparator uses sphere of known radius of curvature that will pass through apex at a designated point of the peripheral cornea.

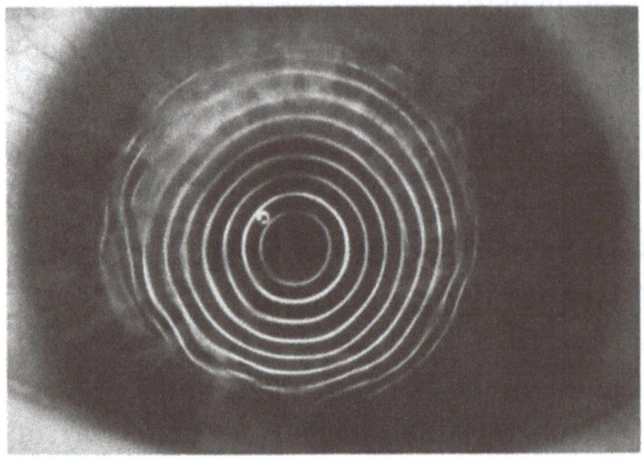

FIGURE 10.6. Keratograph of a corneal transplant showing all nine rings with the "C" in focus. (Courtesy of KERA Corporation, Inc. Santa Clara, California.)

The method of fitting contact lenses with the Corneascope and Comparator is essentially the same regardless of the corneal topography. The steps for fitting are as follows[9]:

1. A Polaroid keratograph of the cornea is taken (Fig. 10.6). All nine Placido rings must be completely visible with the focal point "C" in sharp focus. Precise focusing is important to determine an accurate base curve.
2. The keratograph (backed by the test card) is placed upside down or "C" down into the Comparator (Fig. 10.7).
3. Horizontal and vertical positioning knobs are used to center the green rings of the keratograph relative to the nine black rings on the screen.
4. The magnification knob is used to adjust the image size of the keratograph so that the inside edge of the chosen keratograph ring (ring 8 or 9, in most cases) corresponds to, or is slightly outside, the inside ring edge of the corresponding black Comparator ring (lens ring) in the horizontal meridian (Fig. 10.8). This means that the lens is parallel to K or slightly steeper than K in the horizontal periphery.
5. A minimum clearance of 0.05 mm in the vertical meridian must be provided. This

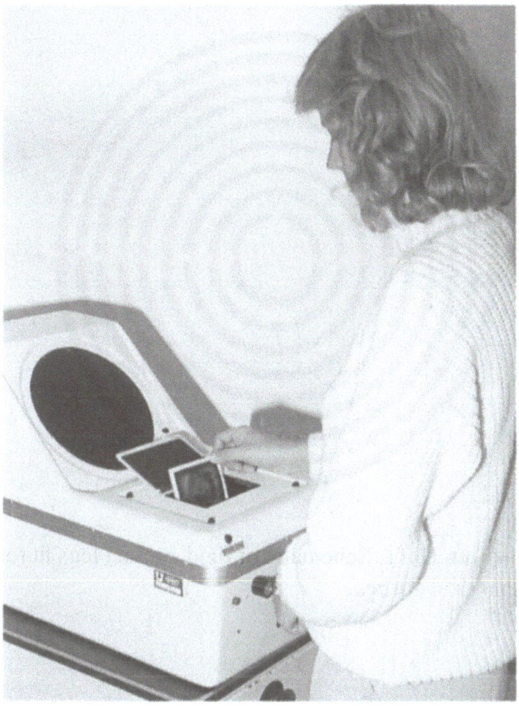

FIGURE 10.7. Backed by the test card, the keratograph is turned upside down (so that the "C" is down) and inserted into the Comparator.

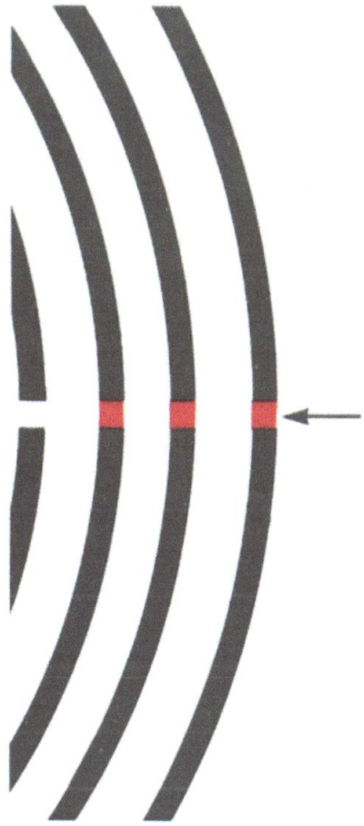

FIGURE 10.8. Schematic demonstrating how inside edge of corneal ring 9 corresponds to inside edge of lens ring 9 (black ring). (Courtesy of KERA Corporation, Inc., Santa Clara, California.)

qualification is met by making sure that the inside edge of the last corneal ring touches the black mark just inside the corresponding black lens ring in the vertical meridian. The approximate base curve of the lens will appear in the window when the base curve button is depressed.

6. The actual lens with appropriate optical zone is placed on the eye and the fluorescein pattern evaluated.

These steps are easy to master with some practice and familiarity with the instruments. Specific clinical examples later in the chapter will illustrate their application.

Figure 10.9 schematically demonstrates a good lens fit. (Note: All illustrations of the Comparator faceplate are of the right eye. The nasal cornea is to the left and the temporal cornea to the right since the Comparator gives

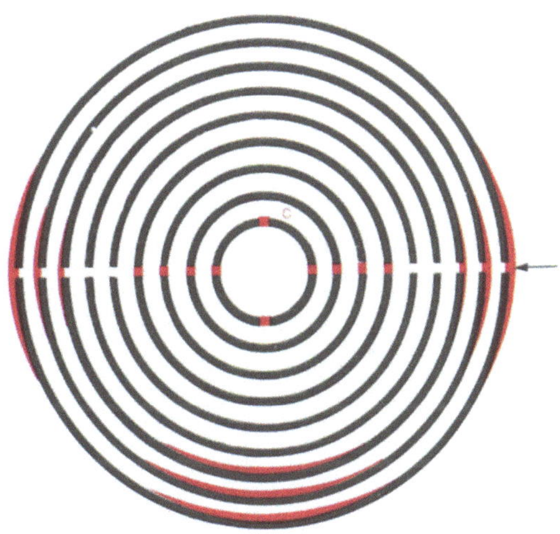

FIGURE 10.9. Schematic of good fit with a hard contact lens. (Courtesy of KERA Corporation, Inc., Santa Clara, California.)

a mirror image of the keratograph.) The corneal rings of the keratograph appear in green on the Comparator faceplate to simulate a fluorescein pattern. They are represented by orange in these illustrations. The corneal rings correspond to the black lens rings superiorly, paralleling the corneal curvature at this point. Inferiorly, the inside of corneal ring 9 touches the black gauge mark indicating that the lens is slightly flatter than the cornea and giving a clearance of 0.05 mm. This clearance is critical for pumping tears beneath the lens with each blink. Lens clearance may be provided superiorly instead of inferiorly in each case. In the horizontal meridian, the black lens rings are slightly steeper than the corneal rings 7, 8, and 9. This provides support and a fulcrum for the necessary vertical rocking motion of the contact.

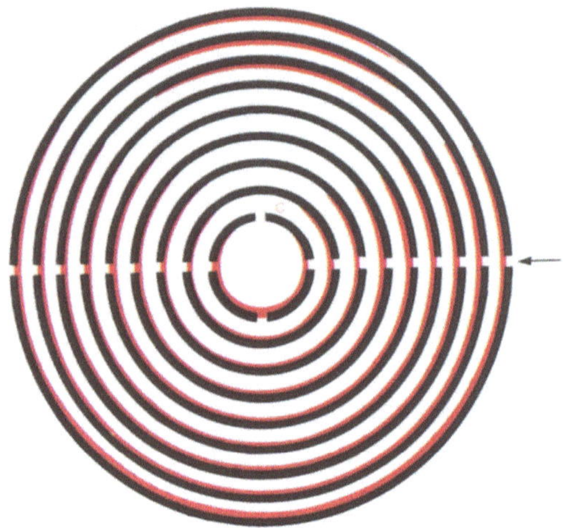

FIGURE 10.11. Schematic of rigid contact lens fit for spherical cornea.

Fitting the "Spherical" Cornea

Occasionally a cornea will be spherical or nearly spherical over the the 40 to 45% of the area encompassed by the nine corneal rings (Fig. 10.10). This is often the case in large-diameter corneas with a more gradual aspheric pattern. The same fitting techniques apply. Again, vertical clearance of 0.05 mm between the optical zone and the cornea must be provided for adequate tear exchange. Figure 10.11 shows that, in order to provide adequate clearance, a contact must be fit slightly flatter than K. All nine corneal rings lie inside the lens rings. Thus, in this case, the lens will bear on the corneal apex rather than at the 3 and 9 o'clock positions.

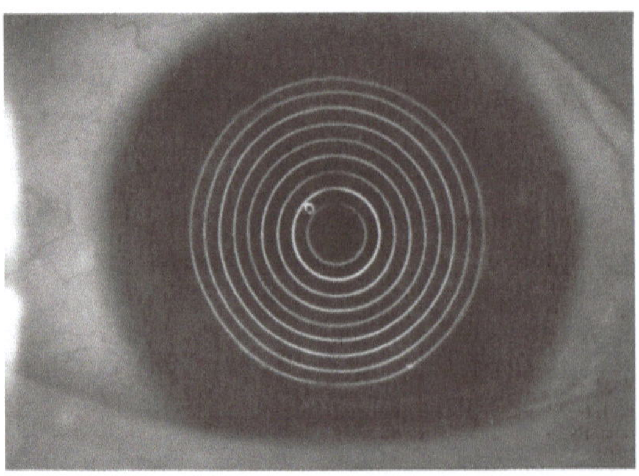

FIGURE 10.10. Cornea with spherical contour within area encompassed by corneal rings. (Courtesy of KERA Corporation, Inc., Santa Clara, California.)

Fitting "With-the-Rule" Astigmatism

With-the-rule astigmatism is the most common form of astigmatism. Fortunately, it is also the most amenable to a good contact lens fit. For our purposes, with-the-rule astigmatism is defined as the condition in which the axis of plus cylinder is within 10° on either side of 90°. Figure 10.12 shows a keratograph of with-the-rule astigmatism where the chord length is shorter (smaller radius of curvature) in the vertical meridian than in the horizontal meridian. This corneal topography is ideal for peripheral bearing in the horizontal meridian with clearance in the vertical meridian (Fig. 10.13). Usually, with-the-rule astigmatism of 3 D or less can be satisfactorily fit with a single curve lens. In many cases, clearance will be greater than 0.05 mm. Higher degrees of astigmatism may require a toric lens to avoid excessive lens movement and rocking.

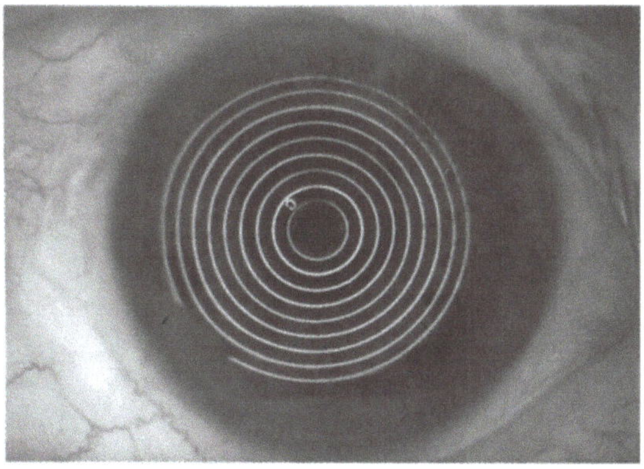

FIGURE 10.12. Keratograph of with-thc-rulc astigmatism. Note steep meridian (short chord) at 90°.

blink and settles temporal to center. The off-center position requires using a larger diameter lens to avoid distortion and blurring created by the blend and peripheral curve. Using the Corneascope and Comparator method of fitting, however, makes the comfortable fitting of a large-diameter lens possible since the optical zone of the larger lens corresponds to the chord length or curvature of the cornea encompassed by the optical zone rather than to the central 3 mm measured by the keratometer.

Fitting "Against-the-Rule" Astigmatism

Regardless of the method chosen to fit rigid contact lenses, comfortably fitting a cornea with against-the-rule astigmatism can be a problem. In this condition, the axis of the plus cylinder is within 10° of the 180° meridian. Figure 10.14 shows the corneal topography of against the rule astigmatism. Hcrc, thc chord length is shorter in the horizontal meridian (steeper base curve) than in the vertical meridian. If the lens is fit to bear at the 3 and 9 o'clock positions, it will be too steep in the vertical meridian (as illustrated in Fig. 10.15), and there is no clearance at the 6 or 12 o'clock positions for tear exchange. The third corneal and lens rings are superimposed indicating that the base curve of the lens is parallel to K if one were to use keratometer readings. In this case, however, the lens must be fit flatter than K to provide adequate clearance in the vertical meridian. The resulting lens will have a flatter base curve relative to the horizontal than to the vertical meridian with bearing on the apex (Fig. 10.16).

Because a lens will tend to position away from the area of steepest lens–cornea relationship, in this case at the 6 and 12 o'clock positions, these lenses invariably position off-center. Since the cornea usually flattens more rapidly nasal to the visual axis due to the positive angle K, it rocks on the apex with each

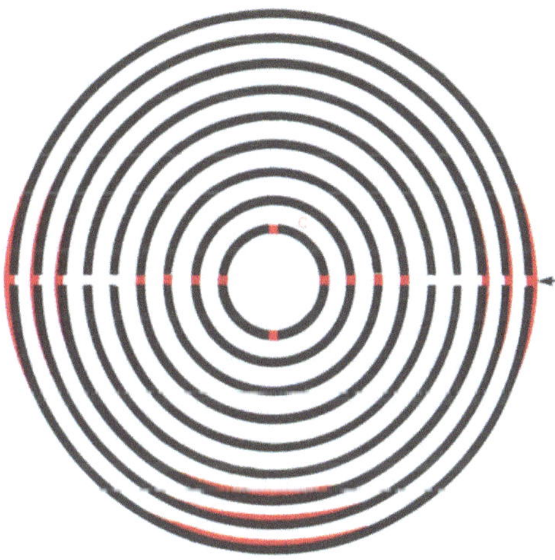

FIGURE 10.13. Schematic of rigid contact lens fit for with-the-rule astigmatism.

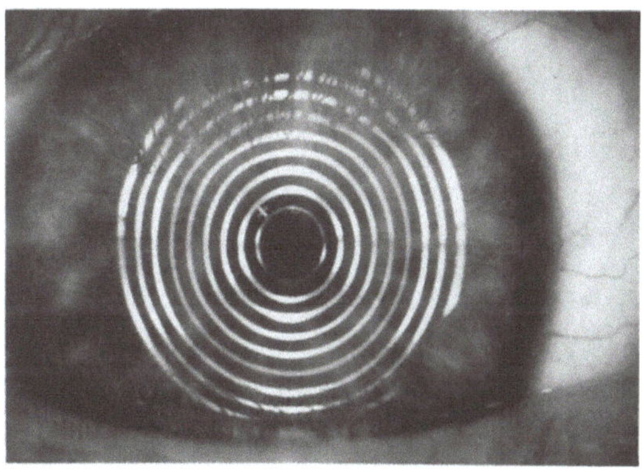

FIGURE 10.14. Keratograph of against-the-rule astigmatism. Note steep meridian (short chord) at 180°.

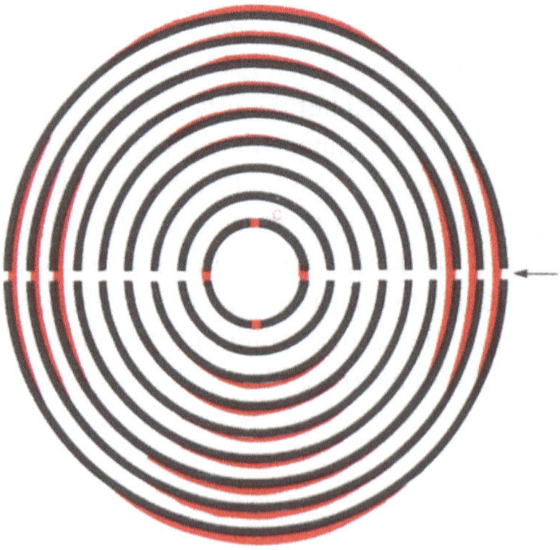

FIGURE 10.15. Schematic of steep rigid contact lens fit in against-the-rule astigmatism.

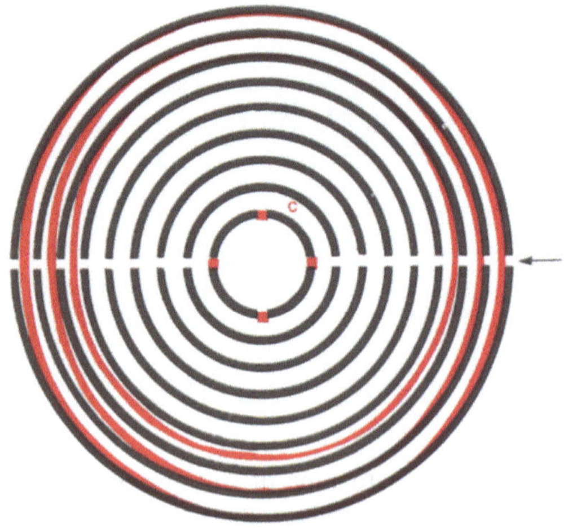

FIGURE 10.16. Schematic of good rigid contact lens fit in against-the-rule astigmatism.

Fitting Keratoconus

Fitting the cornea with regular astimatism can sometimes be difficult. However, fitting a cornea with irregular astigmatism without knowledge of the corneal topography can be virtually a mystical experience. The fitting process is problematic because of the corneal distortion. The evolution of the topographic changes of keratoconus begins with subtle steepening of the inferior temporal midperipheral cornea (Fig. 10.17). The central rings are typically pear-shaped pointing toward the area of steepening. Early in the disease process, the peripheral rings are relatively undistorted. As the condition worsens, the steep area extends circumferentially from the inferior temporal quadrant with flattening of the cornea 180° away in later stages. A completely coned cornea is steep in all quadrants (Fig. 10.18).

Keratometry gives us limited information to accurately fit a hard lens in this situation. The keratometry reading for the vertical meridian is an average between a point on the relatively

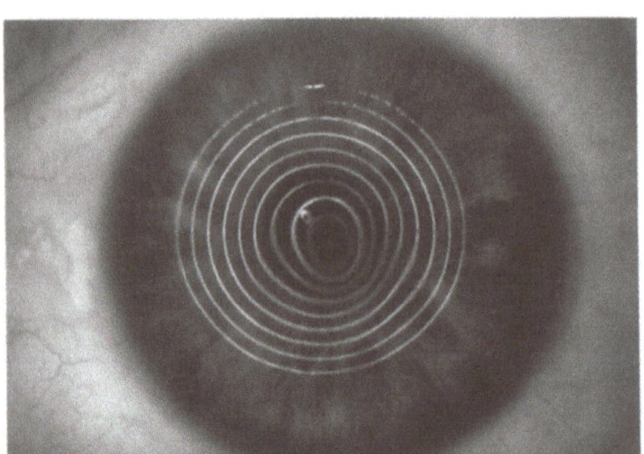

FIGURE 10.17. Keratograph of early keratoconus in a left eye with steepening of the inferior temporal midperipheral cornea.

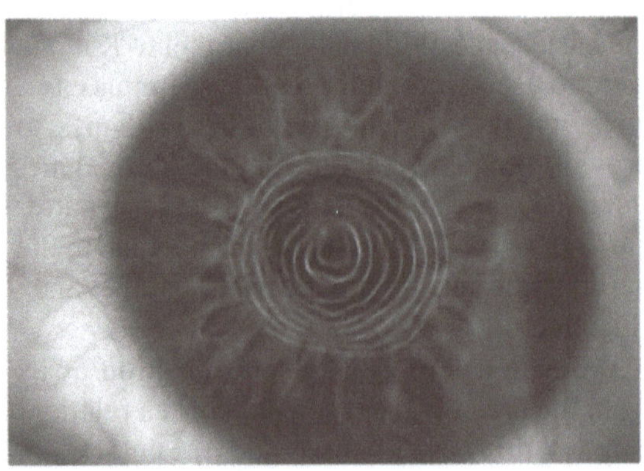

FIGURE 10.18. Advanced keratoconus; entire central cornea is steep. Ring irregularities are due to contact lens compression.

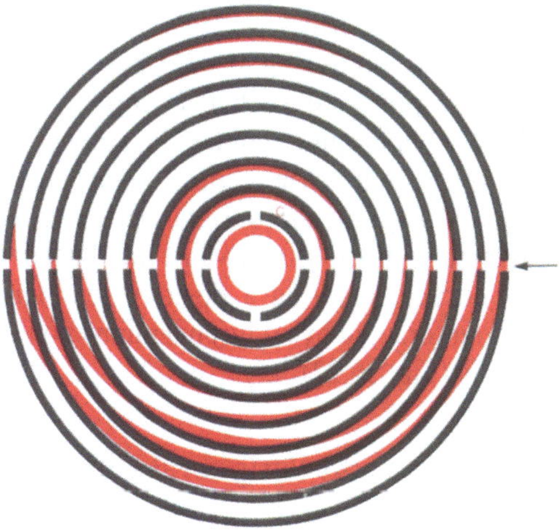

FIGURE 10.19. Schematic of rigid contact lens fit for keratoconus.

unaffected superior cornea and a point on the steepened inferior cornea. The average of these two would indicate that the entire vertical meridian is steep. The trial lens chosen would, therefore, be too steep superiorly and position low with poor movement and poor tear exchange.

The Corneascope and Comparator method of fitting keratoconus is identical to fitting other forms of astigmatism. As stated earlier, the inferior cornea is steeper than the superior cornea. The lens is fit to the superior portion of the ring chosen, ring 9 in this case, and bears on the superior cornea, the apex, and the horizontial periphery. The resulting inferior clearance (Fig. 10.19) facilitates good tear exchange with each blink. Trauma to the apical epithelium, in the author's and another's experience using this fitting method (verbal communication with A.E. Reynolds, O.D., December 1984) is minimized because adequate oxygenation allows for more normal cellular respiration. The lenses should be kept well-polished to avoid unnecessary corneal epithelial trauma.

Fitting the Postsurgical Cornea

Cataract surgery, with modern microsurgical techniques, most often results in minimal astigmatism. Any residual astigmatism usually has an axis of plus cylinder within 20° of the vertical meridian, making contact lens fitting easy. Occasionally, however, wound gape can result in signifcant against-the-rule astigmatism. The principles described previously for fitting against-the-rule astigmatism with a spherical lens should be applied. A toric lens can be attempted for higher degrees of astigmatism. If a satisfactory fit cannot be achieved, surgical correction of the astigmatism may be required.

Surgical manipulation of the cornea usually results in varying degrees of irregular astigmatism. Among corneal transplant patients, residual astigmatism remains the greatest problem in visual rehabilitation. Many approaches to fitting the postkeratoplasty cornea have been described, most concentrating on the use of a rigid lens often larger than the diameter of the graft.[11–15] Because the corneal contour is so vastly different between the graft center and the donor recipient interface (Fig. 10.20), it is necessary to understand the peripheral topography and to fit the flatter surface corresponding to the wound. To illustrate, the keratometry readings corresponding to the third ring of the keratograph in Figure 10.20 are 44.12 by 45.00 D with the steep axis at

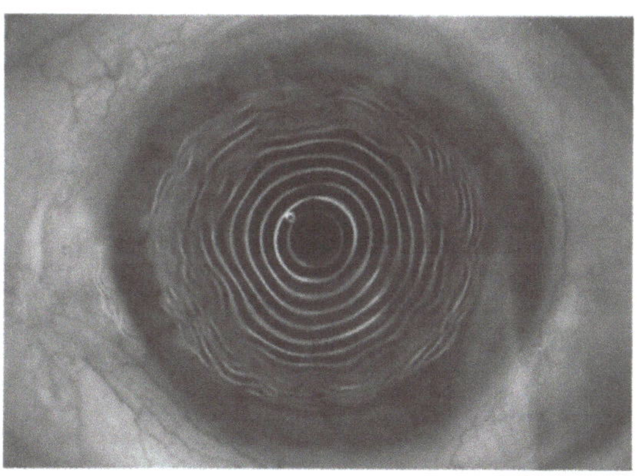

FIGURE 10.20. Keratograph of corneal transplant with sutures in place.

104. Using the keratograph and Comparator method of contact lens fitting to the eighth ring, the recommended base curve is 772 or 43.75 D with an optical zone of 7.7 mm. This contact lens is 0.37 D flatter than a lens fit to the flattest K reading. This feature, combined with the larger total diameter of 8.7 mm allows for free movement over the flatter topography of the wound.

A new lens fitting problem has been seen in those patients with significant residual refractive errors following radial keratotomy surgery. The difficulty in matching the contour of the contact lens to the postradial keratotomy cornea is that there is an exaggerated and opposite relationship between the central and the midperipheral corneal contour. The central cornea is now flatter, and the change in topography from center to periphery is quite abrupt at the midperipheral knee. Conventional fitting techniques based on keratometer readings would end in a very flat fit. Soft contact lenses have been unsatisfactory, resulting in neovascularization of the scars in up to 60% of patients.[16] Rigid lenses are therefore preferable in many cases to avoid this complication and to correct any irregular astigmatism that may be present. Knowledge of the peripheral corneal topography using the keratograph suggests that a steeper fit would be desirable. Figure 10.21 is a keratograph of a cornea after an eight incision radial keratotomy. It graphically demonstrates the exaggerated central flattening produced by the incisions. Keratometry readings are a spherical 37.50 D. Comparator readings at the ninth ring are 795 base curve, which corresponds to a 42.50 D cornea. The peripheral topography requires a steeper fit than is suggested by the central keratometry readings. Using an appropriate optical zone and diameter, this lens will vault the flattened central cornea, creating a positive tear lens that is counteracted by additional minus power in the lens (Fig. 10.22).

Optical Zone and Peripheral Curves

The Corneascope and Comparator derive the base curve by measuring the chord length of the corneal area that the examiner has chosen to fit. Ring 9 is chosen in the majority of cases, unless the topography is unfavorable for an optimal fit. An arrow on the Comparator screen points to Ring 9 indicating that this is the "optical zone ring." When this ring is used for fit, the optical zone equals the base curve (Fig. 10.8). This value is given as a digital display when the optical zone button on the Comparator is pushed. In spherical corneas or

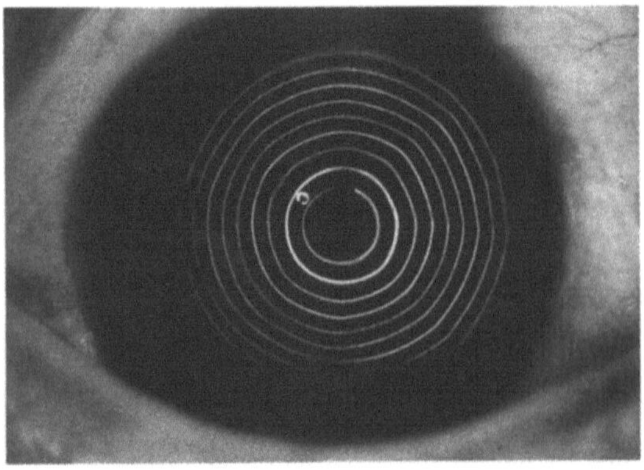

FIGURE 10.21. Keratograph of cornea after radial keratotomy.

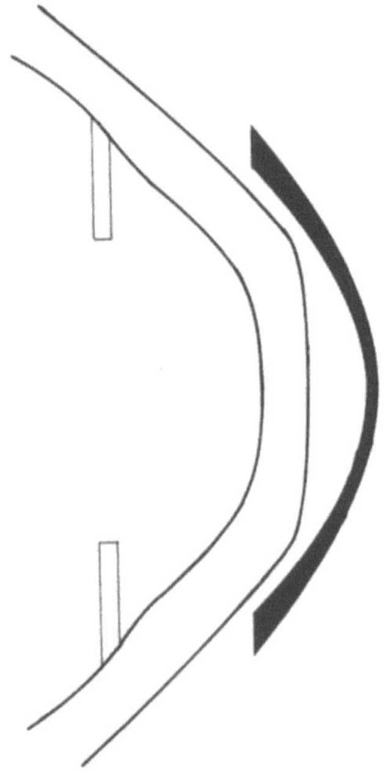

FIGURE 10.22. Contact lens relationship to cornea after radial keratotomy.

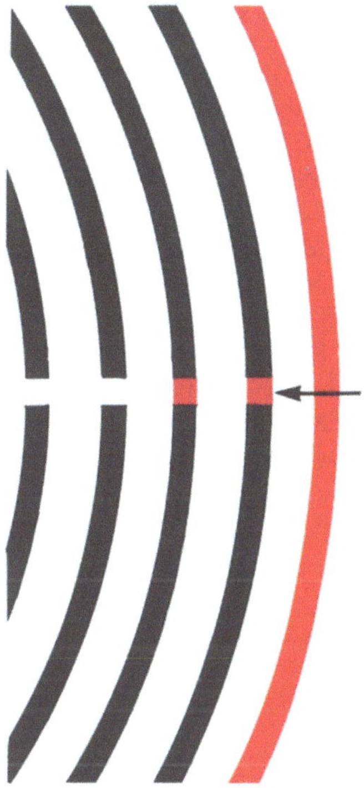

FIGURE 10.23. Correct relationship between optical zone marker and ring 8 to determine the optical zone of the lens. (Courtesy of KERA Corporation, Inc., Santa Barbara, California.)

those with low degree with-the-rule astigmatism, ring 9 in the horizontal meridian is used since this is the flattest corneal meridian that determines the lens fit. In against-the-rule astigmatism or in fitting toric lenses, the corneal ring selected is moved to correspond to the gauge mark inferiorly (since the vertical meridian is now flattest).

When a corneal ring other than ring 9 is used for fit, the base curve is determined in the usual way. For example, if ring 8 is chosen, it is properly aligned with lens ring 8 and the base curve is computed. To determine the optical zone, corneal ring 8 is then enlarged or magnified to correspond to the optical zone ring (Fig. 10.23).

The total lens diameter is usually 1 mm larger than the optical zone allowing for the blend and a peripheral curve 0.4 mm wide. The peripheral curve should be, in most cases, 0.6 mm flatter than the base curve. This allows for upper lid support of the lens and for smooth transit across the peripheral cornea with each blink.

Fitting Procedures for Toric Base Curve Lenses

Using these principles of fitting rigid lenses using the keratograph and Comparator fitting back toric lenses for higher degrees of corneal astigmatism is usually simple. As a rule, if there is more than 2 to 3 D of central corneal astigmatism, a toric fit will prevent excessive rocking. Another way to determine whether a toric lens is indicated is to look at the base curve necessary to provide slight bearing in the horizontal periphery and the curve necessary to provide clearance vertically. If this difference is greater than 0.3 mm, a toric lens should be considered. The two base curves derived above are used to specify the two curves of the lens. The lens power is then determined from the flattest meridian or base curve using calculations or overrefraction. The optical zone corresponds to the steepest base curve and can be derived as described in the section titled Optical Zone and Peripheral Curves.

References

1. Kinoshita JH. Some aspects of the carbohydrate metabolism of the cornea. *Invest Ophthalmol.* 1962;1:178–186.
2. Langham ME. The interrelationship of metabolism and deturgescence of the living cornea. *Invest Ophthalmol.* 1962;1:187–194.
3. de Roetth A Jr. Respiration of the cornea. *Arch Ophthalmol.* 1950;44:666–676.
4. Polse KA, Mandell RB. Critical oxygen tension at the corneal surface. *Arch Ophthalmol.* 1970;84:505–508.
5. Hill RM, Fatt I. How dependent is the cornea on the atmosphere? *J Am Optom Assoc.* 1964;35:873–875.
6. Aukert H: Nahert sich die Hornhautkrummung am meister des Ellipse. *Pfluegers Arch.* 1885;35:597–621.
7. The principle of lens comfort. In: *Instruction Manual for Corneascope and Comparator.* 3rd ed. International Diagnostic Instruments, Ltd, 1980;p VA-1.

8. Rowsey JJ, Isaac M. Corneascopy in keratorefractive surgery. Cornea. 1983;2:133–142.
9. Fitting procedures—Comparator operating instructions. In: *Instruction Manual for Corneoscope and Comparator*. 3rd ed. International Diagnostic Instruments, Ltd, 1980;p. VA-1.
10. Rowsey JJ, Reynolds AE, Brown R. Corneal topography—Corneascope. *Arch Ophthalmol*. 1981;99:1093–1100.
11. Daniel R. Fitting contact lenses after keratoplasty. *Br J Opthalmol*. 1976;60:263–265.
12. Ruben M, Colegrook E. Keratoconus keratoplasty curvatures and contact lens wear. *Br J Ophthalmol*. 1979;63:268–275.
13. Soper JW. Fitting corneal transplants with corneal contact lenses. *International Contact Lens Clinics*. 1976;3:31–35.
14. Casey TA, Mayer RJ. Contact lenses and keratoplasty. In: *Corneal Grafting—Principles and Practice*. Philadelphia: WB Saunders Co, 1984;pp 281–288.
15. Mannis MJ, Zadnik K, Deutch D. Rigid contact lens wear in the corneal transplant patient. *CLAO J*. 1986;12:39–42.
16. Shivitz IA, Russell BM, Arrowshmit PN, et al. Optical correction of postoperative radial keratotomy patients with contact lenses. *CLAO J*. 1986;12:59–62.

11 Corneal Topography in Management of PK Astigmatism*

Richard F. Beatty and David J. Schanzlin

History of Management of Postpenetrating Keratoplasty Astigmatism

In 1869, Snellen[1] suggested that a steep corneal meridian may be flattened by an anterior corneal incision. Bates,[2] in 1894, correctly described the corneal topography results after circumferential corneal relaxing incisions: an increase in radius of curvature of the corneal meridian perpendicular to the circumferential incision. He observed that the closer the incision is to the center of the cornea, the greater the correction of astigmatism. He also noted that the length and depth of the incision influence the change in radius of curvature of the corneal meridian. In 1898, Lans[3] published his results on a series of experiments attempting to reduce astigmatism in rabbit corneas and described a "double-wedge resection" in the cornea. (Fig. 11.1). This procedure caused corneal flattening at the meridian perpendicular to the line of corneal resection. Since the wedge resections were not sutured, he effectively produced peripheral corneal relaxing incisions. However, he failed to realize the relaxing effect of the incisions on corneal topography and thought the corneal flattening was due to wound healing and scar formation (Fig. 11.2). In the 1950s posterior corneal-relaxing incisions were described by Sato in Japan.[4, 5] In his method, a corneal knife was inserted through the limbus and a tangential posterior corneal incision was made through endothelium, Descemet's membrane, and partially through the corneal stroma, through the meridian of steepest corneal power (Fig. 11.3). In 15 eyes undergoing this incision, an average of 2.5 diopters (D) of corneal astigmatism remained in the steep meridian.[5] Subsequently, corneal endothelial decompensation was identified as a universal complication of this procedure.[6]

Troutman,[7] in 1977, described his technique for relaxing incision using a razor-blade knife to dissect into the depth of the corneal wound or adjacent to it, incising half the cornea depth. Incisions were made at both ends of the steep corneal meridian and were 1 clock hour in length—15° on each side of the steepest corneal meridian (Fig. 11.4). He estimated an attainable correction of 3 to 5 D and suggested its use for lower amounts of astigmatism (4 to 5 D). A variation of Troutman's technique was described by Wiedman[8] in which he made relaxing incisions between the limbus and the transplant wound.

Poyales[9] reported a reduction of 4.0 to 5.0 D in astigmatism by using a technique of double concentric corneal trephination and resection of the corneal tissue between the incisions. The cornea was resutured between the trephined circles. Barraquer and Muinos[10] described a scleral resection technique posterior to the corneal limbus and perpendicular to the

* The material in this chapter appeared in substantially modified from as Chapter 9 in Ivan R Schwab, ed, Refractive Keratoplasty, New York:Churchill Livingstone, 1987.

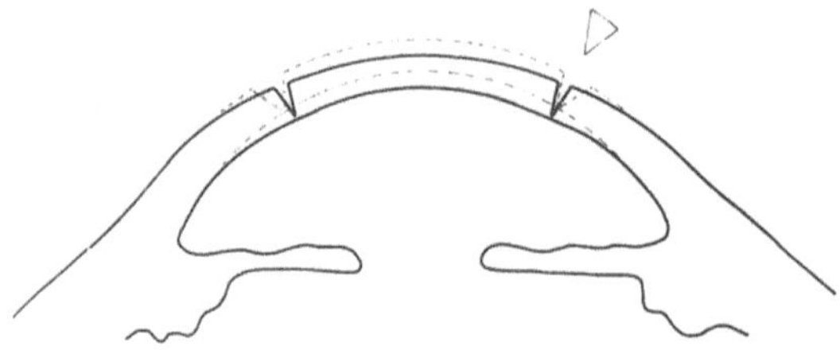

FIGURE 11.1. Double-wedge resection (Lans, 1898).[31]

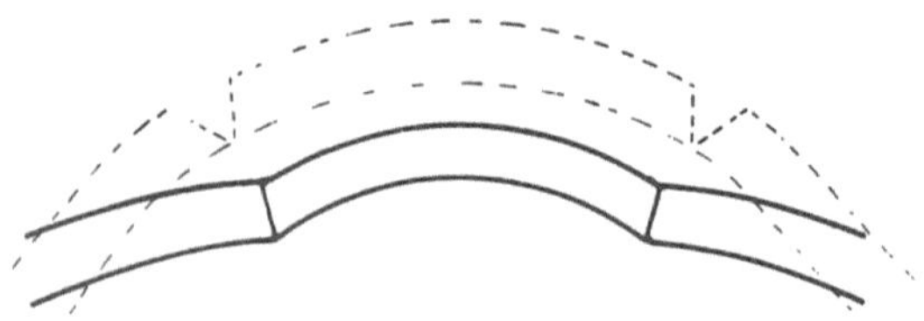

FIGURE 11.2. Cornea flattening after "double wedge resection" proposed to be due to wound healing and scar formation (Lans, 1898).[31]

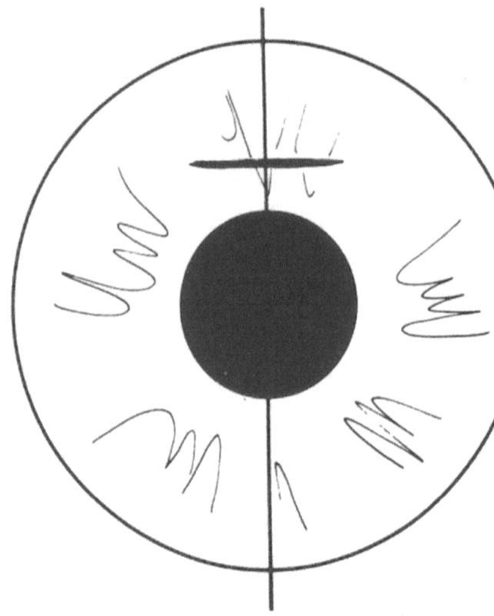

FIGURE 11.3. Posterior half-incision of the cornea perpendicular to the steepest corneal meridian (Sato, 1953).[31]

flattest central corneal meridian (Fig. 11.5). A reduction of astigmatism by 3 to 4 D was accomplished using this lamellar scleral resection. In 1970 Troutman[11] presented a successful treatment of postkeratoplasty astigmatism using corneal wedge resection. He described the excision of a crescentic wedge of tissue at the graft–host interface for a total of 90° circumference. A width of tissue approximately 1.5 mm was excised perpendicular to the flattest central corneal meridian (Fig. 11.6). Suturing of the defect caused steepening of the flattest meridian. An average of 10.3 D of astigmatic correction was obtained (range 6.5 to 15.0 D) using this technique in five eyes.

Refractive Keratoplasty Methods for Penetrating Keratoplasty Astigmatism

Relaxing Incisions

Since Troutman's initial description of corneal relaxing incisions in 1977, others have described similar results for astigmatism after penetrating keratoplasty.[7, 12–17] Troutman and Swinger[12] reported on 4 patients who underwent corneal incision for residual astigmatism following keratoplasty. They used a razor blade set in a blade holder and made a circumferential relaxing incision 60° to 80° in arc

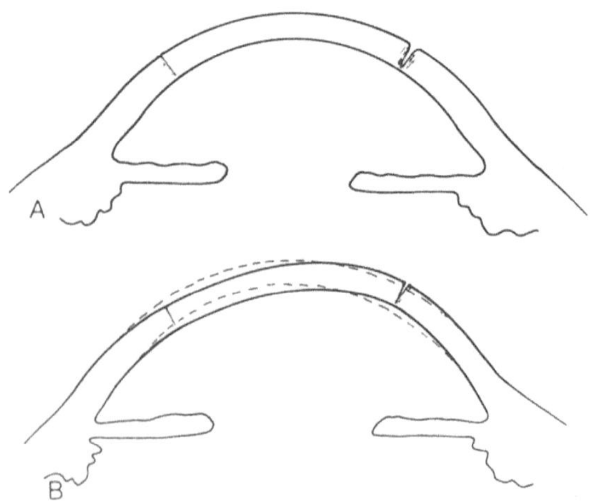

FIGURE 11.4. Troutman relaxing incision. (A) Incision in graft–host interface centered on the steepest central corneal meridian. (B) Effect of single relaxing incision on corneal topography: central corneal flattening with peripheral corneal steepening or bowing.[31]

length, centered on either side of the steepest corneal meridian. The tissue was incised to one-third stromal depth under topical anesthesia at the slit lamp using keratometric observation. They made a second incision at the opposite pole of the steepest meridian if the desired effect was not obtained after the first incision. The patients' eyes were patched for several days postoperatively and treated with topical steroids and antibiotics. One eye was incised so deeply that several 10-0 nylon interrupted sutures were required to prevent a wound dehiscence. Troutman and Swinger observed that the relaxing circumferential incisions caused *flattening* of the steepest corneal meridian perpendicular to the incision and *steepening* of the flatter meridian 90° away. The observed ratio of flattening to steepening was 2:1. An average net change in cylindrical refraction of 8.73 D was observed in their four cases (range 5 to 10.25 D). The vector-corrected astigmatic change averaged 9.35 D (range 5.04 to 15.92 D). No complications were observed in a follow-up period of 4 months.

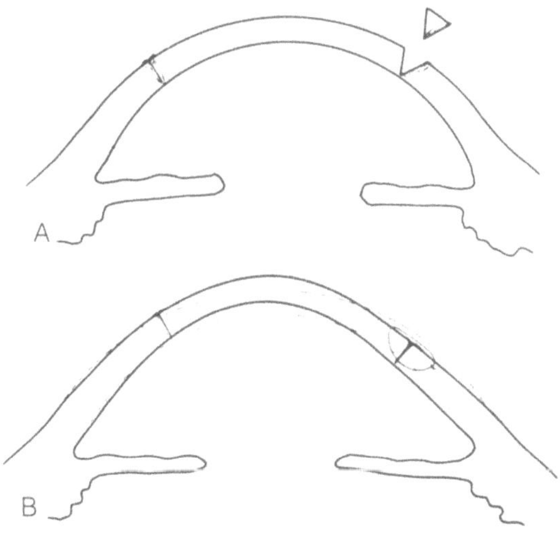

FIGURE 11.6. Troutman wedge resection. (A) Wedge resection at graft–host interface centered on flattest central corneal meridian. (B) Effect of wedge resection on corneal topography: central corneal steepening with peripheral corneal flattening over the sutured wedge resection.[31]

Twenty-six cases of high postkeratoplasty astigmatism were treated with relaxing incisions or wedge resection by Krachmer and Fenzel.[13] They performed relaxing incisions on 16 eyes and wedge resection on 10 eyes. Relaxing incisions were performed as an outpatient procedure at the slit lamp under topical anesthesia. Two incisions 180° apart were made in the keratoplasty wound for a length of 2 clock hours each, bisected by the axis of the steepest meridian. Each incision was one-half to two-thirds deep in the keratoplasty wound using a razor-blade knife. Postoperatively, antibiotic drops were used until the wound reepithelialized, in addition to topical steroid drops 3 to 4 times a day for one week and then tapered. A final refraction was reported in most patients approximately 1 month after surgery. Contact lens fitting was delayed for 2 to 3 months after surgery. Complications included anterior chamber perforation in 2 of the 16 eyes, requiring interrupted 10-O nylon sutures. These two cases subsequently required wedge resections to treat the corneal astigmatism. Average preoperative corneal astigmatism in the relaxing incision group was 10.00 D (range 7.00 to 14.25 D), while postoperative corneal astigmatism averaged 5.75 D (range 1.50 to 11.37 D). The average reduction of corneal astigmatism was 4.25 D for the relaxing incision group. These authors observed a ratio of flattening to steepening of approximately 1:1. The mean postoperative change in spherical

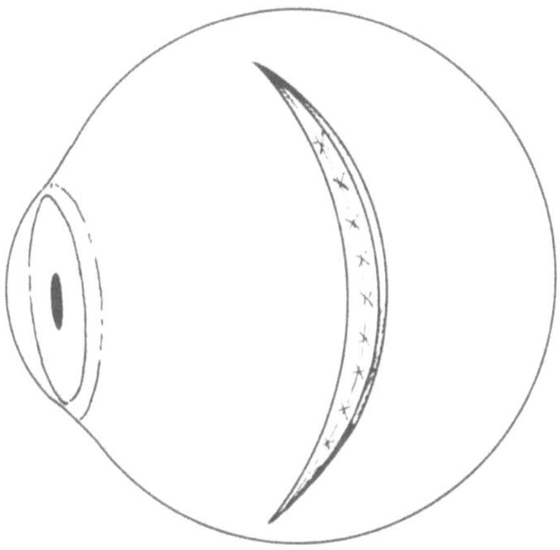

FIGURE 11.5. Scleral resection and resuturing along equator of globe to reduce corneal astigmatism (Barraquer and Muinos, 1956).[31]

equivalent was −0.05 D in the relaxing incision group (range −6.00 to +4.25 D).

Sugar and Kirk[14] reported on 17 patients who underwent relaxing corneal incision surgery for high postkeratoplasty astigmatism. Preoperative keratometric astigmatism varied from 8.05 to 18 D. Surgery was accomplished at the slit lamp under topical anesthesia using a razor-blade fragment. An incision approximately two-thirds corneal depth was made at the graft–host interface. Two incisions 180° apart were made corresponding to the steepest corneal meridian, each spanning 3 clock-hours and bisected by the axis of the steepest corneal meridian. Four patients underwent repeat incisions within 2 weeks of the initial keratotomies because of inadequate depth of the initial incisions. The mean reduction in corneal astigmatism was 7.5 D, with mean postoperative astigmatism by keratometry of 4.95 D. The authors observed corneal steepening in 13 of 15 patients, while the other 2 patients had an overall flattening of the cornea. Krachmer and Ching[15] reviewed a series of 16 radial kertotomy patients and also reported on an additional 48 patients who underwent relaxing incisions. They observed greater astigmatism reduction if the procedure is performed 1 month after all sutures are removed rather than months to years after suture removal.

In 1983, Troutman[16] updated his procedure of corneal relaxing incisions to include the use of compression sutures to retard early healing. He discontinued relaxing incisions at the slit lamp and began using an operating microscope and surgical keratometer. He advocated the placement of two suture loops 90° away from the corneal relaxing incisions, and tightening them to achieve a 50% overcorrection of the preoperative corneal astigmatism. Initially, a slip knot was used in order to adjust the tension of the sutures under keratometric guidance. The compression sutures were removed 60 to 90 days postoperatively, depending on the degree of wound healing and the amount of overcorrection remaining. If sphericity was accomplished with the compression sutures in place, then the sutures were left indefinitely.

Lavery et al.[17] reported results of relaxing incisions on 17 patients with high postkeratoplasty astigmatism. Preoperative astigmatism ranged from 5.63 D to 19.50 D. Using a 3 clock-hour incision placed in the donor–recipient wound, they incised 70 to 90% of the corneal thickness. Flattening in the axis of the relaxing incision was observed in 13 of 17 patients and steepening of the corneal meridian 90° was also noted. Astigmatism was reduced an average of 4.84 D (range 1.75 to 10.50 D) in 12 of 17 patients. Three patients had an increase in astigmatism of 3.42 D (range 2.13 to 5.50 D), which represented an overcorrection. One patient retained the same amount of preoperative astigmatism with a 90° shift in axis. Four of 17 patients sustained a perforation; 3 were microperforations that did not require suturing.

Complications of Corneal Relaxing Incisions

Because the quantitative results of corneal relaxing incisions cannot be predicted, a certain amount of overcorrection and undercorrection is expected. Undercorrection may require a repeat incision or different surgical procedure such as a wedge resection. An overcorrection after relaxing incision may require sutures to repair. Perforations are commonly encountered, particularly when dissecting in the graft–host interface. We have seen that the corneal thickness is difficult to determine preoperatively by wound inspection at the biomicroscope or by pachymetry. Posterior wound gapes are difficult to visualize directly or indirectly by these techniques. As a consequence of dissecting the graft–host interface, a temporary weakening of the graft–host junction occurs until further healing has occurred. However, the healing process may result in a wound that is partial thickness compared to the preoperative wound. In addition, the factor of delayed wound healing must be considered. Histology of radial keratotomy incisions shows complete healing by 5 years. If the cornea is subjected to trauma, this weakened graft–host interface may allow the cornea to rupture at the keratoplasty wound. This may occur with blunt ocular trauma or even eye rubbing. Because of the thinning at the graft–host interface after relaxing incision, a progressive elevation of the donor edge may occur. Other corneal healing problems may complicate the surgery, such as delayed reepithelialization over the wound and corneal melt. An increased rate of corneal graft rejection may be expected with the surgical manipulation of any corneal transplant. For this reason increased topical corticosteroids may be necessary postoperatively for a short time following surgical intervention for astigmatism control.

Wedge Resection

The surgical effect of Troutman's[18] original procedure in 5 eyes was described above. In a subsequent report of 10 eyes, all grafts were clear before wedge resection, measuring astigmatism in excess of 9 D. An average of 11.4 diopters of postkeratoplasty astigmatism was measured prior to wedge resection. A 60° to 90° crescentic wedge of the keratoplasty scar tissue was excised with a greatest width of 1.5 mm centered on the flattest corneal meridian. Monofilament nylon suture (22 μ) was deeply placed to Descemet's membrane to reapproximate the graft edges. Six months after wedge resection and suture removal, astigmatism was less than 6 D with an average of 2.8 D of residual astigmatism. The average flat meridian steepened by +6.50 D combined with an average flattening of −3.00 D of the steep meridian. This represents a ratio of approximately 2:1 steepening to flattening associated with his wedge resections. Myopia was also reduced an average of 2.6 D in 5 of 10 eyes. Troutman[15] preferred corneal wedge resections in myopic corneas with average keratometric reading of greater than 45 D.

Casey et al.[19] reported their results in two patients after a wedge resection done similar to Troutman's technique above and reported astigmatism altered by 3 D.

Kratchmer and Fenzel[13] reported on their series of 10 cases of corneal wedge resection for high postkeratoplasty astigmatism. The average preoperative K reading was 39.37/50.75 D in eyes with an average of 11.50 D of preoperative astigmatism. This decreased postoperatively to 43.00/47.75 D, representing an average 6.75 D reduction in corneal astigmatism over a mean follow-up period of 16 months (range 4 to 43 months). They also noted a trend toward a more myopic spherical equivalent.

In one case involving postkeratoplasty astigmatism of 13 D, Sanders[20] performed a 1 mm wedge resection for 2½ clock-hours down to Descemet's membrane. With sutures still remaining, the postoperative astigmatic error was 2.5 D, providing the patient with uncorrected visual acuity of 20/40 and corrected visual acuity of 20/30.

Van Rij and Vijfvinkel[21] reported their results of wedge resection using razor blades and "V shape knives" to make the crescentic wedge resection. A total of 14 eyes with an average of 11.9 diopters of preoperative astigmatism underwent wedge resection resulting in an average postoperative astigmatism of 5.3 D, an average change of 6.6 D. Sutures remained in place until 3 months after surgery and then were selectively removed one by one depending on the degree of astigmatism control attained.

Lugo et al.[22] reported results of 10 corneal wedge resections with an average preoperative astigmatism of 0.05 D. An average postoperative astigmatism correction of 9.1 D was obtained with an average residual astigmatism of 3.95 D.

Lindstrom and Lavery[23] reviewed their technique of performing wedge resections but did not review specific cases. They preferred to perform wedge resection on eyes with greater than 10 to 15 D of astigmatism. They agreed that a slight increase in myopia or a decrease in hyperopia will occur in eyes undergoing wedge resection for keratoplasty astigmatism. They made a 90° circumferential section of the keratoplasty wound using a diamond micrometer radial keratotomy knife. The diamond knife blade was set at 100% of the thinnest ultrasonic pachymetry reading over or near the graft–host interface. The tissue wedge was excised using the diamond knife and freehand dissection. They resected tissue according to the expected result for an average of 2 D of astigmatism correction to be obtained for each 0.1 mm of tissue excised in the wedge section. They did not perform a paracentesis prior to wound suturing and did not experience difficulty with wound closure. They preferred proline sutures for wound closure because of the indefinite time that they are left in the cornea. Approximately five to seven deeply placed interrupted proline sutures were tightened until an overcorrection of one third to one half of the preoperative cylinder was achieved in the opposite meridian. All sutures were left in place a minimum of 8 weeks and then selectively removed from the steepest corneal meridian to titrate residual astigmatism. If a satisfactory result was achieved, the sutures remained in place indefinitely.

Belmont and Troutman[24] reported on the use of compression sutures for wedge resection and reviewed their technique and results in 13 phakic patients. An average of 10.6 D of astigmatism was present preoperatively, decreasing to 2.0 D at 4 to 6 months. Sutures were subsequently removed in 8 patients with a final mean corneal astigmatism of 2.8 D. Their general rule of tissue resection was 0.67 D of induced steepening in the meridian perpendicular to the resection for each 0.1 mi of corneal tissue resected, while in the meridian 90° away there was an average flattening 0.33 D per millimeter of corneal tissue resected—a 2:1 ratio of steepening to flattening. Under these guidelines, wider tissue resection than anticipated was required for corneal astigmatism less than 10 D. Wedge resections of less than 0.5 mim produced little effect. A smaller resection was required under these guidelines for corneal astigmatism greater than 10 D. The authors cautioned against a wedge resection greater than 1.5 mm in width.

Complications of Wedge Resection

Overcorrection and unpredictability of the surgical result may occur with different methods of quantitating the amount of tissue to be excised, variations between surgical techniques, and healing properties of individual corneas. Graft rejection is possible after surgical manipulation of the cornea by wedge resection at any time in the postoperative period. If the anterior chamber perforation occurs by deliberate paracentesis or accidental corneal perforation, vitreous may come forward in aphakic eyes or iris incarceration may occur in phakic or aphakic eyes. The possibility of endophthalmitis is always present in any corneal penetrating injury or surgical procedure.

Since most surgeons overcorrect 90° to the original axis of astigmatism, patients frequently have visual distortion for a prolonged period after surgery until sutures are removed. As much as 3 to 6 months of postoperative astigmatism and therefore decreased vision may result after wedge resection. Belmont and Troutman[24] have attempted to compensate for this immediate postoperative astigmatism with compression sutures. These are placed across the graft–host junction approximately 60° from each end of the closed wedge-resection wound, creating central corneal steepening in the meridian of the compression sutures.

Wound Revision

Wound revision may be particularly useful in the early postoperative period where a wound uplift has occurred because of early suture removal or loosening. Under topical anesthesia the replacement of interrupted corneal sutures may reapproximate and flatten a graft–host uplift with consequent central corneal steepening along that meridian (Fig. 11.7). High residual astigmatism in the late postoperative period from wound uplift will not be expected to respond to wound revision simply by the replacement of interrupted corneal sutures. Apparent wound flattening by replacement of an interrupted corneal suture is only a temporary phenomenon. Once the suture is removed and tissue compression is released, the wound will tend to resort back to an uplifted configuration with central corneal flattening.

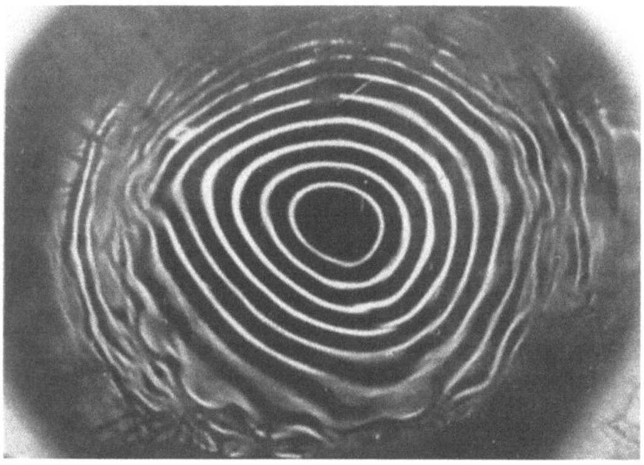

FIGURE 11.7. Corneascope photograph of wound dehiscence at 9:30 o'clock following premature loosening and removal of an interrupted suture from the keratoplasty wound. Keratometry 36.00 × 50.00 × 62 degrees. Replacement of the interrupted suture is indicated along the meridian of central and midperipheral flattening. Note teardrop configuration of mires pointing to wound dehiscence.[31]

Astigmatic Keratoplasty and the Ruiz Procedure

Clinical results with astigmatic keratotomy are quite poor when performed on corneal grafts. The refractive changes are unpredictable, and therefore the procedure is considered unreliable for postkeratoplasty astigmatism.

Thermal Cautery

Thermal cautery has been used in an attempt to resolve residual postkeratoplasty astigmatism by the application of deep nonperforating thermal scars in the meridian corresponding to the flattest corneal meridian.[3, 25–27] The effect of thermal cautery is considered unpredicatable and therefore potentially dangerous.

Repeat Penetrating Keratoplasty

Repeat penetrating keratoplasty has been used in an attempt to manage residual postoperative astigmatism. This appears to be a poor choice for the management of residual astigmatism after keratoplasty in the face of a clear corneal graft. The underlying causes of the residual astigmatism are not resolved by repeating the corneal transplantation. Corneal topography changes will be expected to remain unless compensation in the graft–host wound is made at the time of surgery.

Management of Postpenetrating Keratoplasty Astigmatism

Selective Suture Removal

Selective keratoplasty suture removal can be performed in the immediate or late postoperative period. The type of suture technique dictates the timing of corneal suture removal. With the use of interrupted 10-O nylon sutures, it is customary to wait 3 months before beginning selective suture removal. Sutures are removed prior to this time if they become unraveled or broken or are loose, as evidenced by fluorescein staining and mucous collection. Vascularization up to the corneal wound and progressing into the graft at the point of interrupted suture is also an indication for its removal to prevent further advance of new vessel ingrowth. Selected interrupted sutures are also removed earlier than 3 months for large amounts of astigmatism, although wound uplift and tissue dehiscence may occur. Keratometry and corneascopy are used to determine which suture should be removed. Using a double-running 10-O nylon and 11-O nylon technique, we first place 9-O nylon cardinal sutures followed by a running 10-O nylon suture. The 10-O nylon suture is left in place approximately 3 months before removal in cases of high residual astigmatism (Fig. 11.8). If at 3 months there is no significant corneal astigmatism, then the 10-O nylon suture is left intact. The 11-O nylon suture is left a minimum of 6 months and preferably at least 1 year before its removal. The 11-O nylon suture can compress the wound, and its removal may be necessitated in an attempt to relieve residual

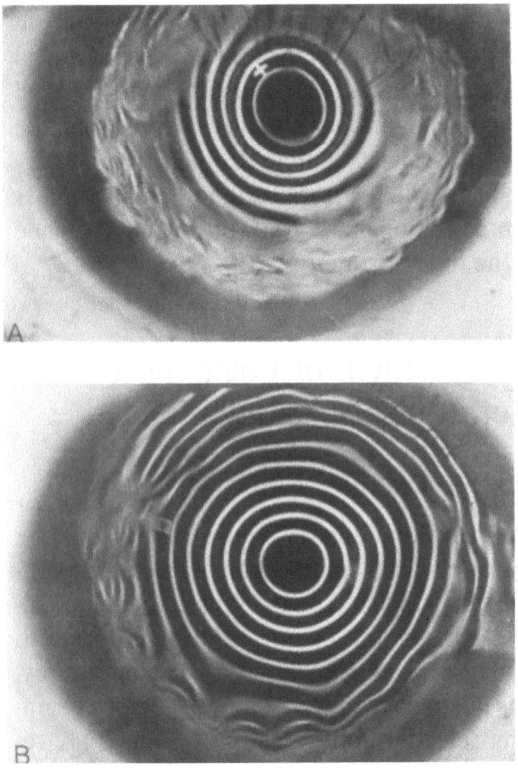

FIGURE 11.8. (A) Corneascope photograph 3½ months after penetrating keratoplasty and extracapsular cataract extraction with posterior chamber intraocular lens implant. Double-running 10-O and 11-O nylon sutures are in place with marked flattening of the corneal graft. Keratometry 38.00 × 39.00 × 20 degrees. V.A. 20/30-1. Removal of the running 10-O nylon suture is indicated to relieve keratoplasty wound compression and allow steepening of the corneal graft. (B) Corneascope photograph 2 months after removal of the running 10-O nylon suture. Keratometry 42.00 × 47.00 × 90 degrees. Refraction −1.50 +3.50 × 90°. V.A. 20/40.[31]

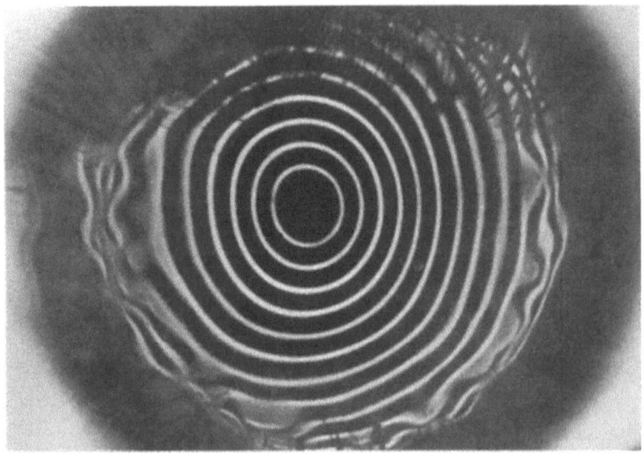

FIGURE 11.9. Corneascope photograph 1 year after penetrating keratoplasty. A running 11-O nylon suture remains in place. Keratometry 46.75 × 52.50 × 180 degrees. Removal of the running 11-O nylon suture is indicated in an attempt to reduce against-the-rule astigmatism.[31]

astigmatism (Figs. 11.9 and 11.10). It should be noted that astigmatism may worsen after selective removal of either 10-O or 11-O nylon suture under these circumstances (Fig. 11.11).

We prefer to use a combined interrupted and running nylon suture technique consisting of interrupted 10-O nylon sutures and a running 11-O nylon suture. The interrupted sutures may be removed at 6 to 8 weeks postoperatively for astigmatism management, leaving the running 11-O nylon suture intact for a minimum of 6 months, but preferably 1 year. If the running suture becomes unraveled or is loose, then it must be removed at an earlier time. In one series of 68 eyes, astigmatism was measured following selective suture removal in penetrating keratoplasties with combined interrupted and running closure.[8] The resulting astigmatic error was reduced to below 3 D in approximately 75% of the cases when 5 to 6 sutures were removed during a postoperative period of 5 months.

The effect of suture removal on corneal topography and astigmatism is generally unpredictable.[27,28] In 10 cases, removal of a running 16 μn (11-O) monofilament nylon suture at 12 months resulted in increased astigmatism of 1.5 D in 7 cases and decreased astigmatism of 1.5 D in 3 cases. The authors concluded that even a running 11-O nylon suture produces some wound tension and therefore distortion at 12 months after surgery. Some patients show increased astigmatism, decreased astigmatism, and even no significant change following suture removal.[27]

Following suture removal in immediate corneal molding effect can be observed, but in general a period of 1 to 2 weeks is required for the donor and recipient corneal tissue to remold and for the topography to stabilize. A minimum follow-up of 2 to 3 weeks is usually necessary to accomplish stabilization of cor-

A
B
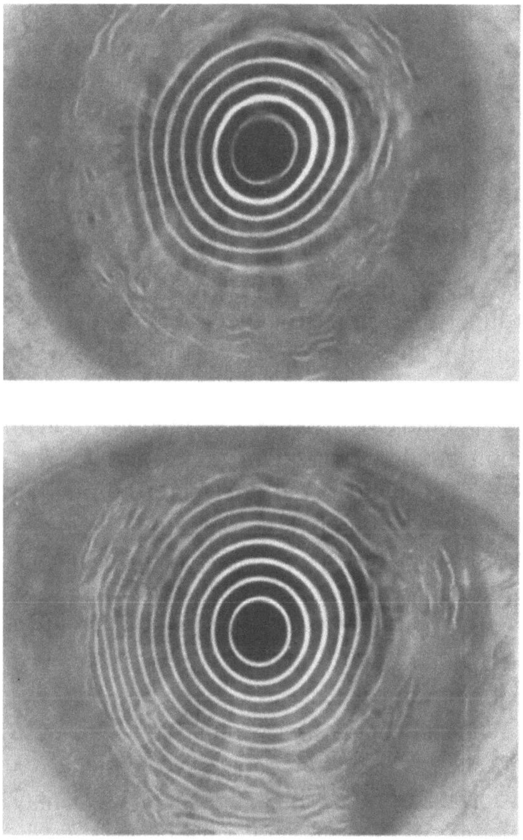

FIGURE 11.10. Corneascope photograph before (A) and after (B) removal of running 11-O nylon suture 1 year following keratoplasty. Wound compression from the 11-O nylon suture has been relieved, allowing central corneal steepening and reduction of astigmatism.[31]

neal topography prior to making a decision for subsequent suture removal.

The hazards of early suture removal are wound uplift and dehiscence. Occasionally the graft–host interface may be resutured to repair the wound dihiscence. One should clinically assess the degree of wound healing at the graft–host junction by the slit-lamp biomicroscope prior to suture removal. Vascularization across the wound and ingrowth of fibrous tissue indicates adhesion between the graft–host wound interfaces.

Contact Lens Molding

Molding of the corneal surface can be accomplished in select cases of postkeratoplasty astigmatism. A graft–host interface dehiscence with wound uplift may mold or flatten down over the wound by the splinting action of a rigid (gas-permeable) contact lens. The lens is fit steeper than the flattest corneal meridian but less than the steepest corneal meridian. If this is attempted in the early postoperative period when wound healing is incomplete or absent, the rigid lens may mechanically mold the wound into a more spherical shape and splint it in this position for wound healing to occur. We have had success using this technique in several patients with moderate amounts of astigmatism due to incomplete wound uplift and graft slippage.

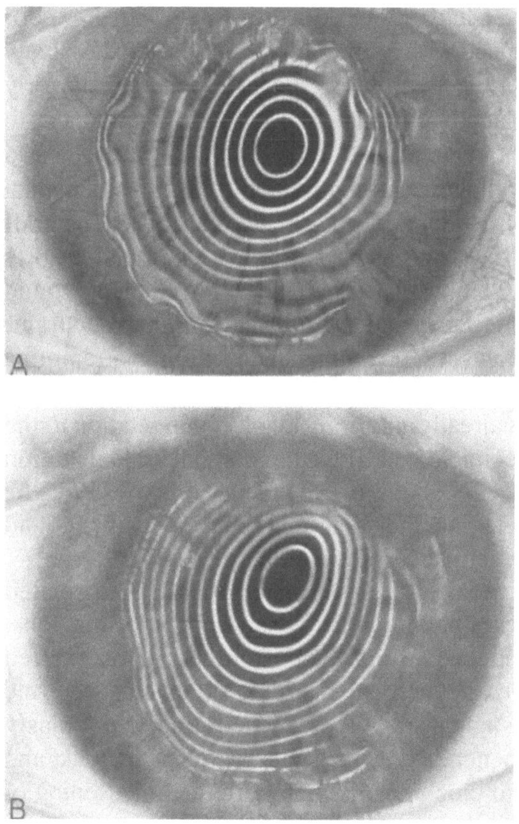

FIGURE 11.11. Corneascope photograph before (A) and after (B) removal of running 11-O nylon suture 1 year following keratoplasty. Note worsening of astigmatism after running suture removal. (A) Keratometry 42.00 × 52.75 × 150 degrees. Refraction −9.00 + 8.00 × 145 degrees V.A. 20/50 −2. (B) Keratometry 41.25 × 60.00 × 45 degrees. Refraction −14.00 +13.00 × 140 degrees. V.A. 20/70.[31]

Relaxing Incisions

Indications for Relaxing Incisions

Rowsey[29] recently reviewed the topographic indications and relative contraindications for relaxing incisions in postkeratoplasty astigmatism. His recommendations are to consider corneal relaxing incisions only after thoroughly reviewing graft and host factors, studying the corneascopy, and after a detailed slit-lamp examination of the graft–host interface. A graft with an excessively steep axis, over 43 D in one quadrant, may undergo a relaxing incision corresponding to that steep quadrant. A flat cornea under 43 D may not be suitable for the flattening effect from circumferential relaxing incisions. Optical distortion and contact lens fitting difficulties have been experienced with corneas that have been excessively flattened. Rowsey suggests that a posteriorly placed graft edge that is too low in respect to the recipient cornea bed may be behaving as a wedge resection producing central steepening of the donor cornea in that meridian. The graft tissue may be repositioned more anteriorly with an incision in the donor–recipient wound interface and resuturing of the quadrant. Rowsey[26] recommended caution in attempting a relaxing incision where the donor graft edge is already anteriorly displaced in relation to the recipient bed. If further corneal graft elevation occurs above the recipient graft bed after the relaxing incision, epithelial breakdown and potential corneal melt may occur.

Against-the-rule astigmatism is associated with poor contact lens centration and lens-induced astigmatism from pressure exerted on the vertical meridian. If against-the-rule astigmatism follows penetrating keratoplasty then relaxing incisions at the 3 o'clock and 9 o'clock position may provide a flattening of the horizontal meridian and correction toward with-the-rule astigmatism. Relaxing incisions should not be performed in a quadrant that previously underwent endothelial cell loss. This may occur with endothelial graft rejection and vitreous or iris adherence to the donor–recipient wound. Severe scarring of Descemet's membrane from previous trauma may prevent the cornea from relaxing adequately underneath a relaxing incision, and this may be a relative contraindication to relaxing incisions.[29]

Operative Technique for Corneal Relaxing Incisions

The preparation of the patient is the same as routinely performed for any other type of intraocular or corneal surgery. We prefer to use an operating room because of the availability of the operating microscope and other instrumentation should they become necessary. The patient is brought to the operating room as an outpatient having had nothing to eat or drink for the previous 8 hr. The patient is placed in the supine position and the operative eye prepped and draped in the routine fashion isolating it in the surgical field. Anesthesia can be accomplished using topical tetracaine 0.5% hydrochloride ophthalmic solution or, in more apprehensive or uncooperative patients, a periorbital or retrobulbar anesthetic block may be administered. General anesthesia is rarely indicated. If general anesthesia or retrobulbar or periobulbar anesthetic block is used, then the optical axis of the eye must be marked prior to administration of the anesthetic. This ensures accuracy of the visual axis for subsequent intraoperative keratotometry and corneascopy.

We routinely bring the clinic chart with the patient to the operating room. The chart contains all of the refractive, keratometric, and corneascopic data, and is available for inspection at all times during the procedure. The corneascope photograph is lined up in the orientation that the surgeon will have when he observes the eye through the microscope. This helps to eliminate any confusion about the position of the corneal astigmatism. Preoperative drawings of the surgical plan, indicating the axis of astigmatism and the proposed axis and length of the incisions, are helpful.

All surgery is performed using an operating microscope with foot-control zoom and focusing. An operating keratometer is desirable for quantitation of the effects of surgery during the time of the operative procedure. A surgical corneascope that can be attached to the operating microscope is useful to observe the topography shifts at various stages of the procedure. If an attachable surgical corneascope is not available then a portable hand-held reusable corneascope can be used.

The patient is asked to fixate on the operating microscope light or on the center of the corneascope or keratometer mires and the visual axis is marked. Observation of the corneascope mires is used to confirm the planned quadrant for surgery. Alternatively, preoperative keratometry is performed just before beginning the surgical procedure to confirm the axis of astigmatism. Pachymetry may be used to measure the corneal thickness over the graft–host wound junction, but reliable measurements may be difficult to achieve because of the irregular nature of many keratoplasty wounds. A combination of visual inspection of the graft–host interface under the operating microscope and pachymetry reading can alert the surgeon to areas of wound thinning with the potential risk for corneal perforation.

We prefer to use a front-cutting diamond knife or microsharp metal blade. Predetermined blade lengths are available for disposable metal knife blades, but we do not prefer to use these in keratoplasty relaxing incisions.

The incision may be made in the graft–host interface or may be made central or peripheral to it. The advantage of making the incision central to the graft–host interface may be a decreased incidence of anterior chamber perforation because of the more uniform thickness of the donor cornea. If the incision is made in the graft–host interface, then careful dissection down through the wound is required in order to decrease the incidence of anterior chamber perforation. Depending on the nature of the postkeratoplasty wound healing, the wound may be poorly healed and easily separated even by blunt dissection with the noncutting edge of the knife. Slow, careful dissection is made through the wound. If a perforation into the anterior chamber occurs, then the procedure must be terminated and the wound resutured using 10-O or 11-0 nylon sutures. Suturing of the corneal wound negates the effect of the operation and produces peripheral corneal flattening over the graft–host interface and central corneal steepening—the opposite of the desired effect.

The initial incision is made circumferentially and bisected by the steepest corneal meridian (Fig. 11.12). The length of the relaxing incision and its depth are titrated depending upon the intraoperative corneoscopic and keratometric changes. Depending on the preoperative parameters, the relaxing incision may only be required on one side of the graft–host interface. If the effect is not sufficient on one side, then a similar dissection is performed 180°, still in the same steep meridian. We routinely perform an incision of 2 clock hours (60°) initially before observing the keratometric and corneascopic changes (Fig. 11.13). Because of expected postoperative wound healing, a reversal of the effect of the relaxing incision may be expected. For this reason an overcorrection is desirable at the time of surgery. Lindstrom and Lavery[23] prefer to overcorrect the patient 30 to 50% of the preoperative cylinder. We recently proposed that there is a region in highly astigmatic corneas where the change in corneal power is maximum, and if a relaxing incision was made in this location, more effective and reliable surgical correction of astigmatism would result. We call this region the inflection zone and performed transverse relaxing inci-

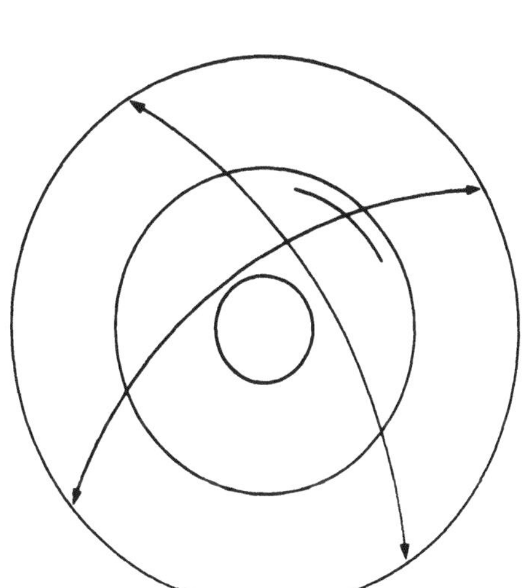

FIGURE 11.12. Relaxing corneal incision inside graft–host interface and 2 clock hours in arc length centered on the steepest central corneal meridian.[31]

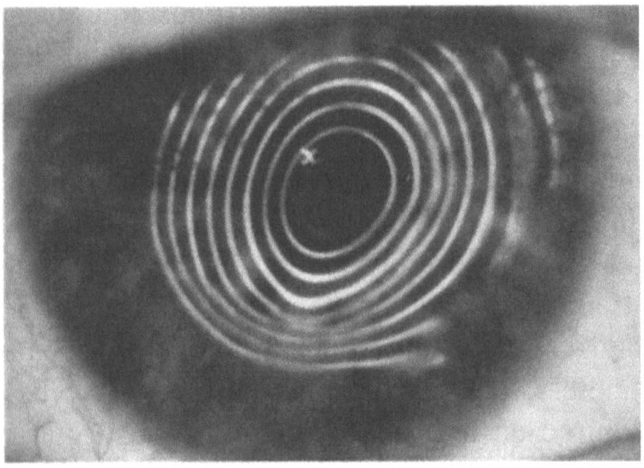

FIGURE 11.13. Corneascope photograph demonstrating inferonasal tissue compression with central corneal steepening. A relaxing corneal incision is indicated in the inferonasal quadrant beginning from 3:30 to 5:30 o'clock. Corneascope photograph is obtained after the initial 2 clock-hour incision to determine whether the incision should be extended or an additional incision added 180° away at the opposite end of the steepest central meridian.[31]

sions in a cadaver eye model to test this hypothesis. Suture-induced astigmatism was reduced 67% with an incision placed at the inflection zone compared to 36% reduction in induced cylinder using incision placement either central or peripheral to this zone ($p < 0.025$). This suggests that relaxing incisions need not be placed solely at the graft–host interface[11] or at some other predetermined position such as 5 mm.[18] Using topographic guidance, a single cut may be more effective when placed at the inflection zone.

Compression sutures are used when a satisfactory result is not achieved by relaxing incisions on both sides of the graft–host junction for at least 90°. The compression sutures are placed in the flattest corneal meridian 90° from the steepest meridian. For astigmatism greater than 8.5 D, compression or augmentation sutures combined with relaxing incision help reduce corneal astigmatism.

The relaxing incisions are irrigated with balanced salt solution on a fine cannula to remove any talc or debris or blood. Cycloplegic antibiotic drops are placed in the eye and the eye patched and shielded in the routine fashion.

After examination on the first day following surgery, topical broad spectrum antibiotic drops are given four times a day. Topical ophthalmic corticosteroids are continued at the preoperative level or increase in frequency for several days postoperatively and thereafter rapidly tapered. The patient is followed in the routine fashion to observe epithelial migration and healing. Immediate postoperative corneoscopy will indicate the potential success or failure of the surgery. If an overcorrection is achieved, then the surgeon must observe serial corneascopic photos and keratometry readings until they stabilize. If undercorrection is achieved, then an insufficient surgical procedure has been performed. Additional relaxing incisions may be necessary at that time, or another surgical procedure may be contemplated. If the desired surgical result is achieved and compression sutures remain in the eye, then the compression sutures are left in place indefinitely. If an overcorrection is present, then the compression sutures are selectively removed in an attempt to relieve the overcorrection.

Wedge Resections

Indications for Wedge Resection

The indication for wedge resection in postkeratoplasty astigmatism is a goal of 10 to 12 D of correction.[29] Lindstrom and Lavery prefer to first perform relaxing incisions in cases with less than 10 to 15 D of postkeratoplasty astigmatism.[30] In cases refractory to this surgical treatment, they perform wedge resections prior to repeating the keratoplasty.

Our approach in postkeratoplasty astigmatism is to analyze the corneascopic image, diagnose the cause of the astigmatism, and therefore directly treat the pathologic process. Our criteria do not include an absolute number of diopters of postoperative astigmatism when determining whether a wedge resection or relaxing incision should be performed. If a large amount of central corneal flattening has occurred from wound gape, then wound revision and wedge resection may be indicated for that meridian. Performing a relaxing incision 90° away would serve only to weaken the wound and result in significant graft flattening, which, in turn, causes difficulty with contact lens fitting. In contrast, wedge resection and wound revision serve to reapproximate tissue and stabilize the wound. The resultant central corneal steepening achieves more physiologic corneal topography.

Olson[30] states that wedge resection is indicated in eyes with a large degree of astigmatism (more than 10 D). He believes the outcome of wedge resection is uncertain in eyes with less than 8 D of astigmatism because of the potential for overcorrection.

Operative Technique for Corneal Wedge Resection

Belmont and Troutman begin a wedge resection by first marking the flatter meridian of the cornea with methylene blue stain on the epithelium.[24] A single razor or diamond blade is used to outline a 90° curvilinear incision centered on the axis mark. This is made "internal or external to the graft scar." A second curvilinear incision is made to include the graft–host interface such that the diameter of the wedge is greatest at the axis of the flattest meridian. Deepening of the wedge incision is performed by freehand dissection and the wedge removed at the depth of the incisions. An alternative technique uses a parallel double-blade diamond knife. This creates two vertical incisions at two-thirds corneal depth straddling the graft–host interface. The tissue is excised using the blade and scissors. Using either technique, the authors recommend a paracentesis to reduce anterior chamber volume and facilitate wound closure. The wound is closed using 8 to 10 interrupted 10-O nylon sutures, beginning at the periphery of the incision and progressing centrally. All sutures are tied initially with double slip knots as previously described.[16] Using the surgical keratometer, the tension on the slip knots is adjusted to achieve an overcorrection of one-half the dioptric power of the original flat astigmatic meridian. The sutures are tied using square knots and buried in the donor tissue.

The wedge resections are performed under retrobulbar anesthesia. A corneal wedge is excised less than 3 clock hours in length, and varies from 1 to 2 mm wide "depending on the amount of preoperative astigmatism." Belmont and Troutman do not use a mathematical quantitative method for determining the amount of tissue to be excised. Suture removal begins 4 to 6 weeks postoperatively and continues for several months. If a satisfactory refractive result is obtained, sutures are left in place.

Wound Revision/Compression Suture (Corneal Tuck) for Postkeratoplasty Astigmatism

Lindstrom and Lavery[23] describe the wound revision/compression suture technique as "essentially a hybrid of the relaxing incision and wedge resection." They state "we have found this technique useful for correcting as much as 4–6 diopters of residual astigmatism following relaxing incision when a repeat of the relaxing incision was not felt prudent and a wedge resection was expected to produce an overcorrection." Their technique is performed under retrobulbar anesthesia. The flatter meridian is identified and a dissection to three-fourths to seven-eighths depth is made in the graft–host interface, in the same manner as for relaxing incisions. From this point on the technique is similar to a wedge resection "except (that) no tissue is excised." Suture tension is adjusted to achieve one-third to one-half overcorrection of the pre-existing astigmatism. Selective suture removal begins at 2 months.

Rowsey[29] reviewed the corneal tuck for postcataract astigmatism and found variable results. He stated that the results of the procedure are variable and the long-term effects are unknown.

Approximation of the wound edges is first done with 1 or 2 centrally placed interrupted

8-O silk sutures. Placement of 10-O nylon sutures begins peripherally and progresses centrally to complete the wound closure, and then the silk sutures are removed. Intraoperative corneoscopy and keratometry are performed to determine the overall effect. If an undercorrection occurs, then a wider wedge excision can be done. An overcorrection of one-third to one-half of the preoperative cylinder is desirable but sometimes not possible to achieve. Merely overtightening the nylon sutures may give an apparent effect at the time of operation, but a permanent tissue compression does not necessarily occur after suture removal. A paracentesis is not routinely performed, because wedge resection is essentially an extraocular procedure. All suture knots are buried in the host corneal stroma and the eye is patched.

Patients are maintained on postoperative topical antibiotics and corticosteroids. The antibiotics are discontinued after 2 weeks and the corticosteroids are tapered toward the preoperative maintenance level. Refraction, keratometry, and photokeratoscopy are performed at each follow-up visit. Selective suture removal begins at 8 weeks postoperatively if an undesirable overcorrection is present. Selective suture removal allows relative steepening of the wound interface with central flattening in the meridian of the cut suture. If an adequate astigmatism correction has been achieved, then the remaining sutures are left in place indefinitely (see Fig. 11.14). With the eventual hydrolysis of nylon after 2 years, however, corneal topography may change if wound healing with tissue compression is not complete.

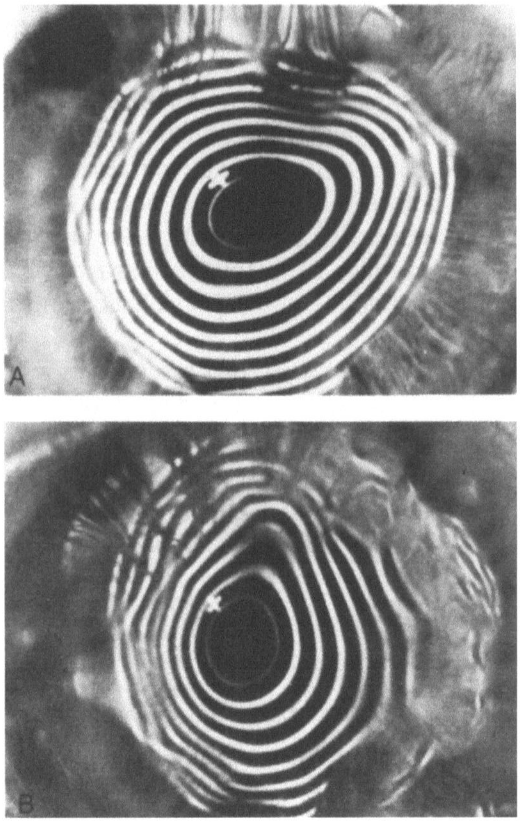

FIGURE 11.14. Corneascope photograph before (A) and after (B) wedge resection. (A) The peripheral corneal topography is abnormal from 12:30 to 3:30 o'clock and accounts for the excessively flattened central corneal topography oriented in the corresponding meridian. (B) Wedge resection has been performed for 90° from 12:30 through 3:30 o'clock, resulting in central steepening of the previously flat corneal meridian and reduction of astigmatism.[31]

Summary

For almost 100 years the concept of surgically altering the anterior refractive surface of the eye has been investigated as a way of correcting spherical and astigmatic refractive errors. The procedures of corneal incision, corneal tissue excision, and corneal suturing have evolved by theory, laboratory investigation, and clinical experience. It is only recently that attention has been focused on these techniques in their application to corneal refractive errors after penetrating keratoplasty. Troutman, in the 1970s, first popularized the corneal relaxing incision and wedge resection as a way of managing postpenetrating keratoplasty astigmatism. We have followed the evolution of these procedures through the experience of numerous investigators, and have reviewed the complications encountered. Consequently, we have adopted the following guidelines for the use of corneal relaxing incisions and wedge resections in postpenetrating keratoplasty.

Corneal relaxing incisions and wedge resections are indicated in the eyes with postkeratoplasty astigmatism that cannot be visually rehabilitated by spectacles or contact lenses. Instead of relying on an absolute amount of astigmatism that can be corrected by each of these procedures, we believe that analysis of the corneal topography, with special emphasis to the graft–host interface will determine the procedure of choice.

If wound compression is associated with central corneal steepening along the same meridian, then a relaxing incision is indicated just inside the graft–host interface for an arc length of 60°. Corneal topography is again analyzed, this time by intraoperative corneascopy, to determine if the relaxing incision should be deeper, or greater arc length, or repeated 180° away along the same meridian. In eyes uncorrectable by relaxing incisions, wedge resections may be attempted before consideration of repeat keratoplasty.

When wound dehiscence or slippage is associated with central corneal flattening along the same meridian, a wedge resection of 90° of the wound will produce flattening over the wound and central corneal steepening perpendicular to the wedge resection. An initial overcorrection of the astigmatism is desirable; this can be titrated in the postoperative period by selective suture removal.

Modifications of these procedures for special circumstances have led to development of the concepts of wound revision and compression sutures, or a combination of these two techniques (corneal tuck). Wound revision with resuturing is useful for early wound dehiscence or slippage that may follow premature suture removal. Compression sutures are useful to reduce postoperative astigmatism immediately following relaxing incisions and wedge resections when purposeful overcorrection of the initial astigmatism has been produced. After selective suture removal in wedge resections and the healing of relaxing incisions, the compression sutures may be removed depending on the nature of the astigmatism and the corneal topography.

Overcorrection and undercorrection remain significant problems associated with corneal relaxing incisions and wedge resections. Besides the unpredictable nature of these procedures, other complications may occur, such as corneal perforation, melting, infection, or graft rejection reaction. The procedures are limited to the extent that the corneal topography is able to be adjusted without compromising its physiologic functions. Still, prevention of postpenetrating keratoplasty astigmatism remains the best method of management.

References

1. Snellen H. Die Richtung der Hauptmeridiane des astigmatischen Auges. *Albrecht von Graefes Arch Klin Exp Ophthalmol.* 1869; 15:199–207.
2. Bates WH. A suggestion of an operation to correct astigmatism. *Arch Ophthalmol.* 1894;23:9–13.
3. Lans LJ. Experimentelle Untersuchungen über Entstehung von Astigmatismus durch nicht-perforirende Corneawunden. *Albrecht von Graefes Arch Ophthalmol.* 1898;45:117–152.
4. Sato T. Posterior incision of cornea; surgical treatment for conical cornea and astigmatism. *Am J Ophthalmol.* 1950;33:943–948.
5. Sato T. Posterior half-incision of cornea for astigmatism; operative procedures and results of the improved tangent method. *Am J Ophthalmol.* 1953;36:462–466.
6. Akiyama K, Tanaka M, Kanai A, Nakajima A. Problems arising from Sato's radial keratotomy procedure in Japan. *CLAO J.* 1984;10:179–184.
7. Troutman RC. *Microsurgery of the Anterior Segment of the Eye.* St Louis: CV Mosby, 1977;p 286.
8. Wiedman M. Cylinders into spheres: astigmatic cornea repair. Read before the Tenth Corneal Research Conference. Boston, June 17, 1977.
9. Poyales J. Actas 1 Congreos Oftalmologico Latino, Rome, 1953.
10. Barraquer J, Muinos A. Lamellar scleral resection: indications and technique. *Am J Ophthalmol.* 1956;41:92.
11. Troutman RC. *III Symposium of the International Ophthalmic Microsurgery Study Group,* Mexico. Basel: Karger, 1970.
12. Troutman RC, Swinger C. Relaxing incision for control of postoperative astigmatism following keratoplasty. *Ophthalmic Surg.* 1980;11:117–120.
13. Krachmer JH, Fenzel RE. Surgical correction of high postkeratoplasty astigmatism. *Arch Ophthalmol.* 1980;98:1400–1402.
14. Sugar J, Kirk AK. Relaxing keratotomy for

postkeratoplasty high astigmatism. *Ophthalmic Surg*. 1983;14:156–158.
15. Krachmer JH, Ching SST. Relaxing corneal incisions for postkeratoplasty astigmatism. *Int Ophthalmol Clin*. 1983;23:153–157.
16. Troutman RC. Corneal wedge resections and relaxing incisions for postkeratoplasty astigmatism. *Int Ophthalmol Clin*. 1983;23:166–168.
17. Lavery GW, Lindstrom RL, Hofer LA, et al. The surgical management of corneal astigmatism after penetrating keratoplasty. *Ophthalmic Surg*. 1985;16:165–169.
18. Troutman RC. Microsurgical control of corneal astigmatism in cataract and keratoplasty. *Trans Am Acad Ophthalmol Otolaryngol*. 1973; 77:563–572.
19. Casey TA, Werb A, Rerrie J. *Trans Ophthal Soc UK*. 1974;94:127.
20. Sanders N. Wedge resection in host cornea to correct postkeratoplasty astigmatism. *Ophthalmic Surg*. 1979;10:53–54.
21. Van Rij G, Vijfvinkel G. Correction of postkeratoplasty astigmatism by razor blade and v-shaped knife wedge resection. *Ophthalmic Surg*. 1983;14:406–410.
22. Lugo M, Donnenfeld, ED, Arentsen JJ. Corneal wedge resection for high astigmatism following penetrating keratoplasty. *Ophthalmic Surg*. 1987;18:650–653.
23. Lindstrom RL, Lavery GW. Correction of postkeratoplasty astigmatism. In: Sanders DR, Hofman RF, Salz JJ, eds, *Refractive Corneal Surgery*. Thorofare, NJ: Slack, 1986;p 215.
24. Belmont SC, Troutman RC. Compensating compression sutures in wedge resection. *J Refract Surgery*. 1985;1:104–107.
25. O'Connor R. Corneal cautery for high myopic astigmatism. *Am J Ophthalmol*. 1933;16: 337.
26. Rowsey JJ, Doss JD. Preliminary report of Los Alamos keratoplasty technique. *Ophthalmology*. 1981;88:755.
27. Perlman EM. An analysis and interpretation of refractive errors after penetrating keratoplasty. *Ophthalmology*. 1981;88:39–45.
28. Stainer GA, Perl T, Binder PS. Controlled reduction of postkeratoplasty astigmatism. *Ophthalmology*. 1982;89:668–676.
29. Rowsey JJ. Review: current concepts in astigmatism surgery. *J Refract Surgery*. 1986;2:85–94.
30. Olson RJ. Modulation of postkeratoplasty astigmatism by surgical and suturing techniques. *Int Ophthal Clin*. 1983;23:137–151.
31. Beatty RF, Schanzlin DJ. Wedge resection and relaxing incisions. In: Schwab IR, ed, *Refractive Keratoplasty*. New York: Churchill Livingstone, 1987;ch 9.

12
The Corneal Modeling System

Peter J. McDonnell

Measures of corneal topography can be obtained using the keratometer and photokeratoscope, the uses and limitation of which have been reviewed elsewhere in this book. The keratometer assumes that the cornea is spherical or spherocylindrical, and measures only a small percentage of the anterior corneal surface. The photokeratoscope samples a greater portion of the corneal surface, but deviations from spherical topography must be fairly pronounced before visual inspection alone will be informative. Despite the limitations of these two instruments, both have proven extremely useful clinically. With the advent of "the era of refractive surgery," however, has arisen a need for instrumentation that will allow rapid qualitative as well as quantitative assessment of the topography of the entire cornea; the Corneal Modeling System (CMS)[1] (Computed Anatomy, New York) was designed to fill this need. An improved photokeratoscope that spans almost the entire corneal surface is combined with the computer-assisted analysis of the photokeratoscope images pioneered by Dingeldein and Klyce.[2]

The human cornea is an anisotropic multilayered three-dimensional structure. Over the last two decades, numerous investigators have worked to refine the measurement anterior curvature.[3–9] During this same time period, optical, and then ultrasonic pachymeters have been developed for use in the evaluation of corneal thickness. The Corneal Modeling System is unique because it integrates corneal curvature and thickness measurements in a continuous mathematical model of the human cornea. The implications of such an achievement are major in terms of advancing our knowledge of corneal topography in general, as well as its surgical modification. In particular, the development of such a model might well be an important step in terms of successful numerical modeling (finite element analysis) of the human cornea.

Topographic Data

Data acquisition involves use of a cylindrical photokeratoscope that generates a 32-ring image covering virtually the entire cornea from its apex to the limbus (Fig. 12.1). The image of the reflected rings is acquired by the system in one thirtieth of a second using real time digital video. The photokeratoscope rings are then successively digitized and topographic data points are extracted in polar coordinates using 256 radial lines scanning across the 32 rings. On a typical photokeratoscope image, this generates an average of 7000 data points. These data are then used to generate continuous mathematical functions describing the anterior corneal surface.

The topographic data may then be represented in a variety of ways, including wire mesh models. Clinically, the most useful representation to the clinician is the color-coded map. With the so-called absolute scale (Fig. 12.2), all maps are directly comparable, with each color representing a preset range of cur-

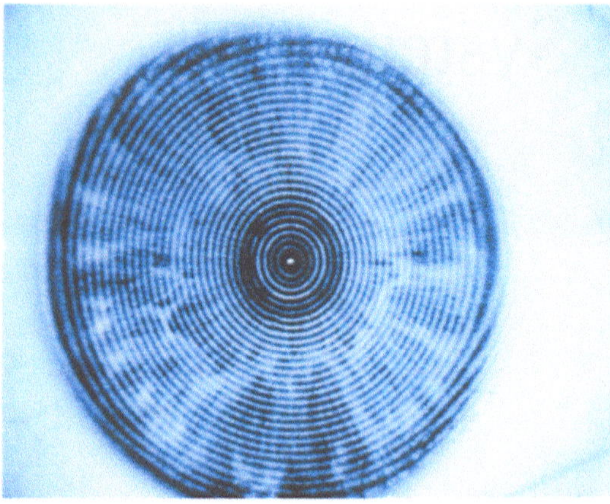

FIGURE 12.1. CMS photokeratoscope generates 32-ring image covering cornea from apex to limbus.

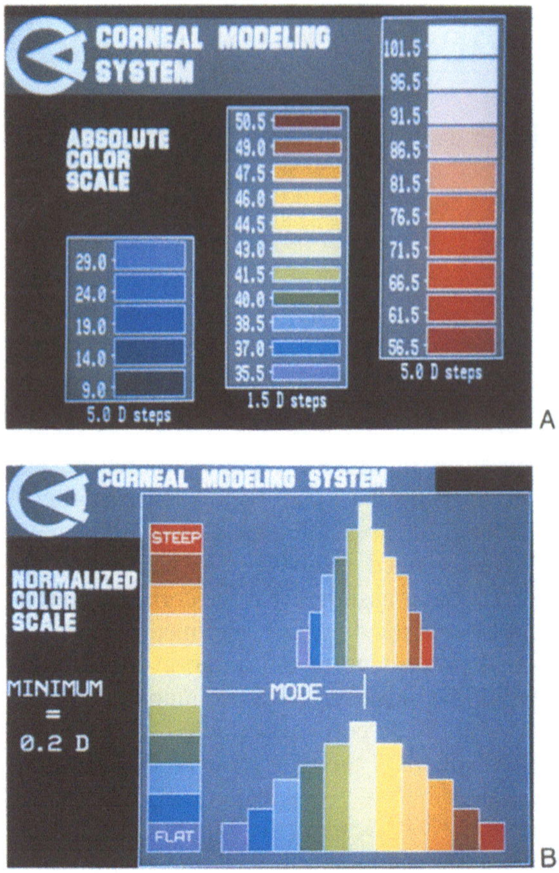

FIGURE 12.2. (A) With absolute color scale, each color represent a 1.5 D range between 35.5 and 50.5 D. Outside of this range, color changes represent steps of 5 D. (B) With the normalized color scale, 11 separate colors are used to represent the range of curvatures present on any particular cornea.

vatures. Within the so-called normalized scale, 11 separate colors are used to represent the range of curvatures present on any particular cornea. Thus, depending on the difference between the steepest and flattest regions, the steps between colors may be quite small or rather large. In our experience, the absolute scale is satisfactory in most clinical situations and has the advantage of allowing direct comparison of different examinations because the curvatures corresponding to each color are the same. The normalized scale may be useful in selected situations, including looking at regional variations in corneal power as the dioptric intervals are often much smaller than with the absolute scale.

The interactive cursor can be moved to any location on the surface of the topographic display; as this is done, the distance of the cursor from the corneal apex, as well as the axis in which the cursor is located, are displayed on the upper right of the screen. Specific quantitative information of local corneal power at any point is thus available to the examiner. For hard copies of the examinations, photographs can be taken of the screen image using Polaroid instant film or 35 mm film.

Accuracy and Reproducibility

Hannush and Waring[10] compared the CMS with the KERA Corneascope (KERA Corp, Torrance, CA) and with the Bausch and Lomb keratometer (Rochester, NY). Using calibrated steel balls, they found that results using the CMS were as accurate and as reproducible as were those of the Bausch and Lomb keratometer. The corneascope, according to these authors, was less accurate and showed only fair reproducibility. A subsequent study by these same authors in human eyes indicated that the standard deviation of measurement of corneal power at any particular point using the Corneal Modeling System was 0.2 D, a value about twice that achieved with the keratometer, and slightly better than that achieved with the corneascope.[11] We have repeated this study in normal subjects as well as individuals after radial keratotomy, and confirmed a standard deviation of about ±0.2 D.[12]

Examination of the Normal Cornea

As noted previously in this text, the normal cornea demonstrates asphericity, being steepest centrally and with progressive flattening toward the periphery. The magnitude of this flattening may be up to 5 to 7 D (Fig. 12.3).

Naturally Occurring Astigmatism

With the CMS, astigmatism is typically reflected by the presence of a band of relative corneal steepening that may or may not be narrowed centrally to have a dumb-bell type of configuration. Although this relative corneal steepening is frequently symmetrically distributed around the corneal apex (Fig. 12.4), there may be steepening located primarily in one meridian, with very little steepening in the meridian 180° away (Fig. 12.5). Also, the steepest and flattest axes of the cornea may not always be orthogonal, as would be expected in spherocylindrical optics. This "asymmetrically distributed astigmatism" has potentially important implications in the surgical correction of such astigmatic errors.

Diurnal Changes in Corneal Curvature

The examination of normal unoperated eyes confirms previous findings by others[13, 14] that the cornea, on average, tends to steepen slightly from morning to evening. We examined the local curvature at nine locations on the cornea (corneal apex and superior, inferior, nasal, and temporal corneas 1.5 and 3 mm peripheral to the corneal apex) (Fig. 12.6). A new finding in this study[12] was a horizontal disparity in the diurnal changes occurring from morning to evening. In these normal eyes, the temporal cornea tended to flatten slightly in the evening (mean of −0.1 diopters at 1.5mm and −0.2 D at 3.0 mm from the corneal apex), while the nasal cornea tended to steepen (mean of 0.6 D at both 1.5 and 3 mm from the corneal apex) ($p<0.05$). The flattening observed temporally was unique to this quadrant, as the superior, inferior, and nasal cornea all showed steepening. The magnitude and direction of diurnal changes did not correlate with patient age or sex. Possible explanations for topographic changes include variations in corneal

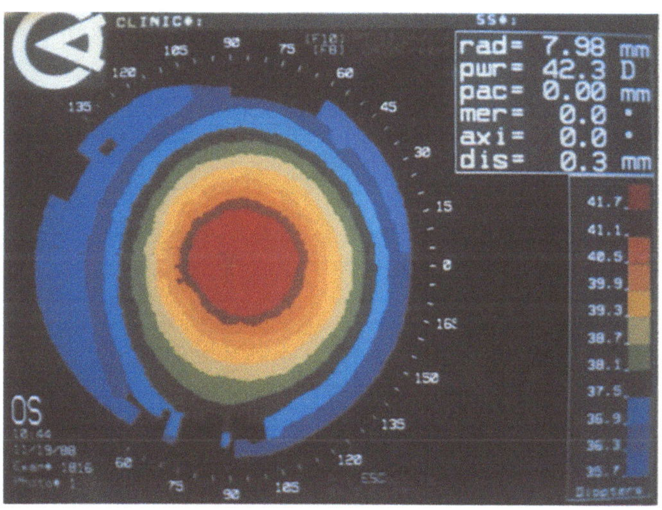

FIGURE 12.3. Color-coded topographic map of normal unoperated cornea without astigmatism demonstrating progressive flattening from corneal apex toward the peripheral cornea.

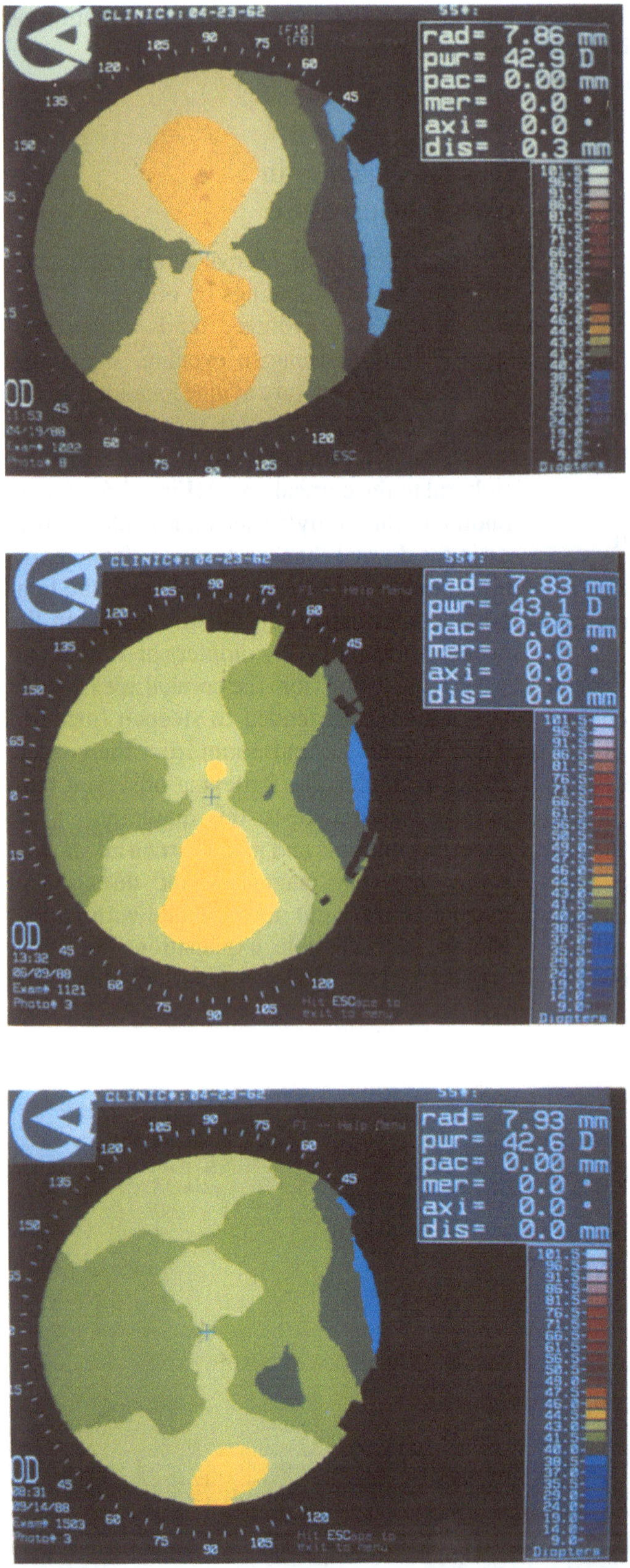

A

B

C

FIGURE 12.4. (A) Color-coded map of cornea with 4.5 D of naturally occurring keratometric astigmatism. (B) Same cornea as in (A) following single keratotomy incision in the 100° axis. Most of the superior steepening is now absent, with little change inferiorly. (C) Same cornea as in (B) following subsequent inferior keratotomy incision demonstrating reduction in inferior steepening.

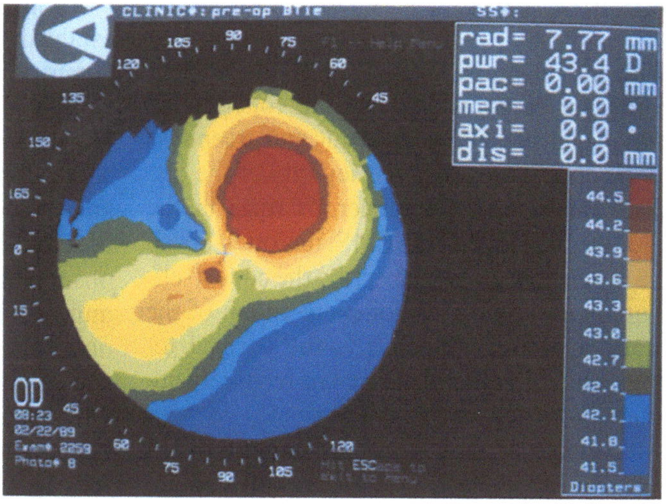

FIGURE 12.5. Color-coded map of cornea with 5.5 D of naturally occurring keratometric astigmatism. Steepening can be seen to be asymmetrically distributed about the visual axis, with greater steepening in the superonasal quadrant than in the inferotemperol quadrant.

hydration, lid pressure, or accommodation during the day.

Contact Lens-Induced Corneal Topographic Changes

Using the Corneal Modeling System, contact lens-induced corneal warpage can be quantitated and followed. Wilson and co-workers[15] demonstrated that these contact-lens-induced corneal topographic changes may take 6 months or more to resolve completely. A specific finding of note by these authors was the fact that contact lenses that are decentered superiorly have a tendency to produce an inferior corneal steepening that may suggest a mild form of keratoconus. It is therefore incumbent upon the clinician, whenever possible, to examine patients after they have been out of their contact lenses for at least 6 weeks. Failure to do so might lead to the erroneous diagnosis of keratoconus, or to inappropriate surgical intervention, such as keratotomy for correction of apparent astigmatism which might in fact be due to a reversible contact lens-induced corneal change.

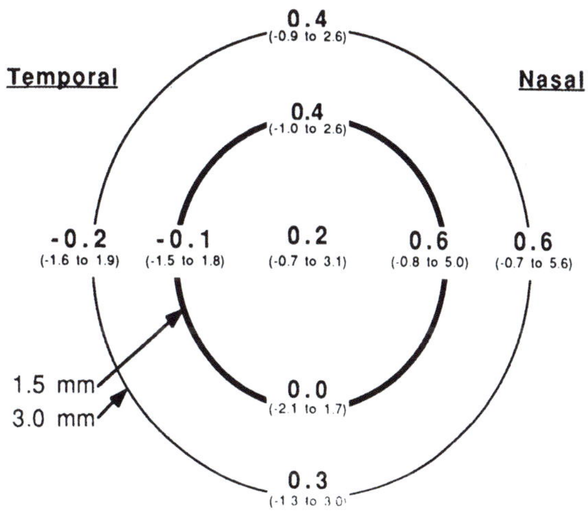

FIGURE 12.6. Mean change in diopters at the nine locations on the normal cornea. Ranges of the fluctuations are shown in parentheses.

Keratoconus

With keratoconus, steepening of the inferior cornea is demonstrated on the topographic maps (Fig. 12.7). The diameter and steepness of the cone varies with the severity of the disease. Because of the numerous rings in the photokeratoscope of the CMS, it is often possible for the rings to circumscribe the cone itself, thereby describing the complete extent of the protruding cone. Superiorly, the corneal topography is frequently normal or relatively unaffected.

Potential applications of the data provided by the CMS include assistance with contact lens fitting and planning the surgical correction of keratoconus, either with penetrating keratoplasty or epikeratophakia. Contact lenses are frequently necessary for visual rehabilitation after penetrating keratoplasty for keratoconus, and Kaufman has suggested that this may, in part, reflect a failure of the surgeon to excise all of the ectatic corneal tissue at the time of penetrating keratoplasty or to totally circumscribe the cone with an epikeratophakia lenticule if this procedure is performed. Preoperative topographic mapping, such as that provided by the CMS, might help guide the surgeon in planning surgical intervention, with specific attention to excising or circumscribing all the ectatic cornea, if possible.

An instructive application of the CMS is in establishing the inheritance pattern of keratoconus. It is typically reported that keratoconus is familial in only about 6 to 8% of cases.[16, 17] Others have described what appear to be autosomal dominant inheritance patterns, although an autosomal recessive pattern has been proposed also. One possible explanation for these observations is that keratoconus may have multiple different etiologies, inheritance being only one. Alternatively, the "keratoconus gene" may have incomplete penetrance and variable expressivity, such that our usual techniques of diagnosing this condition will not detect an abnormality in a family member who has the keratoconus gene but who does not have overt clinical disease. To address this issue, Rabinowitz and co-workers[18] used the CMS to examine the family members of patients with keratoconus, and demonstrated in each large family that some members appear to be affected by mild forms of the disease without overt clinical signs (apical protrusion and thinning, epithelial iron line, Vogt's striae, retinoscopic or photokeratoscopic abnormalities). These mild or abortive forms of keratoconus, called "keratoconus fruste" by Amsler,[19] exhibit central steepening, asymmetry in central corneal power between the two eyes, and greater steepening inferior to the corneal apex than above (Fig. 12.8). Examina-

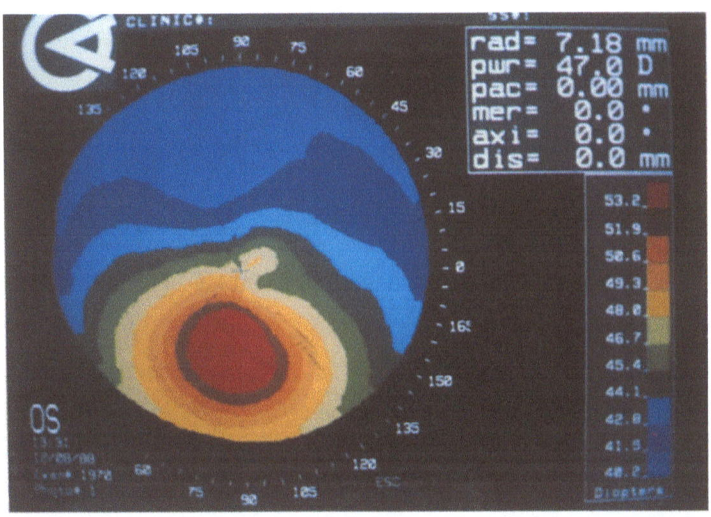

FIGURE 12.7. Color-coded map of keratoconus demonstrates steepening of inferior cornea with relatively normal superior peripheral curvatures.

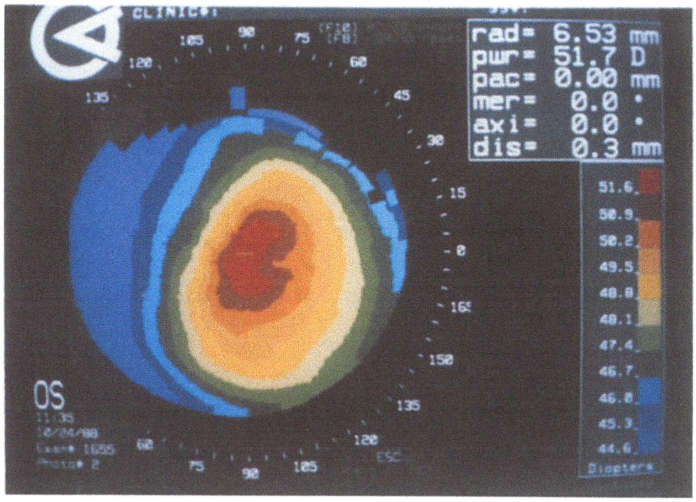

FIGURE 12.8. Mild form of keratoconus fruste in biomicroscopically normal cornea of family member of patient with keratoconus. This cornea shows central steepening (51.7 D), with greater steepening below the corneal apex than above; there is asymmetry in central corneal power between the two eyes. Keratometry revealed only 0.5 D of astigmatism.

tion of five families of patients with keratoconous in each case has revealed the presence of family members with these topographic abnormalities but without overt clinical disease (Fig. 12.9). These preliminary data suggest that keratoconus is, in many instances, inherited in an autosomal dominant manner. These findings may facilitate linkage analysis studies that may help identify the gene(s) responsible for this condition.

Contact Lens Fitting and Keratoconus

With the topographic map of keratoconus, it possible to describe these corneas in terms of cone diameter, steepness of the cone, and the more normal peripheral curvatures. Contact lenses may then be fit using this information.[20] One technique is to use lenses such as the Soper or McGuire lenses with steep central curvatures to vault the central cone and flatter peripheral base curves to match the more normal peripheral corneal curvature. Alternatively, as described by Bronstein and Reynolds,[21] who used the photokeratoscope, lenses with base curves matching the superior normal curvature can be used to fit mild-to-moderate cases of keratoconus. It is possible in the fitting of these corneas with markedly distorted topography that the CMS computer-generated mathematical model of the anterior corneal curvature could be used as a template for a computer-controlled contact lens lathe that could create lenses to match the corneal topography of specific individuals.

Topographic Analysis and Refractive Surgery

Radial Keratotomy

The CMS confirms the previous observations of Rowsey and co-authors[6, 22] with regard to the effects of radial keratotomy on corneal topography. Preoperatively, the normal cornea is aspheric, being steepest in the center and with progressive flattening towards the periphery. After radial keratotomy, the reverse situation exists, with the central cornea being flattest and with steepening towards the periphery (Fig. 12.10). After radial keratotomy, zones of central corneal flattening are typically centered around the corneal apex. We have observed three basic configurations to these optical zones: round or oval, bandlike, and dumbbell or split optical zones (Fig. 12.11). The round optical zone is that kind most frequently encountered.[23]

In some patients with round optical zones, we have noted smaller flat optical zones within

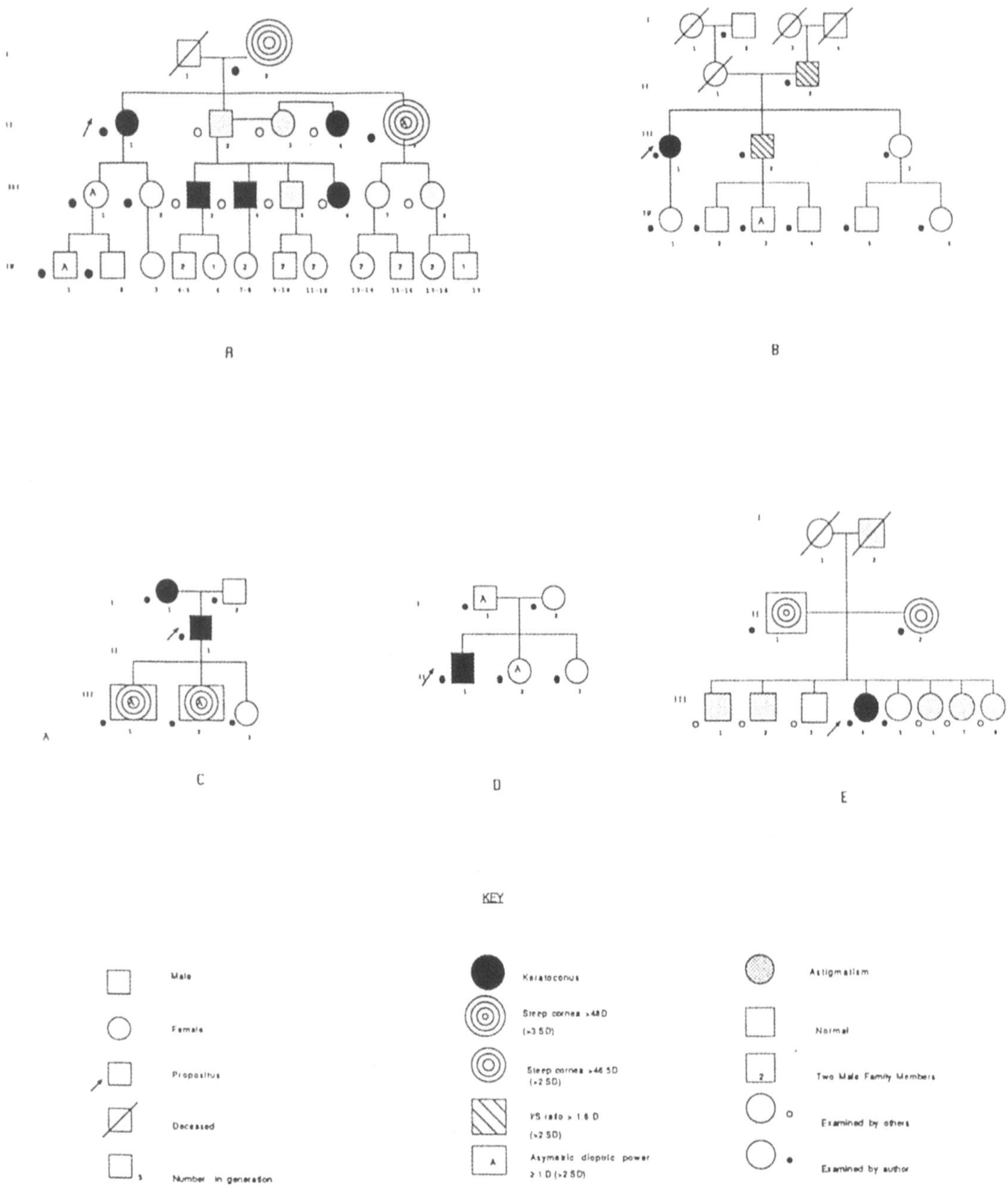

FIGURE 12.9. Kindred of patients with keratoconus. With computer-assisted topographic modeling, apparently affected individuals can be identified who have no evidence of overt clinical disease.

the larger roughly circular optical zone (Fig. 12.12). Typically, these small flatter optical zones are located inferior to the corneal apex. Patients with such multifocal corneas may enjoy both excellent distance and near visual acuity, a situation that we believe to resemble that of a multifocal contact lens[24] or intraocular lens. Wilson and Klyce suggested the analogy of a progressive addition bifocal because of the continuously changing curvatures along the corneal surface.[25, 26] Such a multifocal cornea may explain why patients with re-

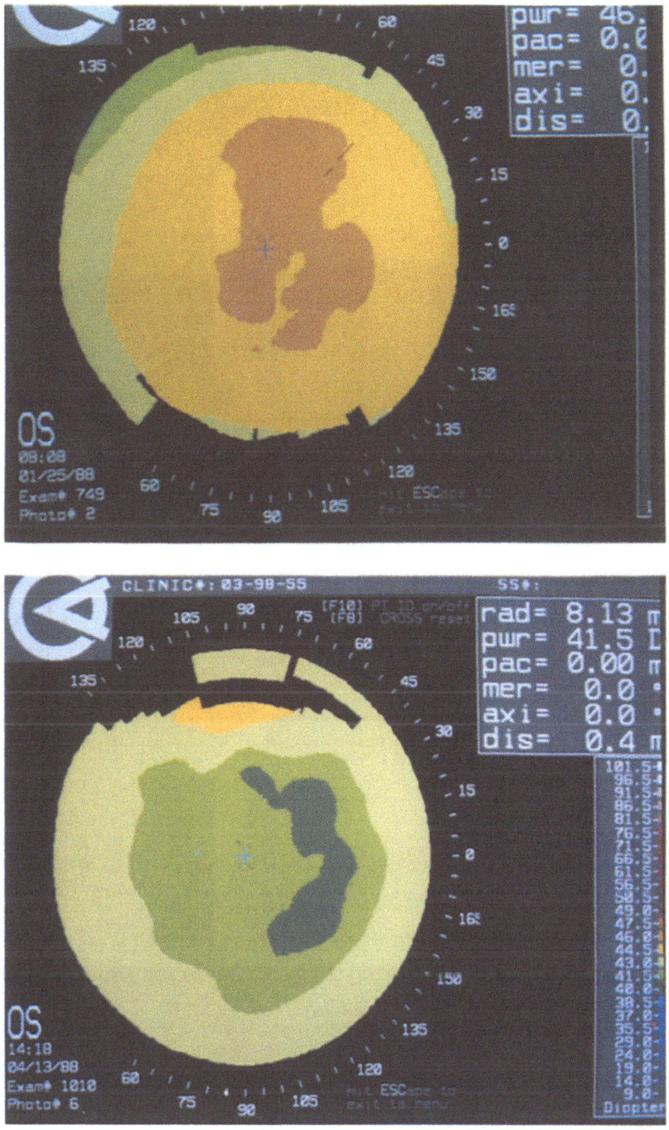

A

B

FIGURE 12.10. (A) Preoperative cornea with mild amount of with-the-rule astigmatism. Cornea is aspheric with progressive flattening from apex to periphery. (B) Same cornea as (A) following 4-incision radial keratotomy. Central cornea is now flattened disproportionately relative to periphery, such that central corneas is now the flattest, rather than steepest region of the cornea.

sidual myopic refractive errors after radial keratotomy can have better visual acuity than do individuals with a similar refractive error who have not had surgery. Santos and associates,[27] and Waring and associates[28] suggested that patients who have undergone radial keratotomy may have better visual acuity than expected based on their refraction because of the increased spherical aberration of the paracentral cornea, which produces a larger blur circle on the retina. At least some of these patients have been demonstrated, with the CMS, to have a greater flattening inferior to the corneal apex, which explains the excellent distance acuity, while the steeper superior region would explain the good unaided near acuity. These patients that we have observed typically do complain of mild monocular diplopia; this is a common occurrence also in patients wearing bifocal contact lenses, and is attributed to a prismatic effect at the junction of the two optical zones.[29] Thus, in some patients a bifocal or multifocal cornea may have the disadvantage of causing monocular diplopia and degradation of the retinal image. Dingeldein et al.[30] performed computer-assisted analysis of photokeratoscope images and found that focal dispersion analysis with ray tracing may be an accurate predictor of best-corrected spectacle acuity. The "surface regularity index" de-

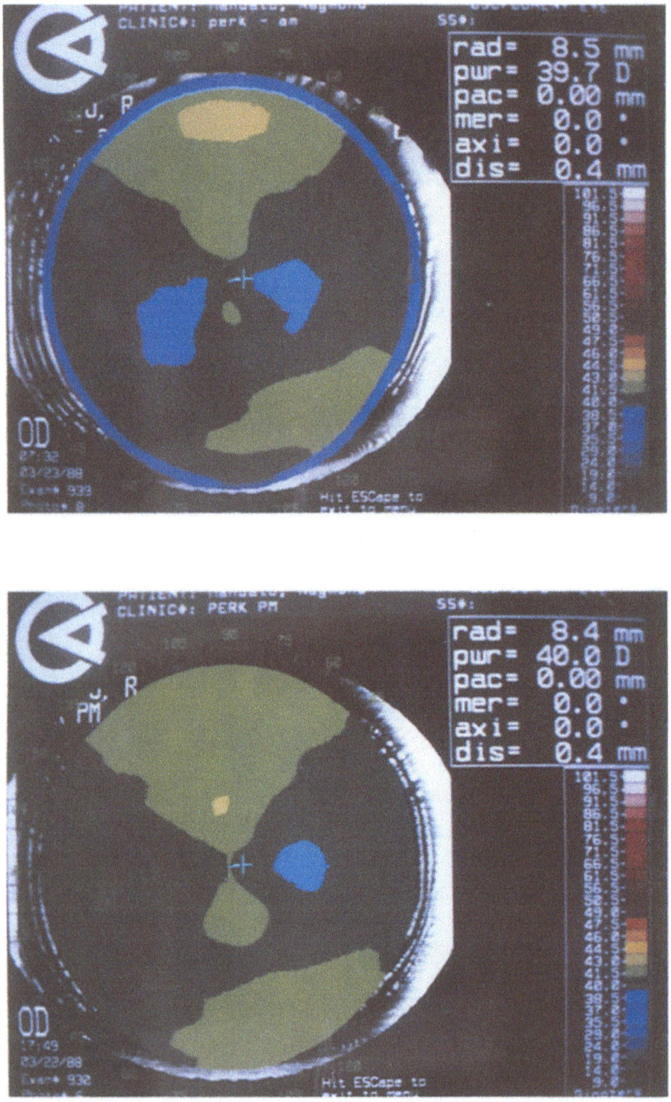

A

B

FIGURE 12.11. (A) Morning examination of cornea 6 years after 8-incision radial keratotomy. Dark band indicating region of corneal flattening extends across the interpalpebral zone, with narrowing centrally. Two small, flatter islands are seen on either side of corneal apex. (B) Evening examination of same cornea shown in (A). Central cornea is now steepened and flat islands on either side of corneal apex have decreased in size or disappeared. This patient reports decrease in uncorrected visual acuity from morning to evening.

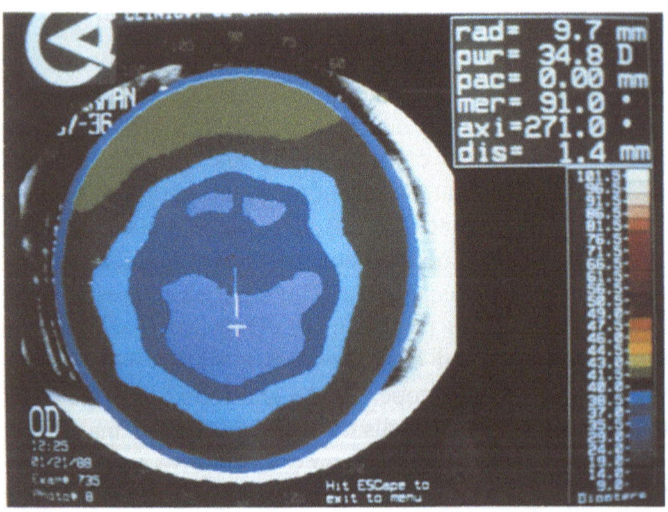

C

FIGURE 12.12. Map of cornea 3 years after 8-incision radial keratotomy demonstrates large, roughly spherical optical zone encompassing flatter zone inferior to corneal apex. Corneal power within this flatter zone is 34.8 D. Steeper cornea centrally measures 37.8 D.

scribed by these authors may be a measure of the degradation of the retinal image that occurs in some patients with multifocal corneas after radial keratotomy and other refractive surgical procedures, following trauma, or in the presence of inherent corneal topographic abnormalities such as keratoconus.

The lack of correlation between changes in uncorrected visual acuity, spherical equivalent, keratometry, and intraocular pressure from morning to evening has been documented uniformly in studies that have examined the possible relationships between these variables.[31–33] In the large series of PERK Study patients, Schanzlin et al.[33] found that the changes in keratometry did not correlate with changes in refractive error. This discrepancy does not mean that diurnal refractive changes are not due to changes in topography; rather the keratometer, because it measures only the average curvatûre of the central 3 mm of the cornea, may not provide a sufficiently detailed picture of the diurnal changes occurring in the corneal topography.

After radial keratotomy, central flat optical zones are created that can be characterized as round, oval or band like, or dumbbell shaped or split.[23] The dumbbell form of optical zone is associated with larger amounts of refractive and keratometric astigmatism than are the round or band like zone.[34] We correlated the shape of the optical zone with the presence or absence of diurnal variation (fluctuation) of visual acuity. Of eyes with symptomatic diurnal fluctuation of visual acuity, 90% had dumbbell shaped or split optical zones (Fig. 12.11), and only 1 in 10 had round optical zones. Of eyes without symptomatic diurnal fluctuation in visual acuity, in our experience only round or bandlike optical zones are encountered. Thus, the presence of a split or dumbbell-shaped optical zone after radial keratotomy suggests that the patient is likely to experience diurnal fluctuation in visual acuity.

The explanation for the variation in appearances of the flat optical zones after radial keratotomy is not obvious. This variation occurs despite the fact that our patients were operated on according to the same technique, with creation of radial incisions with a diamond blade set to 100% of the thinnest of the paracentral corneal thicknesses measured intraoperatively. The variations in optical zone shape cannot be attributed to any recognized intra- or postoperative complications, such as microperforations or incorrect marking of the visual axis. It is possible that relatively minor variations in incision depth, not appreciable with biomicroscopy, might be responsible for these local variations in curvature.

Following radial keratotomy, we have measured local diurnal changes in corneal curvature centrally and at 1.5 and 3.0 mm superiorly, nasally, and temporally from the corneal apex. The magnitude of diurnal fluctuation was greater in eyes after radial keratotomy than in normal unoperated corneas,[12] and these topographic changes have been shown to persist, in some eyes, for up to six years after radial keratotomy.[35]

Contact Lens Fitting After Radial Keratotomy

The postradial kėratotomy eye presents a unique challenge in terms of contact lens fitting. Unlike the normal cornea that progressively flattens from center to periphery, the cornea after radial keratotomy shows exactly the opposite progression, namely steepening from center to periphery due to the disproportionate flattening that occurs centrally with this procedure.[22, 36, 37] We have used the CMS to measure the superior midperipheral curvature, about 3.5 mm superior to the corneal apex. We then select a rigid gas-permeable contact lens having a base curve equivalent to the anterior corneal curvature at this point. We have been almost uniformly successful in fitting patients using this technique.[37] The contact lens vaults the flatter central cornea resulting in a plus tear lens, and as a result a minus correction is uniformly required in these patients (Fig. 12.13).

Myopic Keratomileusis and Myopic Epikeratophakia

Although visual distortion is a common complaint after refractive surgery, the reasons for this complication are not always ascertained. Maguire and co-workers[38] examined this phenomenon after myopic keratomi-

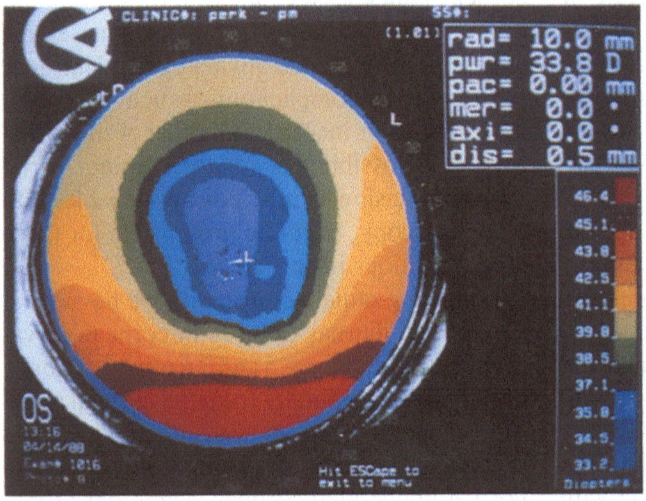

A

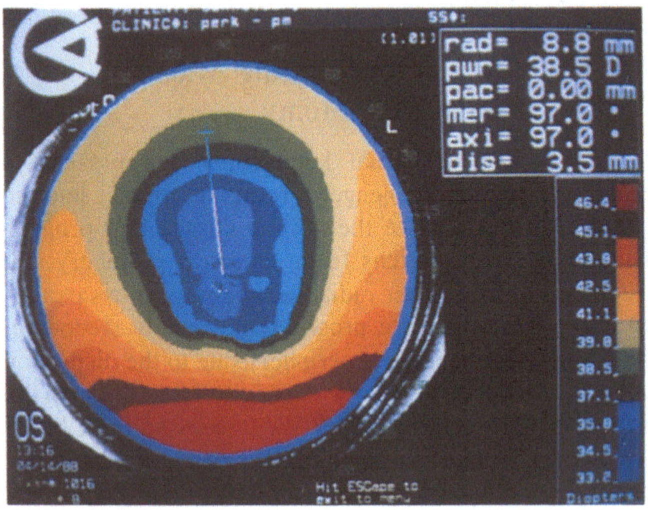

B

FIGURE 12.13. (A) Computerized corneal topography of eye overcorrected after radial keratotomy. Central corneal power is about 33.8 D. (B) Same cornea as in (A). Cursor is 3.5 mm above center of visual axis, where corneal power is about 38.5 D. (C) Rigid gas-permeable contact lens with base curve of 38.5 D. Lens is located superiorly, with superior edge beneath upper lid. Fluorescein pattern demonstrates vaulting of lens over centrally flattened cornea. (D) Schematic illustration of lens fit with base curve equal to midperipheral curvature. Central pooling of tears results from vaulting of extremely flattened central cornea. (Reprinted with permission from McDonnell PJ, Garbus JJ, Caroline P, and Yoshinaga P. Corneal Topography as an aid in fitting contact lenses after radial keratotomy. *Ophthalmology*, in press.)

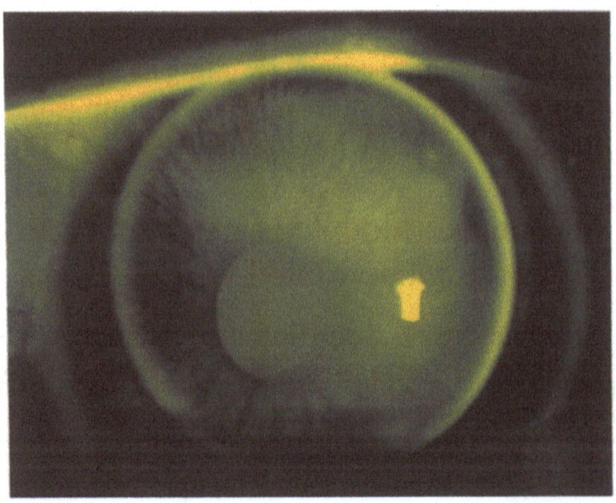

C

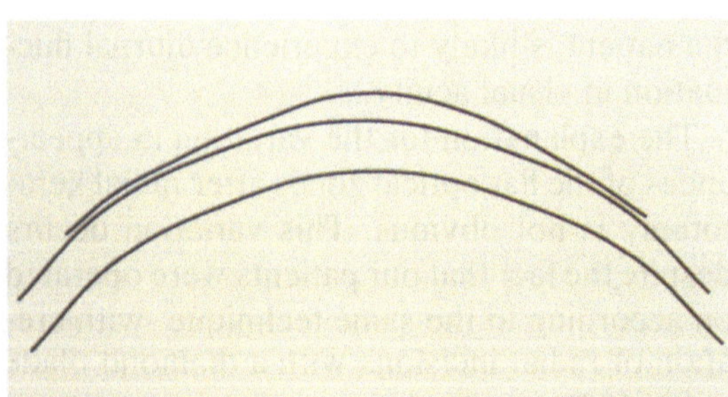

D

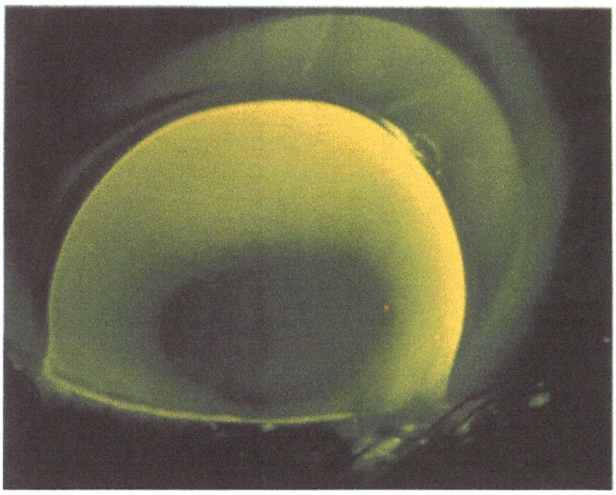

E

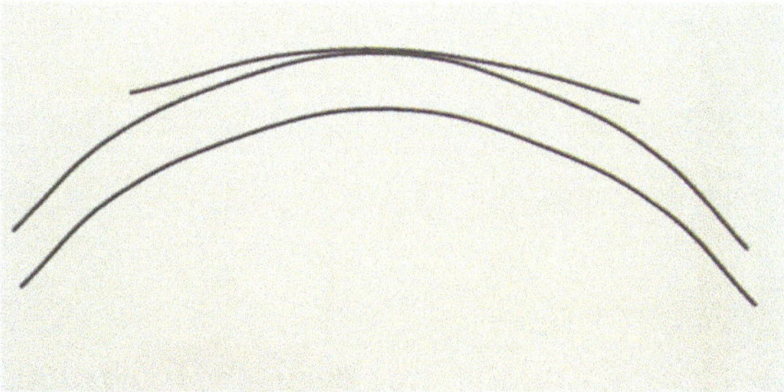

F

FIGURE 12.13. (E) Lens fit "on K" with central bearing, peripheral edge left, decentration, and discomfort. (F) Schematic illustration of lens fit "on K" with base curve equal to central keratometry readings. Edge lift results in discomfort and lens decentration with blink. (Reprinted with permission from McDonnell PJ, Garbus JJ, Caroline P, and Yoshinaga P. Corneal topography as an aid in fitting contact lenses after radial keratotomy. *Ophthalmology*, in press.)

leusis; Fig. 12.14 illustrates the right eye of a 26-year-old woman with unsatisfactory spectacle-corrected visual acuity 9 months after refractive surgery. Biomicroscopy revealed no scarring in the visual axis, and good visual acuity was obtainable with a hard contact lens. Topographic analysis using the Klyce system revealed a steady increase in corneal power across each meridian, indicating that the cornea has the properties of a multifocal lens whose optical performance would not be adequate except under intense illumination, which would cause the pupil to simulate a pinhole.

Computer-assisted topographic analysis has been used also to evaluate the topography of patients undergoing epikeratophakia for myopia.[39] Analysis of the keratoscope photographs of seven patients revealed several interesting findings. First, the optical zone, designed to be 6 mm in diameter, was often much smaller. Fig. 12.15 is from a patient whose predicted postoperative central curvature was 38.5 D. Although this flattening was achieved centrally, the zone of flattening was less than 6 mm, and in fact measured only about 3 mm. Second, graft decentration limited the visual result in some patients (Fig. 12.16), a problem exacerbated by the smaller than expected central zones of flattening.

Local Corneal Topographic Changes Due to Intersecting Corneal Incisions

The intersection of incisions in the cornea has been noted to result in marked gaping of the incision edges, with resultant delays in the healing of these incisions. A particular problem induced by these intersecting incisions is marked irregular astigmatism.[40] With the CMS, one can readily appreciate the marked corneal flattening that occurs over the area of the intersecting incisions, with local flattened areas having curvatures of 29 D or less (Fig. 12.17). In these patients, rigid contact lens fitting is typically necessary to restore good postoperative visual acuity. Unfortunately, it is in this subgroup of patients that a lens fitting is most difficult due to the marked local variations in anterior corneal curvature.

Surgically Induced Astigmatism and Its Surgical Correction

Postsurgical astigmatism, in contrast to naturally occurring astigmatism, is usually asymmetrically distributed about the corneal apex (Figs. 12.17 and 12.18). By this is meant that while there is typically a predominant axis of the steepening, the amount of steepening in the

A

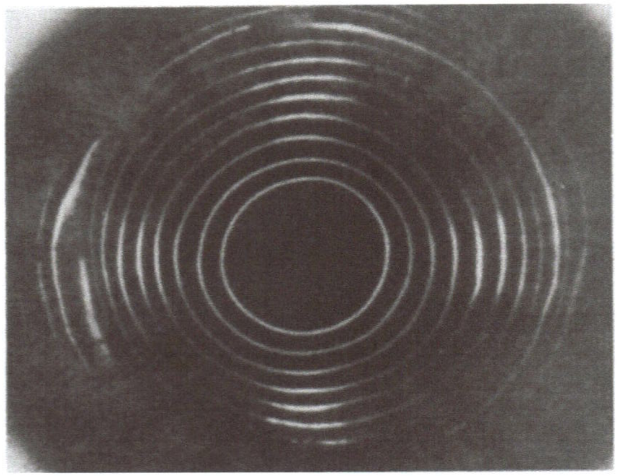

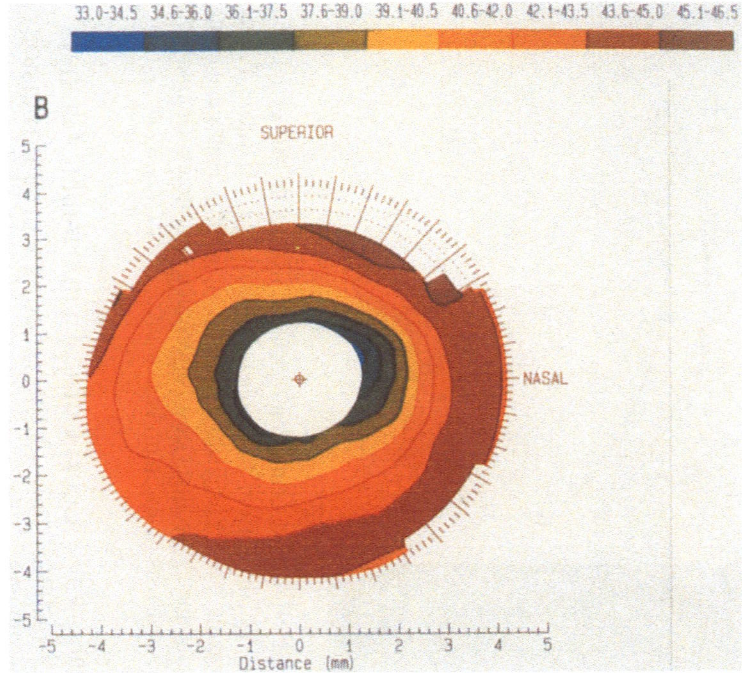

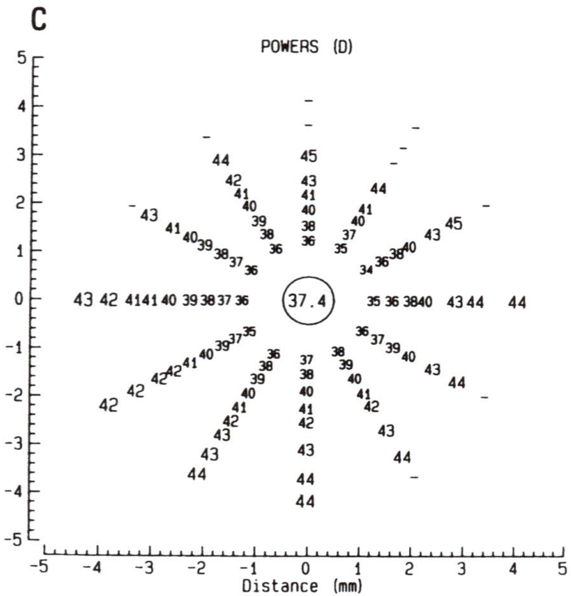

FIGURE 12.14. (A) Photokeratograph analysis of the right eye of a 26-year-old woman 9 months following myopic keratomileusis. Spectacle correction of −6.50 + 4.50 × 155° improved her uncorrected visual acuity of 20/200 to 20/40. Keratometry readings were 37.5/39.5 at 10°. Hard contact lens correction improved her vision to 20/20. (B) Color-coded analysis of the photokeratograph shown in (A). Concentric irregular bands of progressively higher power surround fixation. (C) Surface power plot of (A). Note that the powers surrounding fixation range from 34 to 37 D. (Reprinted from Maguire LJ, Klyce SD, Sawelson H, McDonald MB, Kaufman HE. Visual distortion after myopic keratomileusis. Computer analysis of keratoscope photographs. *Ophthalmic Surg*. 1987; 18:352–356.)

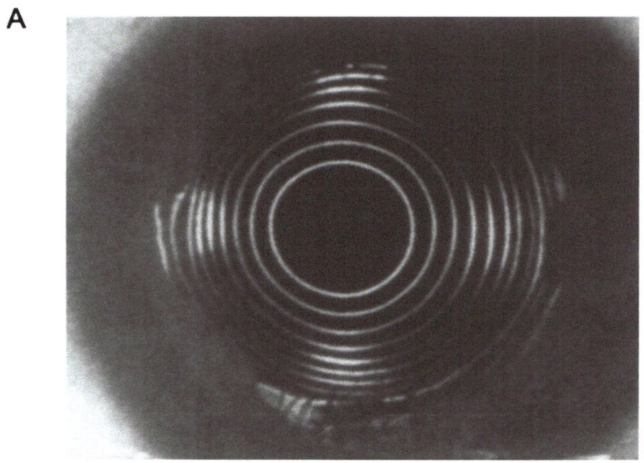

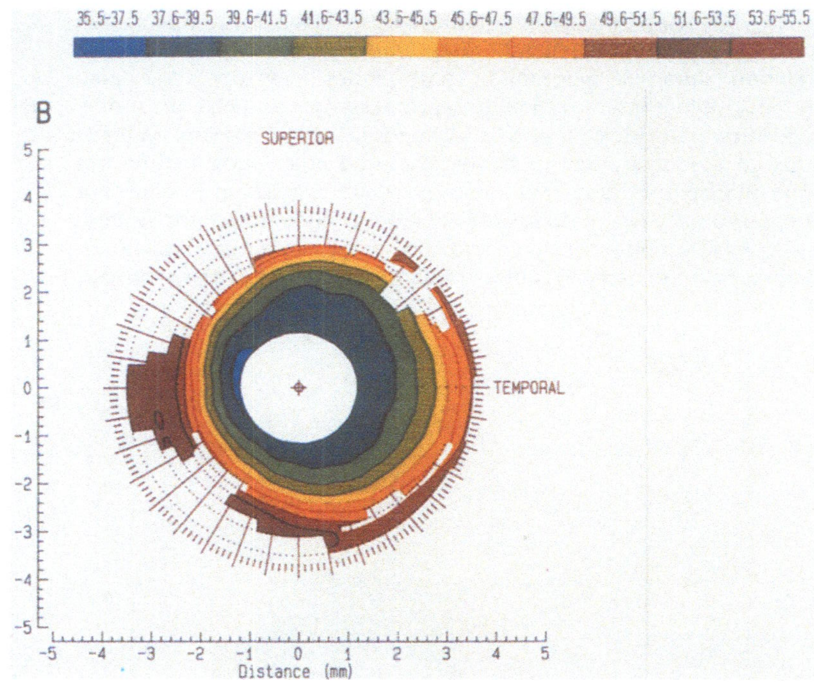

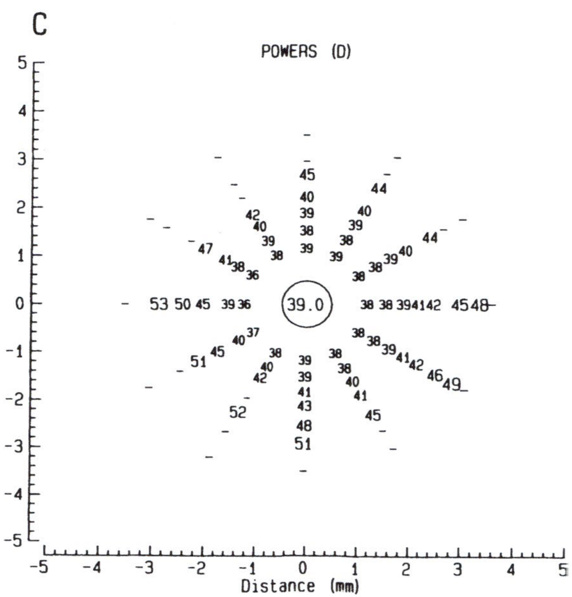

FIGURE 12.15. (A) Photokeratograph of the left eye of a patient 8 months following epikeratophakia for myopia. Uncorrected visual acuity was 20/25. (B) Contour map analysis of (A). The central zone of power covers an area 3.8 × 3.6 mm. Bands of progressively higher powers are present concentric to this zone. The optical zone is clearly <6 mm, the intended size of the optical zone. (C) Surface power analysis of (B). (Reprinted with permission from Maguire LJ, Klyce SD, Singer DE, McDonald MB, Kaufman HE. Corneal topography in myopic patients undergoing epikeratophakia. *Am J Ophthalmol*. 1987;103: 404–416.)

A

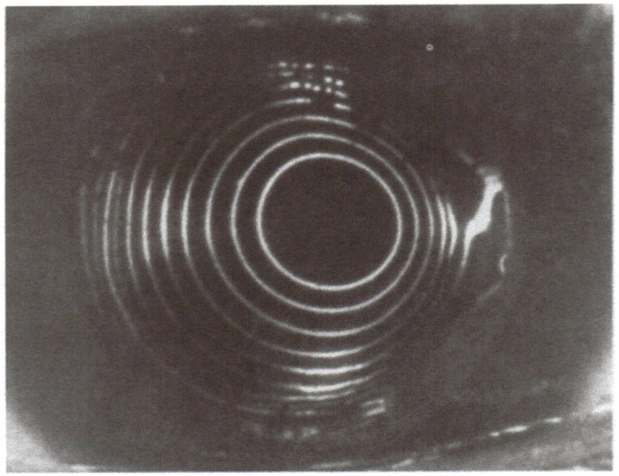

B

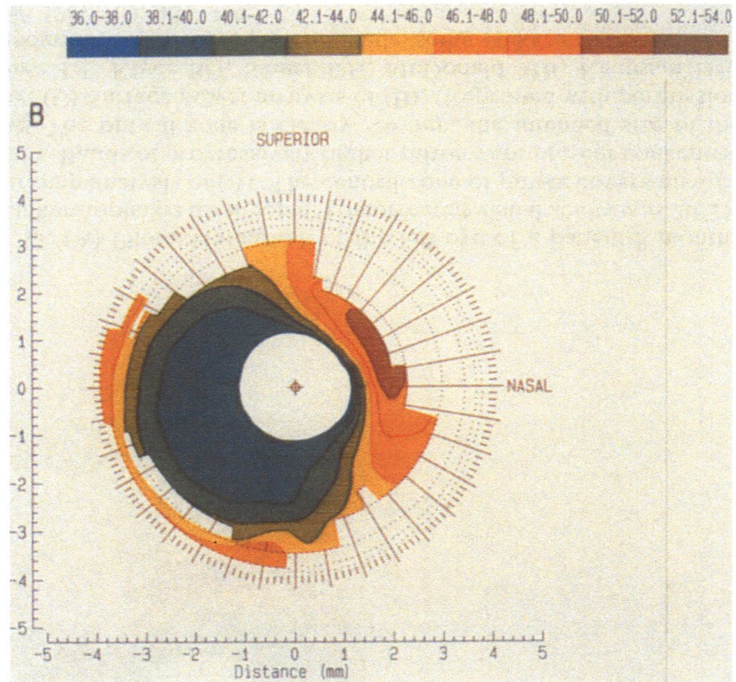

C

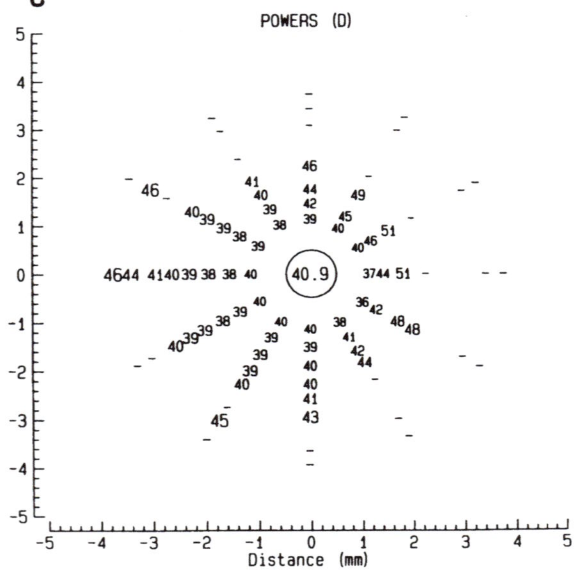

FIGURE 12.16 (A) Photokeratograph of the right eye of the same patient represented in Figure 12.15. Uncorrected visual acuity was 20/25 2 ½ months following epikeratophakia for myopia. (B) Color-coded contour map of the right cornea. Note the inferotemporal decentration of the optical zone. The power of the graft rapidly increases superonasally. Surface power plot analysis of (A). (Reprinted with permission from Maguire LJ, Klyce SD, Singer DE, McDonald MB, Kaufman HE. Corneal topography in myopic patients undergoing epikeratophakia. *Am J Ophthalmol*. 1987;103:404–416.) (C) Surface power plot of the cornea represented in Figure 12.17A.

FIGURE 12.17. (A) Cornea after combined radial and astigmatic keratotomy with intersection of incisions demonstrating wide incisions filled with included epithelium. (B) Color-coded topographic map of cornea with intersecting incisions in three meridians illustrates a profound flattening over each site of intersection.

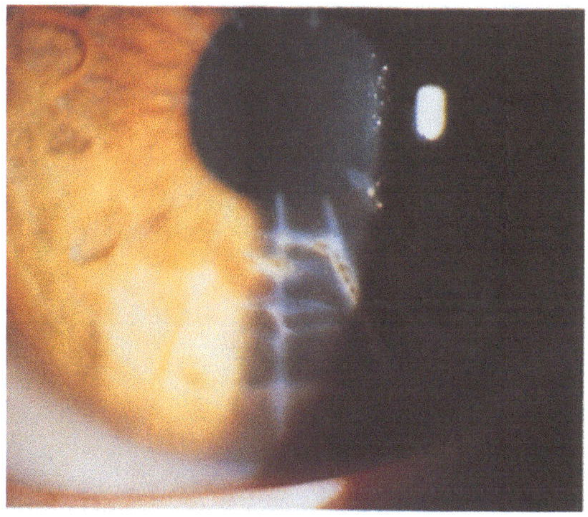

A

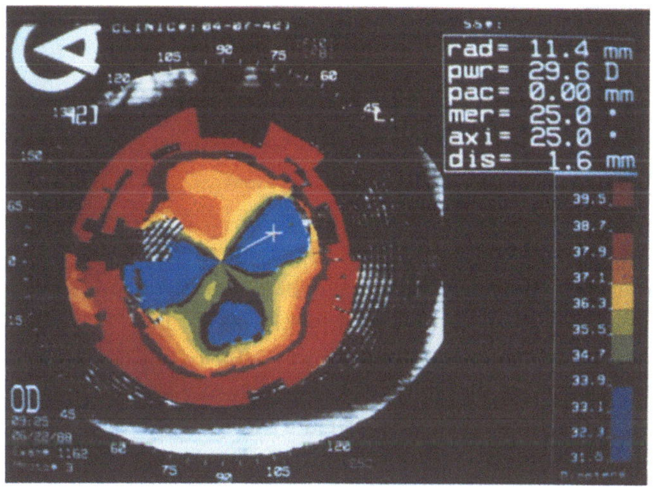

B

two meridians opposite or nearly opposite one another may be very asymmetric. For example, in a postsurgical eye with marked with-the-rule astigmatism, the cornea may show an extensive amount of steepening inferior to the visual axis, with little steepening superiorly. Unlike the keratometer, the CMS does not assume that the meridians of steepening will be exactly 180° apart, and, in fact, in some instances this assumption can be seen to be invalid. It may be that this type of information will be crucial in the planning of astigmatism-reducing procedures.

Astigmatic keratotomy is often effective in reducing the local corneal steepening in the meridian in which the incision is created, with relatively minor changes in the axis 180° away (Fig. 12.4). Thus, in some patients surgery may be most appropriately limited to a single quadrant, and in other patients surgery might be performed in two quadrants, but a greater amount of surgery will be performed in the quadrant with the greatest amount of local corneal steepening. We are currently involved in a prospective study of surgery for postpenetrating keratoplasty astigmatism designed to test the hypothesis that the results of surgery will be enhanced by basing the procedure on a knowledge of the preoperative topographical map. It may be that a large multicenter clinical trail will ultimately be required to conlusively show whether surgery designed on the basis of preoperative topography will significantly improve the results of surgery.

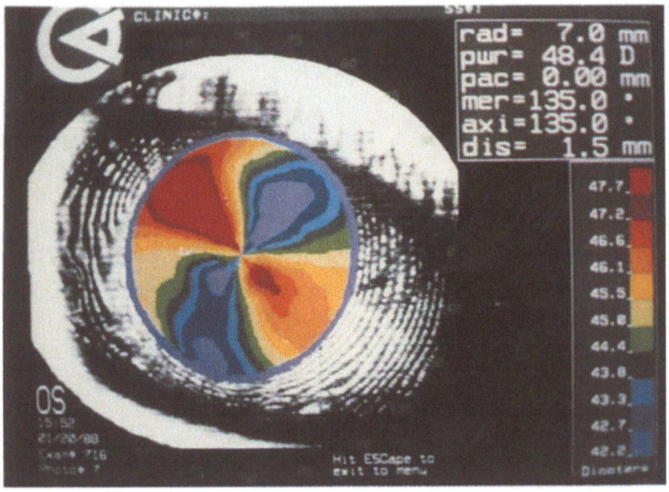

FIGURE 12.18. Patient with 5.5 D of keratometric astigmatism after penetrating keratoplasty. Corneal steepening and flattening are asymmetrically distributed about the corneal apex, with greatest steepening in the superonasal quadrant and relatively less steepening in inferotemporal quadrant. Patient was successfully managed with rigid gas-permeable contact lens.

Pachymetry with the Corneal Modeling System

Optical pachymetry was first used clinically for assessing corneal thickness, but has been replaced with ultrasonic pachymetry as the latter has been shown to have less intra- and interobserver variability. The CMS obtains pachymetric data of the cornea by acquiring a series of optical cross sections of the cornea using a dual beam scanning laser slit lamp (Fig. 12.19). A typical analysis uses a total of 14 optical cross sections acquired on seven video frames using real time digital video. These cross-sectional images result in approximately 12,000 data points for pachymetric analysis. Continuous mathematical functions are generated to fit the anterior and posterior curves. The spatial separation of the surfaces is precisely defined. As with the topographic maps, the cursor may be moved along the various slit images, thereby allowing the examiner to determine local corneal thicknesses.

A major potential advantage of the laser pachymeter is that it is a noncontact technique that does not require corneal anesthesia. It is known that corneal anesthetics, such as proparacaine hydrochloride, will disrupt the surface epithelium and can potentially affect the measurement. Furthermore, with the large pachymetry probes, the precise location where the measurement is being taken may be uncertain and it may be difficult to repeat measurements due to variability and of probe placement.

Laser Pachymeter: Intra- and Interobserver Variability

We compared the laser pachymeter of the CMS with two different ultrasonic pachymeters. In terms of intra- and interobserver variability, the results with the laser pachymeter were as good as or superior to those obtained with the ultrasonic devices.[41] The actual corneal thickness measurements obtained with the CMS were comparable to the readings obtained with the ultrasonic pachymeter. The computer-assisted laser pachymeter avoids the subjectivity that is necessary in determining the end point by optical pachymeters, and thus seems to be a potentially useful device for clinical and research use.

Summary

The ability of the Corneal Modeling System to incorporate curvature and thickness data into a single mathematical construct of the cornea is

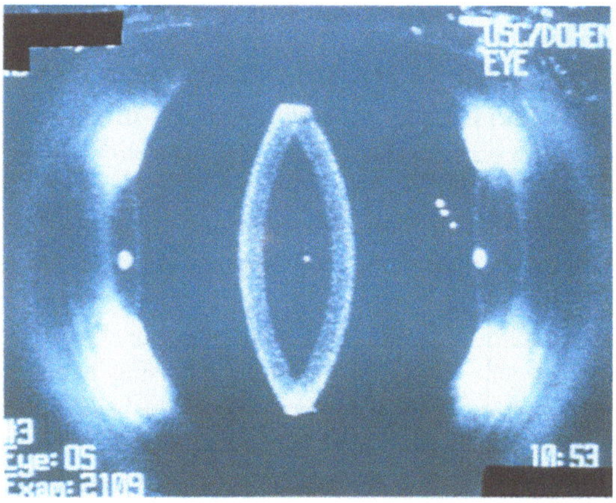

FIGURE 12.19. Dual beam scanning lasar slit-lamp optical cross-sections of cornea. Continuous mathematical functions are generated to fit anterior and posterior curves, thereby allowing examiner to determine local corneal thickness along the slit image.

an important achievement. As experience with this instrument is gained, a number of important issues in corneal topography can be addressed, such as the possible influence on corneal topography of diurnal changes in corneal thickness due to hydration and the relationship of corneal thickness in general to changes in corneal shape. Computer assisted topographic measurement devices will undoubtedly play a particularly important role in the design and evaluation of current and future refractive procedures.

References

1. Gormley DJ, Gersten M, Koplin RS, et al. Corneal modeling. *Cornea.* 1988;7:30–35.
2. Dingeldein SA, Klyce ST. Imaging of the cornea. *Cornea.* 1988;7:170–182.
3. Ludlam WM, Wittenberg S. Measurements of the ocular dioptric elements utilizing photographic methods. Part II. Cornea—theoretical considerations, *Am J Optom Arch Am Acad Optom.* 1966;43:249–267.
4. Ludlam, WM, Wittenberg S, Rosenthal J, et al. Photographic analysis of the ocular dioptric components. *Am J Optom Arch Am Acad Optom.* 1967;44:276–296.
5. Kuyama H, Sasamoto K, Maruyama S, et al. A new photokeratometer for contact lens in clinic. *J Jpn CL Soc.* 1979;80–84.
6. Rowsey JJ, Reynolds AE, Brown R. Corneal topography, corneascope. *Arch Ophthalmol.* 1981;99:1093–1100.
7. Doss JD, Hutson RL, Rowsey JJ, et al. Method for calculation of corneal profile and power distribution. *Arch Ophthalmol.* 1981;99:1261–1265.
8. Klyce SD. Computer-assisted corneal topography: high-resolution graphic presentation and analysis of keratoscopy. *Invest Ophthalmol Vis Sci.* 1984;25:1426–1435.
9. Mandell RB, St Helen R. Mathematical model of the corneal contour. *Br J Physiol Opt.* 1971;26:183–197.
10. Hannush SB, Waring GO III. Computer assisted corneal topography: accuracy and reproducibility with three instruments. *Invest Ophthalmol Vis Sci.* 29(suppl):1988;389.
11. Hannush SB, Waring GO III, Crawford SL, et al. Reproducibility of corneal topographic measurements with keratometry, photokeratoscopy, and corneal modeling. *Ophthalmology.* 1988;95(suppl):163.
12. Gritz D, Nobe J, McDonnell PJ. Diurnal variation in corneal topography. In press.
13. Kiely PM, Carney LG, Smith G. Diurnal variations of corneal topography and thickness. *Am J Optom Arch Am Acad Optom.* 1970;47:892–899.
14. Reynolds D, Poynter HL III. Diurnal variation in central corneal curvature. *Am J Optom Arch Am Acad Optom.* 1970;47:892–899.
15. Lin DTC, Wilson SE, Dlyce SD, et al. Post keratoplasty corneal topographic changes following suture removal quantified by the Corneal Modeling System. *Invest Ophthalmol Vis Sci.* 1989;30(suppl):188.
16. Franceschetti A, Lisch K, Klein D. Zwei eineilige zwillingspaare mit konkordantem keratokonus. *Klin Monatsbl Augenheilkd.* 1958;133:15–30.
17. Kennedy RH, Bourne WM, Dyer JA. A 48-year

clinical and epidemiologic study of keratoconus. *Am J Ophthalmol.* 1986;101:267–273.
18. Rabinowitz YS, Garbus J, McDonnell PH. Corneal topography in family members of patients with keratoconus. *Arch Ophthalmol.* 1990; 108:365–371.
19. Amsler M. Kératocône classique et keratocone fruste: arguments unitaires. *Ophthalmologica.* 1946;111:96.
20. Mohamedi P, McDonnell PJ, Garbus JJ. Contact lens fitting in keratoconus using a computerized corneal topographic analysis system. *Ophthalmology.* 1988;95(suppl)174.
21. Bronstein L, Reynolds AE. Keratoconus: changes with contact lenses. *Contact Lens Forum.* 1989;6:13–23.
22. Rowsey JJ, Balyeat HD, Monlux R, et al. Prospective evaluation of radial keratotomy: photokeratoscope corneal topography. *Ophthalmology.* 1988;95:322–334.
23. McDonnell PJ, Garbus JJ. Corneal topographic changes after radial keratotomy. *Ophthalmology.* 1989;96:45–49.
24. McDonnell PJ, Garbus J, Lopez P. Topographic analysis and visual acuity after radial keratotomy. *Am J Ophthalmol.* 1988;106:692–695.
25. Wilson SE, Klyce SD. Topographic analysis and visual acuity after radial keratotomy (correspondence to editor). *Am J Ophthalmol.* 1989;107:436–437.
26. McDonnell PJ, Garbus JJ, Lopez PF. Topographic analysis and visual acuity after radial keratotomy (reply to editor). *Am J Ophthalmol.* 1989;107:437–437.
27. Santos VR, Waring GO III, Lynn MJ, et al. Relationship between refractive error and visual acuity in the Prospective Evaluation of Radial Keratotomy (PERK) study. *Arch Ophthalmol.* 1987;105:86–92.
28. Waring GO III, Lynn, MJ, Culbertson W, et al. Three-year results of the Prospective Evaluation of Radial Keratotomy (PERK) study. *Ophthalmology.* 1987;94:1339–1354.
29. Erickson P, Robboy M. Performance characteristics of a hydrophilic concentric bifocal contact lens. *Am J Optom Physiol Optics.* 1985;62:702–708.
30. Dingeldein SA, Pittman SD, Wang J, et al. Analysis of corneal topographic data. ARVO Abstracts. *Invest Ophthalmol Vis Sci.* 1988;29 (suppl):389.
31. Fish LA, McDonnell PJ, Garbus J. Does the magnitude of diurnal fluctuation in visual acuity after radial keratotomy change with time? *Ophthalmology.* 1988;95(suppl):162.
32. Busin M, Arffa RC, McDonald MB, et al. Change in corneal curvature with elevation of intraocular pressure after radial keratotomy in the primate eye. *CLAO J.* 1988;14:110–112.
33. Schanzlin DJ, Santos VR, Waring GO III, et al. Diurnal change in refraction, corneal curvature, visual acuity, and intraocular pressure after radial keratotomy in the PERK study. *Ophthalmology.* 1986;93:167–175.
34. McDonnell PH, McClusky DJ, Garbus J. Corneal topography and fluctuating visual acuity after radial keratotomy. *Ophthalmology.* 1989;96:665–670.
35. McDonnell PJ, Fish LA, Garbus JJ. Persistence of diurnal fluctuation after radial keratotomy. *Refract Corneal Surg.* 1989;5:89–93.
36. Shivitz IA, Arrowsmith PN, Russell BM. Contact lenses in the treatment of patients with overcorrected radial keratotomy. *Ophthalmology.* 1987;94:899–903.
37. McDonnell PJ, Garbus JJ, Caroline PJ, et al. Computerized analysis of corneal topography as an aid in fitting contact lenses after radial keratotomy. *Ophthalmology,* in press.
38. Maguire LJ, Klyce SD, Sawelson H, et al. Visual distortion after myopic keratomileusis, Computer analysis of keratoscope photographs. *Ophthalmic Surg.* 1987;18:352–356.
39. Maguire LJ, Klyce SD, Singer DE, et al. Corneal topography in myopic patients undergoing epikeratophakia. *Am J Ophthalmol.* 1987; 103:404–416.
40. McDonnell PJ, Caroline PJ, Salz J. Irregular astigmatism after radial and astigmatic keratotomy. *Am J Ophthalmol.* 1989;107:42–46.
41. Gritz DC, Garbus JJ, Gauderman WJ, et al. Computer-assisted laser pachymetry: comparison with two ultrasonic pachymeters and its evaluation of normal corneal thickness and diurnal variation in thickness. *Invest Ophthalmol Vis Sci.* 1989;30(suppl):218.

13

Photogrammetric Index Method (PIM) System of Astigmatism Analysis and Its Use in Surgery for Astigmatism*

Kenneth L. Cohen and Nancy K. Tripoli

History of the Photogrammetric Index Method

Keratorefractive surgical practice has led to a need for corneal measurement that can evaluate surgical techniques. Surgical results have been quantitated by refraction, a measure of the net diopter power of the eye, and keratometry, which estimates corneal curvature in an annular region approximately 3 mm from an undefined corneal center. Keratometry fits the complex curvature of the cornea to a spherocylindrical model and does not respect irregular astigmatism. To meet needs for measurement that respects the irregularities of a large corneal surface region, developers of computer-based keratoscopes sought to increase the accuracy of corneal curvature estimates. Corneal curvature is calculated at many locations around the cornea according to analysis of reflected Placido ring patterns. The records produced by these efforts, diopter charts or texture- or color-coded maps, offer increasingly detailed data about individual corneas.[1-3] However, progress has been slower to synthesize corneal topographic data into information that can more effectively analyze keratorefractive surgical results.

Investigations of astigmatism have been especially inhibited by the lack of a uniform schema for depicting corneal topography of patient groups and comparing corneal shape changes over time. Each keratoscope record of a patient's corneal shape at a point in time produced a map or chart. Comparisons between keratoscope records consisted of anecdotal observations.[4] Understanding how the corneal shape responds to surgery was advanced through examining individual keratoscope records and noticing similarities and differences in the appearance of Placido ring patterns, diopter charts, or map patterns.

The Photogrammetric Index Method (PIM) was developed to allow evaluation of corneal astigmatism over time in groups of subjects.[5] It is based on the commonsense observations that a circular Placido ring describes a cornea with no astigmatism, that an elliptical ring describes regular corneal astigmatism, and that a ring whose shape deviates from both a circle and an ellipse describes irregular astigmatism. Therefore, a mathematical depiction of the shapes of rings can describe the quantity and nature of corneal astigmatism. Unlike keratometry, PIM does not force-fit the corneal shape to a spherocylindrical model. Its analysis of ring shape constitutes indexing of corneal shape irregularities. PIM does not measure corneal power.

The PIM Indices

Corneal astigmatism is the difference in corneal curvature between two meridians.[6] Regular astigmatism is corneal curvature that

* Supported in part by NEI RO1-EY05374, the North Carolina Lions Foundation for the Blind, Inc., and Research to Prevent Blindness, Inc.

changes gradually by a uniform increment from one meridian to the next, and irregular astigmatism is unequal, incremental curvature change from one meridian to the next.[6] PIM infers corneal surface symmetry from Placido ring shape. For the annular corneal region that reflects a Placido ring, a circular ring implies no corneal curvature change from one meridian to the next. Inequality of ring width in different directions implies dissimilar corneal curvature along different corneal meridians. An elliptical ring implies uniform, incremental curvature change from one meridian to the next. A ring shape that is not a circle or an ellipse implies perturbations of unequal curvature change from one meridian to the next.

A Placido ring can be mathematically described as a closed loop that is geometrically more or less like a circle. PIM measures the width of the ring along selected meridians. A computer routine simulates placing the ring between parallel rulers, measuring its width, rotating the ring a preselected number of degrees, measuring again, and rotating again until intervals from 0° to 180° have been measured (Fig. 13.1). To define the exact location of the chord that is the ring width measurement, a line perpendicular to the rulers is extended from the point at which the first ruler touches the ring to the opposite ruler, and the process repeated for the second ruler. The chord is a line segment perpendicular to the parallel rulers and midway between the points where the rings touch the rulers. From among measurements along 36 meridians, the shortest and longest chords are selected. PIM indices are based on the lengths, intersections, and directions of these maxima and minima.

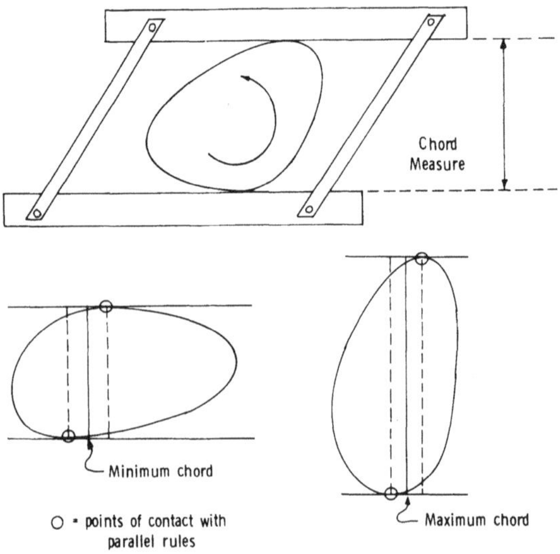

FIGURE 13.1. The width of a ring is measured along selected meridians. A computer routine simulates placing the ring between parallel rulers, measuring its width, rotating the ring a preselected number of degrees, measuring again, and rotating again until intervals from 0° through 180° have been measured. To define the exact location of the chord which is the ring width measurement, a line perpendicular to the rulers is extended from the point at which a ruler touches the ring to the opposite ruler and the process repeated for the other ruler. The chord is a line segment perpendicular to the parallel rulers and midway between the points where the rings touch the rulers. From among measurements along the selected meridians, the maximum and minimum chords are selected. (From Ref. 5, with permission.)

PIM quantitates corneal shape from the shortest and longest chords. Their lengths are the maximum and minimum ring widths. Their directions are presumed to be the principal astigmatic meridians. Four PIM indices are calculated for each ring. The index, eccentricity (E), is the minimum chord length divided by the maximum chord length (Fig. 13.2). E values imply the magnitude of astigmatism in a ring's annular region. If the ring is a circle, chord lengths are the same along all the meridians, and the value of E is 1.0. The more elliptical the ring, the lower is the value of E. The eccentricity index does not describe irregularities in ring shape. The additional indices, R_o and R_a, depict the angular differences between the directions of the maximum and minimum chords and the horizontal meridian, thus describing the directions of the principal meridians.

Values for A, SM_o, and SM_a for the same ring assess the regularity of the astigmatism. Angularity (A) is the acute angle between the directions of the maximum and minimum chords and has the maximum value of 90° (Fig. 13.2). Symmetry is measured using the line segments formed by the intersection of the major and minor chords. Major symmetry (SM_o)

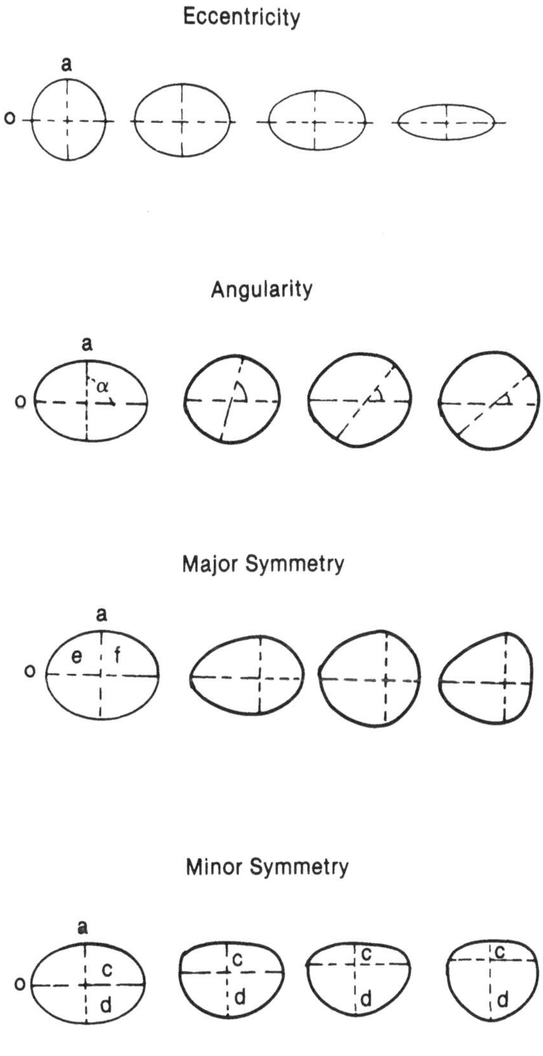

FIGURE 13.2. Schematics of the ring indices. Eccentricity (E), is the minimum chord length (a) divided by the maximum chord length (o). If the ring is a circle, chord lengths are the same along all the meridians, and the value of E is 1.0. The more elliptical the ring, the lower is the value of E. Angularity (A) is the acute angle (α) between the directions of the maximum and minimum chords. Symmetry is measured using the line segments. Major symmetry (SM_o) is the shorter length (f) divided by the longer length (e) of the maximum chord segments (o) formed by intersection with the minor chord (a). Minor symmetry (SM_a) is the shorter length (c) divided by the longer length (d) of the minimum chord segments (a) formed by intersection with the major chord (o). (From Ref. 5, with permission.)

is the shorter divided by the longer line segment of the maximum chord (Fig. 13.2). Minor symmetry (SM_a) is the shorter divided by the longer line segment of the minimum chord (Fig. 13.2). When A, SM_o, and SM_a are all close to 1.0, the ring is elliptical. Lower values imply rings that are not circles or ellipses.

The clinical significance of the astigmatic characteristics assessed by A, SM_o, and SM_a increases as astigmatism increases. When E is very close to 1.0 indicating little or no astigmatism, the ring widths in all meridians are close to equal. When there is no astigmatism, there are no principal meridians. Valucs for thc A index, which depend on the directions of the maximum and minimum chords, become random. Values for SM_o and SM_a, however, are high because widths of a nearly circular ring are likely to pass through the ring's center. A low E value and a high A value for a ring describe principal meridians at 90° to each other as is characteristic of regular astigmatism. However, the same ring may have low SM_o and SM_a values, indicating irregular astigmatism. Taken together, the PIM ring indices describe the astigmatic characteristics of a ring's annular region.

The E, A, R, and SM indices describe each ring separately. Other indices measure relationships between rings and describe qualities of the entire corneal area enclosed by the keratograph. PIM analysis includes indices that describe the consistency of the chord directions from central to peripheral cornea and the tendency of chords to pass through a common location.[5] The whole cornea index, trend (T), is the Spearman rank correlation between ring numbers and the values of each ring index. Although each of the ring indices, E, A, SM_o, and SM_a, can be used to compute a separate T value for each cornea, we have used only T of eccentricity and T of angularity. When T of eccentricity is high and positive, peripheral rings are more nearly circular than central rings since E values increase as ring numbers increase (Fig. 13.3). A highly negative T of eccentricity indicates that central rings are more nearly circular than peripheral rings. Likewise, a highly positive or negative T of angularity indicates that astigmatism is more

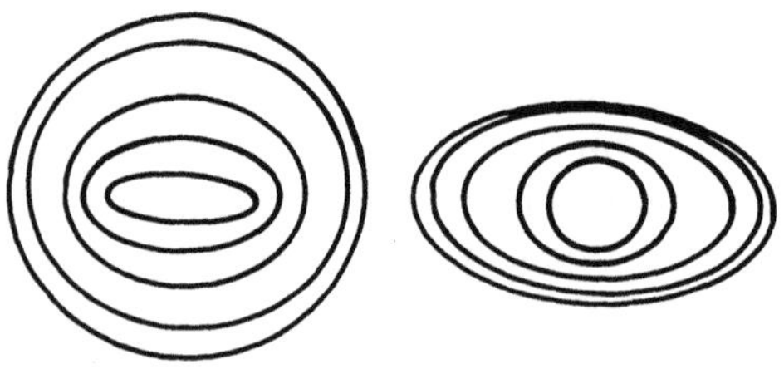

T of E = +1.0 T of E = −1.0

FIGURE 13.3. Examples of trend (T) of eccentricity. Trend of eccentricity is the Spearman rank correlation between ring numbers and eccentricity values. When *T* of eccentricity is high and positive, peripheral rings are more nearly circular than central rings. A highly negative *T* of eccentricity indicates that central rings are more nearly circular than peripheral rings. (From Ref. 5, with permission.)

regular in either the peripheral or central cornea respectively.

Validation of the PIM Indices

PIM indices were validated by measuring the nine-ring CorneaScope ring patterns of 30 eyes from 20 adult subjects who were placed in three clinically determined groups of ten eyes each.[5] A symmetrical (S) group had equal horizontal and vertical keratometric readings. In a regular (R) astigmatic group, the vertical exceeded the horizontal keratometric readings by more than 0.5 D, and the direction of the vertical principal meridians ranged between 85° and 95°. A keratoconic (K) group had a diagnosis of keratoconus based on standard clinical criteria.

Where possible, expected differences between the groups were predicted. The central corneal area measured by the keratometer is usually enclosed by the central three CorneaScope rings. Keratometric differences between S and R groups were used to predict differences in the larger area encompassed by all CorneaScope rings. These predictions assumed that the directions of the maximum and minimum chords would correspond to the principal keratometric meridians. S-group corneas, which had no measurable keratometric meridians, were expected to produce circular rings, R-group corneas elliptical rings, and K-group corneas irregular rings.

S-group rings were predicted to have *E* values near 1.0, R-group *E* values were predicted to be less than 1.0, and K-group *E* values were predicted to be the closest to zero. A values were predicted to be closer to 90° in the R group than in the S group, where the directions of principal meridians would be artifactual and therefore, random. *A* values were also predicted to be closer to 90° in the R group than in the K group because keratoconic corneas frequently exhibit irregular astigmatism. *SM* values for the S and R groups were expected to be near 1.0, and the *SM* values for the irregularly astigmatic K group were expected to be low to reflect disparate chord segments. No predictions were formulated for the T index.

Our findings are summarized in Table 13.1. As predicted, PIM ring index values described the circular rings of the S group with a tight set

TABLE 13.1. Results of photogrammetric index method (PIM) validation study.

Index	Prediction for means	Results
Eccentricity	S > R > K	Supported ($p = 6.0 \times 10^{-7}$)
Angularity	S < R	Supported ($p = 3.9 \times 10^{-3}$)
	K < R	Not supported ($p = 3.6 \times 10^{-1}$)
Symmetry major	S > K < R	Supported ($p = 2.6 \times 10^{-2}$)
Symmetry minor	S > K < R	Supported ($p = 2.0 \times 10^{-2}$)
Trend eccentricity	No prediction	Mean Spearman *r* for K group = 0.862 ($p = 1.0 \times 10^{-3}$)
Trend angularity	No prediction	Mean Spearman *r* for K group = −0.289 ($p = 1.4 \times 10^{-2}$)

S = symmetrical group, R = regularly astigmatic group, and K = keratoconic group.
From Ref. 5, with permission.

of E values close to 1.0 and higher than either the R group or the K groups (Fig. 13.4). The S group A values varied greatly and were farther from 90° than was seen in the R group (Fig. 13.5). The S group SM_o and SM_a values were higher than in the K group (Fig. 13.6). Also as predicted, the R group had E values lower than the S group but higher than the K group, had the highest A values of any group, and had higher SM_o and SM_a values than found in the K group. As predicted, the K group had the lowest E values and SM_o and SM_a values of any group. Contrary to prediction, A values were no higher in the R group than in the K group, indicating that the principal meridians were as likely to be orthogonal in the K group as in the R group. Although no predictions were made for T indices, T of E and T of A were significantly elevated and positive for the K group.

Hypotheses based on the commonsense observation that corneas with no keratometric astigmatism should have circular rings and keratometrically determined regularly astigmatic corneas should have elliptical rings were confirmed. In fact, the amount of astigmatism documented by the keratometer was highly correlated with the mean E value for each cornea in the R group ($r = -0.90$).

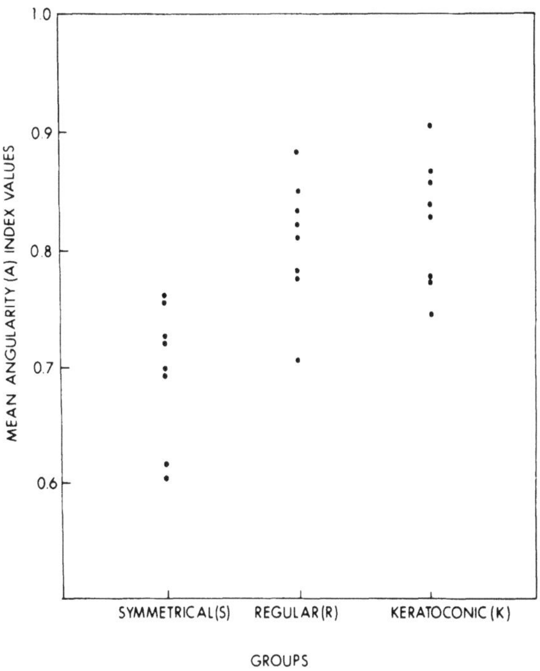

FIGURE 13.5. Mean angularity (A) values for each ring for symmetrical (S), regular (R), and keratoconic (K) groups. (From Ref. 5, with permission.)

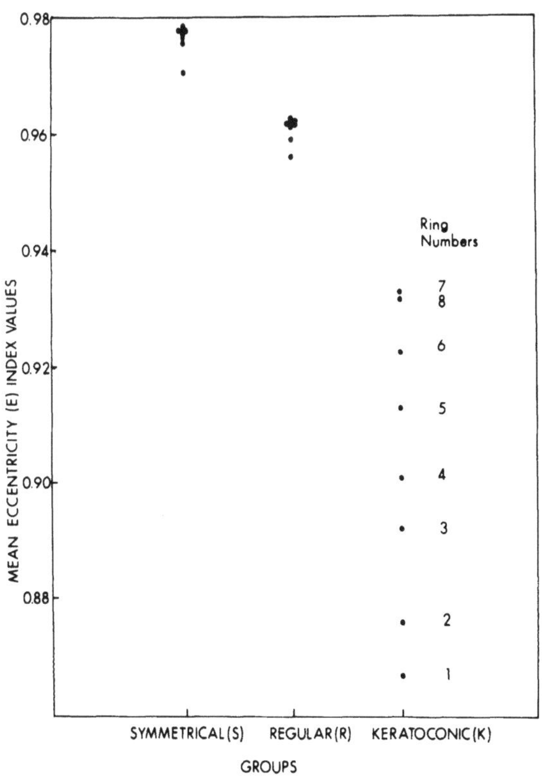

FIGURE 13.4. Mean eccentricity (E) values for each ring for symmetrical (S), regular (R), and keratoconic (K) groups. (From Ref. 5, with permission.)

Of special interest is the description of keratoconic astigmatism that emerged from PIM evaluation of the K group corneas. These corneas had oblique astigmatism, and their rings were asymmetrical.[6] However, the principal meridians intersected as close to 90° as those of regularly astigmatic corneas, although the directions of the meridians were more variable. In keratoconic corneas, the peripheral cornea had less astigmatism than the central cornea. Although it appeared that the peripheral cornea had less orthogonal principal meridians than the center, this was artifactual. The closer to circular peripheral rings of keratoconic corneas reduced the precision of locating maximum and minimum chords, and thus the intersections of the principal meridians were less likely to be orthogonal.

The PIM validation exercise demonstrated

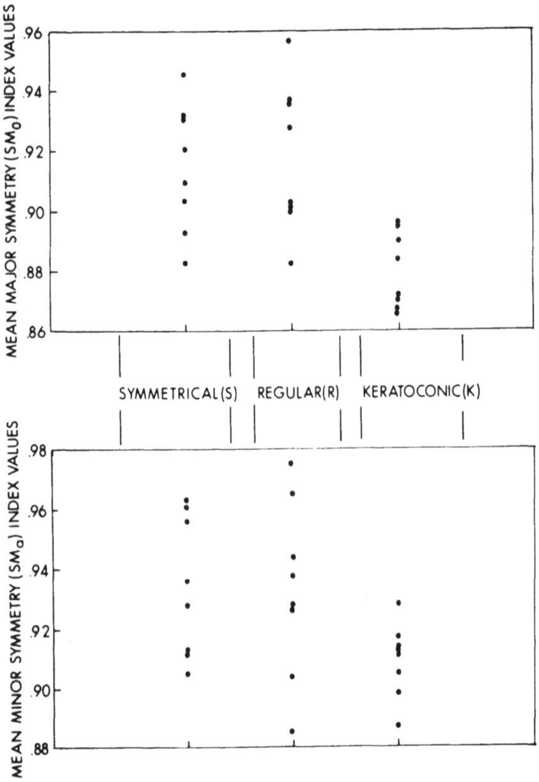

FIGURE 13.6. Mean symmetry values for each ring for symmetrical (S), regular (R), and keratoconic (K) groups. (A) Major symmetry (SM_o). (B) Minor symmetry (SM_a). (From Ref. 5, with permission.)

the usefulness of corneal indices that quantitate characteristics of groups of corneas. Keratoconic corneas are said to be "steep," "astigmatic," and "irregularly shaped." The PIM description of 10 keratoconic corneas clearly defined their average differences from regularly astigmatic and symmetrical corneas. The ability to compare groups of corneal topographic records is critical to the study of astigmatism.

Although PIM was validated using the nine-ring CorneaScope, its use is not restricted to that instrument. Any Placido ring pattern can be similarly quantitated. However, the ring reflections of other instruments may depict different annular regions of the corneal surface. Therefore, specific information and conclusions reported herein need to be adapted to these differences between instruments.

Use of PIM to Study Keratorefractive Surgery for Astigmatism

Development of a Laboratory Model of Arcuate Keratotomy

Arcuate keratotomy is a useful keratorefractive procedure to reduce corneal astigmatism. Arcuate keratotomy placed in the steepest corneal meridian flattens the steepest and steepens the flattest corneal meridians to reduce astigmatism. However, published clinical studies report variable outcomes.[7–11] Duffey et al. suggested that quantitative data from cadaver eyes after keratorefractive surgery could be used to predict clinical results.[12] To standardize and define arcuate keratotomy as a clinically useful keratorefractive procedure, the PIM eccentricity measure of ring circularity was used to model induced astigmatism in cadaver eyes.[13]

Arcuate keratotomy was performed around each of four clear zones with diameters of 3, 5, 7, and 9 mm. Each cornea received two 30° symmetrical, circumferential keratotomies, one beginning at 12 o'clock and proceeding to 1 o'clock and one beginning at 6 o'clock and proceeding to 7 o'clock. These keratotomies were extended for a total of 60°, to 2 o'clock and 8 o'clock respectively, and then for a total of 90° to 3 o'clock and 9 o'clock respectively (Fig. 13.7). Using a nine-ring CorneaScope, keratographs were taken before any keratotomy, after the initial 30° keratotomies, and after extending the keratotomies to 60° and 90°.

Central to the keratotomies, rings that were circular preoperatively became oval. Along a meridian connecting the keratotomy midpoints, ring widths increased indicating corneal flattening, and 90° away ring widths decreased indicating corneal steepening. PIM E was calculated for all rings on all keratographs. The change in E, induced astigmatism, was computed as 1.0, the E value of a ring whose shape is a circle, minus the average E value for the experimental condition. A Central Corneal Eccentricity Model of induced astigmatism,

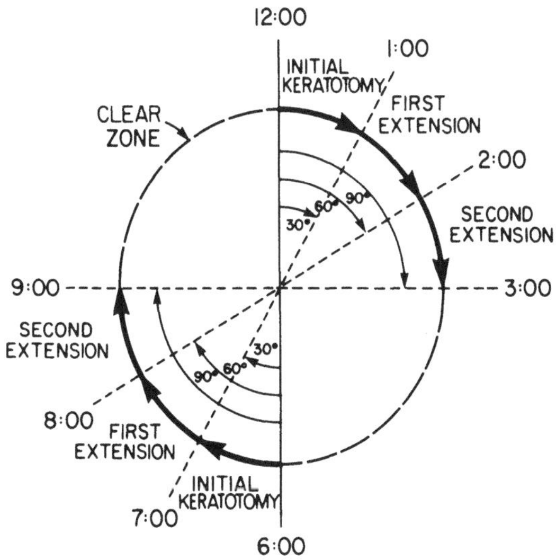

FIGURE 13.7. Surgical procedure for the laboratory model. Each cornea received two 30° symmetrical, circumferential keratotomies, one beginning at 12 o'clock and proceeding to 1 o'clock and one beginning at 6 o'clock and proceeding to 7 o'clock. These keratotomies were extended for a total of 60°, to 2 o'clock and 8 o'clock respectively, and then for a total of 90° to 3 o'clock and 9 o'clock respectively. (From Ref. 13, with permission.)

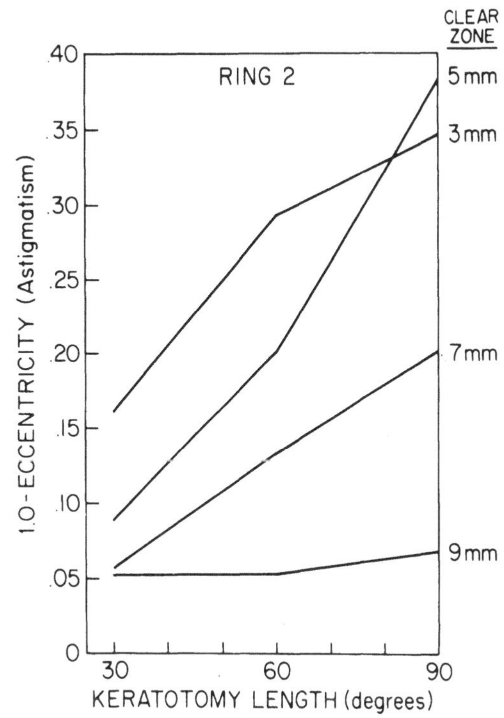

FIGURE 13.8. The Central Corneal Eccentricity Model. A model of the change in Eccentricity, induced astigmatism, for the second CorneaScope ring was constructed. The amount of induced astigmatism was graphed against each keratotomy length for 3, 5, 7, and 9-mm clear zones. Increased keratotomy length induced greater astigmatism, and a smaller clear zone resulted in greater astigmatism except for 90° keratotomies using a 3-mm clear zone. (From Ref. 14, with permission.)

the change in E for the central, second CorneaScope ring was constructed (Fig. 13.8).[14] The centermost keratoscopic ring that could be processed was used because it was most likely to represent the central cornea and was least affected by unhealed cadaver eye corneal surface discontinuities. The amount of induced astigmatism was graphed against each keratotomy length for clear zones of 3, 5, 7, and 9 mm. Points for the same clear zone were connected to allow interpolation of the astigmatism that would be induced by intermediate keratotomy lengths.

Use of the Laboratory Model to Design Arcuate Keratotomy

The Central Corneal Eccentricity Model of arcuate keratotomy was used to correct disabling astigmatism. The objective was to choose keratotomy lengths by comparing keratoscope ring ovality induced by arcuate keratotomy in cadaver eyes to the keratoscope ring ovality of patients in order to produce circular keratoscope rings in the visually important central cornea.

Correcting Corneal Astigmatism that Resulted from Perforating Trauma

The keratographs of three patients whose corneal astigmatism resulted from perforating trauma were processed by PIM (Table 13.2). To compute the correction needed to produce an E of 1.0, E values of the patients' second rings were subtracted from 1.0, and this value was called A_C. A_C for each patient was located on the ordinate of the model (Fig. 13.8). The

TABLE 13.2. Preoperative and postoperative data for penetrating corneal trauma patients who had arcuate keratotomy designed by PIM analysis.

Patient 1

Preoperative values

Keratometry: 41.00/44.50 × 80° | Refraction: −0.25 + 2.75 @ 70° | Astigmatism: 3.50 D

			PIM indices			
Ring	Eccentricity	Angularity	Major symmetry	Minor symmetry	Steepest meridian (°)	Flattest meridian (°)
2	0.885	80	0.971	0.926	65	165
3	0.927	55	0.926	0.959	90	145
4	0.925	85	0.923	0.900	85	170
5	0.928	90	0.894	0.968	75	165
6	0.933	55	0.904	0.913	105	160
7	0.941	85	0.842	0.938	75	160
8	0.946	70	0.915	0.933	85	155
9	0.940	80	0.922	0.983	70	150

Postoperative values 26 months following surgery

Keratometry: 41.50/44.00 × 75° | Refraction: 1.75 + 2.00 @ 70° | Astigmatism: 2.5 D

			PIM indices			
Ring	Eccentricity	Angularity	Major symmetry	Minor symmetry	Steepest meridian (°)	Flattest meridian (°)
2	0.933	85	0.962	0.888	90	5
3	0.929	50	0.988	0.976	45	175
4	0.947	70	0.962	0.811	60	170
5	0.949	80	0.838	0.912	70	170
6	0.951	90	0.947	0.874	65	155
7	0.951	75	0.938	0.951	55	130
8	0.944	90	0.896	0.975	60	150
9	0.939	50	0.907	0.785	70	120

Patient 2

Preoperative values

Keratometry: 37.62/42.62 × 120° | Refraction: + 11.25 + 4.25 @ 115° | Astigmatism: 5.00 D

			PIM indices			
Ring	Eccentricity	Angularity	Major symmetry	Minor symmetry	Steepest meridian (°)	Flattest meridian (°)
2	0.837	75	0.913	0.892	110	5
3	0.846	80	0.970	0.863	90	10
4	0.850	80	0.810	0.908	115	15
5	0.838	75	0.830	0.720	115	10
6	0.884	80	0.834	0.753	105	5
7	0.924	85	0.788	0.837	115	30
8	0.919	85	0.918	0.646	95	0
9	0.915	75	0.698	0.688	100	175

Postoperative values 14 months following surgery

Keratometry: 43.75/40.75 × 120° | Refraction: + 11.75 + 2.50 @ 130° | Astigmatism: 3.0 D

			PIM indices			
Ring	Eccentricity	Angularity	Major symmetry	Minor symmetry	Steepest meridian (°)	Flattest meridian (°)
2	0.924	85	0.942	0.915	115	30
3	0.901	85	0.975	0.986	120	35
4	0.915	65	0.780	0.787	145	30
5	0.914	70	0.900	0.869	135	25

TABLE 13.2. *Continued.*

			PIM indices			
Ring	Eccentricity	Angularity	Major symmetry	Minor symmetry	Steepest meridian (°)	Flattest meridian (°)
6	0.936	40	0.828	0.821	65	25
7	0.940	70	0.806	0.680	130	20
8	0.946	55	0.928	0.950	120	175
9	0.930	75	0.950	0.963	110	5

Patient 3

Preoperative values

Keratometry: 42.00/46.10 × 86° Refraction: −11.75 + 4.25 @ 100° Astigmatism: 3.1 D

			PIM indices			
Ring	Eccentricity	Angularity	Major symmetry	Minor symmetry	Steepest meridian (°)	Flattest meridian (°)
2	0.800	75	0.895	0.812	65	170
3	0.889	70	0.871	0.770	70	140
4	0.942	60	0.833	0.921	80	20
5	0.961	85	0.930	0.968	75	170
6	0.961	50	0.930	0.852	135	5
7	0.976	70	0.782	0.938	140	70
8	0.960	60	0.838	0.731	110	50
9	0.940	70	0.934	0.754	110	40

Postoperative values 7 months following surgery

Keratometry: 46.75 × 45.75 × 90° Refraction: −12.50 + 1.25 @ 135° Astigmatism: 1.0 D

			PIM indices			
Ring	Eccentricity	Angularity	Major symmetry	Minor symmetry	Steepest meridian (°)	Flattest meridian (°)
2	0.916	65	0.956	0.927	145	80
3	0.955	65	0.910	0.778	5	70
4	0.969	50	0.962	0.989	110	160
5	0.953	60	0.842	0.707	110	50
6	0.944	75	0.899	0.966	105	30
7	0.930	80	0.882	0.918	105	25
8	0.937	75	0.993	0.965	125	20
9	0.926	70	0.958	0.893	120	10

keratotomy length that had induced the same amount of astigmatism in cadaver eyes as a patient's A_c was read from the abscissa, one length corresponding to each clear zone. The steepest corneal meridian, on which the keratotomies would be centered, was felt to be best represented by the entire corneal area recorded by the keratoscope, and was located as the mean R_a value, the mean direction of the shortest ring chords, from all measured rings. Keratotomies were performed with a diamond knife blade length set at 100% of thinnest corneal thickness determined by intraoperative ultrasonic pachymetry in the region to be incised.

For the first patient, who had 3.5 D of keratometric astigmatism, the Central Corneal Eccentricity Model recommended 37° keratotomies around a 5-mm clear zone or 52.5° keratotomies around a 7-mm clear zone.[14] The patient's measurement values are shown in Table 13.2, and keratographs are seen in Fig. 13.9a. High *SM* values and consistent directions of the major and minor meridians for all

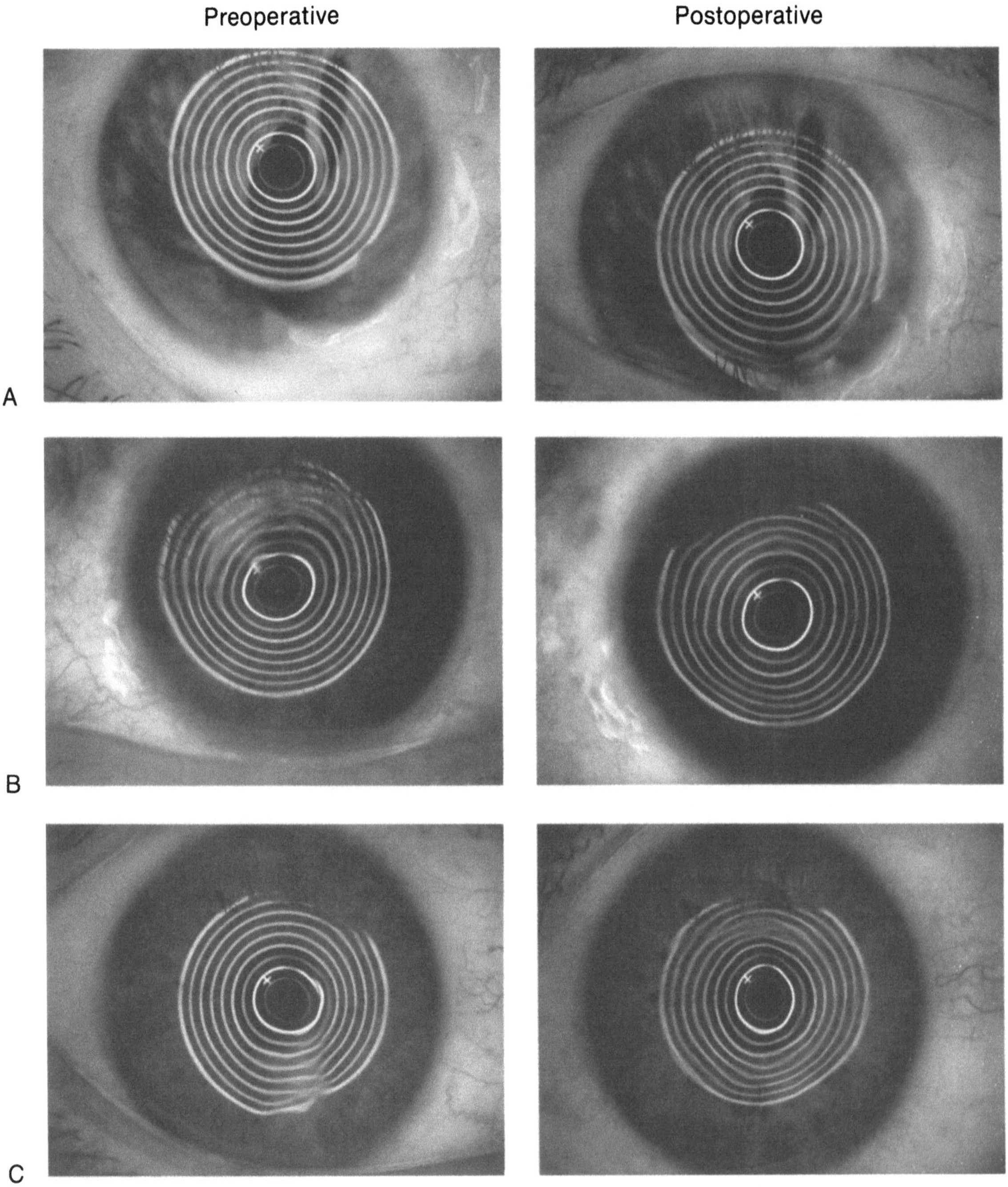

FIGURE 13.9. Preoperative and postoperative nine-ring CorneaScope photographs of three patients (A, B, and C) who had corneal astigmatism from perforating trauma. Length and position of arcuate keratotomies were based on the Central Corneal Eccentricity Model.

rings suggested a favorable outcome for symmetrical, arcuate keratotomies. To minimize the risk of overcorrection in this initial use of the model, 40° keratotomies were performed around a 7-mm clear zone. Keratotomies straddled the average steepest corneal meridian. Postkeratotomy measurement showed 2.5 D of keratometric astigmatism (29% improved), and the second ring E value was 41.5% improved 26 months after surgery. The postkeratotomy and prekeratotomy principal meridians as identified by PIM were the same, indicating that the cornea was undercorrected.

The second patient had 5 D of keratometric astigmatism. Although the directions of the major and minor meridians were consistent throughout all rings, low SM_a values indicated irregular astigmatism. The patient's PIM values are shown in Table 13.2, and keratographs are seen in Figure 13.9b. The Central Corneal Eccentricity Model recommended 50° keratotomies around a 5-mm clear zone or 70° keratotomies around a 7-mm clear zone. A 7-mm clear zone was selected to avoid incision through the traumatic corneal scar, and keratotomies straddled the average steepest meridian. Postkeratotomy measurement showed 3 D of keratometric astigmatism (40° improved), and the second ring E 53.4% improved 14 months after surgery. Low postkeratotomy, SM_a values suggested that arcuate keratotomy was less effective in flattening the region surrounding the corneal scar.

The surgical design for the third patient illustrates application of a wider range of information available from PIM. The patient had a vertical corneal scar from 2 o'clock to 5 o'clock that passed close to the corneal center. Preoperative keratometric astigmatism was 3.1 D. The patient's PIM values are shown in Table 13.2, and keratographs are seen in Figure 13.9C. The model recommended 60° keratotomies around a 5-mm clear zone or 85° keratotomies around a 7-mm clear zone. The average directions of principal meridians for the four most central CorneaScope rings were 73° (steepest) and 170° (flattest), and these values were 124° and 40°, respectively, for the four most peripheral rings. The average steepest meridian for all rings was at 98°. Differences between central and peripheral corneal shapes suggested that symmetrical keratotomies could increase corneal asymmetry. To flatten the steepest corneal meridian in the central cornea, a 60° keratotomy was performed around a 5-mm clear zone centered on the 70° meridian. In the inferior cornea, a 60° keratotomy was performed around a 7-mm clear zone and centered on the 90° meridian. This was a compromise between centering the keratotomy on the steepest peripheral meridian, 124°, and incising through the scar. Postkeratotomy measurement showed 1 D of keratometric astigmatism (68% improved), and the second ring E value was 58% improved seven months after surgery.

Correcting Postkeratoplasty Astigmatism

The postkeratoplasty astigmatism of seven eyes of seven patients was corrected by arcuate keratotomy based on the Central Corneal Eccentricity Model in a prospective study.[15] The 5-mm clear zone data for cadaver eyes was used as a model to reduce postkeratoplasty astigmatism. Although a 7-mm clear zone would more closely approximate the diameter of most keratoplasty wounds, the 7-mm data required longer keratotomy lengths that could increase the risk of the procedure. Keratotomies were performed in the keratoplasty wound using a diamond knife whose blade length was set to 100% of minimum corneal thickness determined by intraoperative ultrasonic pachymetry in the region to be incised. Keratotomies were centered on the average steepest corneal meridian for all rings calculated by PIM. Keratotomies were performed a mean of 22.6 months (range 17.7 to 28.9 months) after keratoplasty and a mean of 5.5 months (range 3.0 to 10.7 months) after suture removal. Arcuate keratotomy length ranged from 50° to 80°. The patients were followed up for a mean of 7.0 months (range 2.0 to 18.4 months).

The results of this study compare favorably with astigmatism correction reported in other studies and illustrate the use of PIM to design arcuate keratotomy surgery.[7–11] Prekeratotomy, postkeratotomy, change, percent change, and axis change in keratometric astigmatism for each eye are shown in Table 13.3. Prekeratotomy keratometric astigmatism was 9.27 D ± 2.14 D (mean ± s.d.), postkeratotomy astigmatism was 2.75 D ± 2.25 D, change in astigmatism was −6.25 D ± 2.71 D, mean percent change in astigmatism was −69.8% (range −36.4% to −100.0%), and mean axis change was 17.5° (range 0° to 45°). No eyes were overcorrected. The cornea (patient 2) with the largest change in keratometric axis had 1.12 D residual astigmatism and −88.8% change in astigmatism. Preoperative

TABLE 13.3. Preoperative and postoperative keratometric data for penetrating keratoplasty patients who had acuate keratotomies designed by PIM analysis.

Patient	Preoperative corneal astigmatism (D)	Residual astigmatism (D)	Net decrease in corneal astigmatism (D)	Decrease in corneal astigmatism (% of preoperative)	Change in keratometric axis (°)
1	9.87	2.50	−7.37	−74.7	0.0
2	10.00	1.12	−8.88	−88.8	45.0
3	10.88	5.50	−5.38	−49.5	15.0
4	4.50	1.75	−2.75	−61.1	35.0
5	9.87	0.00	−9.87	−100.0	n/a
6	10.13	2.25	−7.88	−77.8	5.0
7	9.63	6.12	−3.51	−36.4	5.0
Mean	9.27	2.75	−6.52	−69.8	17.5

n/a = not applicable

and postoperative keratographs of this patient's cornea are shown in Figure 13.10.

Prekeratotomy, postkeratotomy, change, and percent change in E are shown in Table 13.4. Also shown is the change in E as a percent of the change needed to produce a circular ring (100 times the net change in E divided by the quantity 1.0 minus preoperative E). Prekeratotomy E was 0.794 ± 0.071 (mean ± s.d), postkeratotomy E was 0.915 ± 0.053, change in E was 0.121 ± 0.067, and percent change in E was 58.5% (range 24.3% to 85.4%). All corneas had decreased keratometric astigmatism and increased E values. Arcuate keratotomy length was positively correlated with change in E (Spearman $r = 0.85$, $p < 0.05$).

Best spectacle corrected preoperative and postoperative visual acuity ranged from 20/20 to 20/60 and from 20/15 to 20/50, respectively. Five patients had improved postoperative visual acuity. In patients 1 and 7, the preoperative and postoperative visual acuities were equal. The mean change in preoperative spherical equivalent was −0.411 D (range +3.00 to −3.75 D).

Because the knife blade length was set at 100% of intraoperatively determined keratoplasty wound thickness, five eyes had intraoperative perforations. Four eyes had no wound leak at 24 hr after surgery, and one eye had a wound leak that sealed at 48 hr after surgery. When compared to other studies, our perforation rate was the highest reported.[7–11] The eye that had the longest keratotomy, 80° (patient 6), had a transiently elevated donor

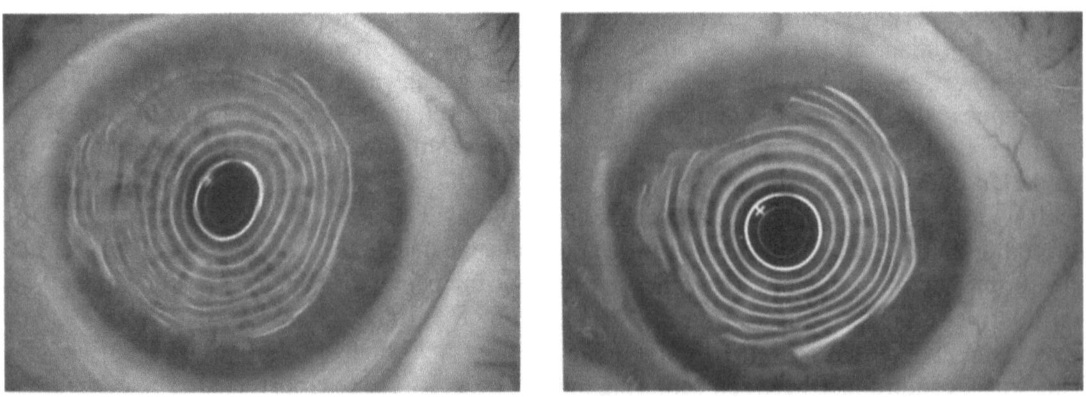

FIGURE 13.10. Preoperative (left) and postoperative (right) nine-ring CorneaScope photographs of a patient with postkeratoplasty keratometric astigmatism of 10 D (patient 2).

TABLE 13.4. Preoperative and postoperative photogrammetric index method (PIM) eccentricity *(E)* results for the central second corneascopic ring for penetrating keratoplasty patients who had arcuate keratotomies designed by PIM analysis.

Patient number	Preoperative eccentricity	Postoperative eccentricity	Net change eccentricity	Change eccentricity as % of needed change
1	0.782	0.913	0.132	60.6
2	0.781	0.968	0.187	85.4
3	0.760	0.836	0.076	31.7
4	0.899	0.959	0.060	59.4
5	0.841	0.968	0.127	79.9
6	0.673	0.898	0.225	68.8
7	0.819	0.863	0.044	24.3
Mean	0.794	0.915	0.121	58.5

keratoplasty edge. To obtain maximum effect from the keratotomies, no corneas were sutured. A recent finite element mathematical model of the corneal response to arcuate keratotomy suggested that blade length may be shortened to 70% of corneal thickness and maximum response still be obtained.[16]

Mire ovality as defined by PIM *E*, a crude estimate of corneal symmetry, is a corneal topography feature metric. This metric was used to define a cadaver eye model, and the model was used to determine keratotomy length and/or clear zone size of arcuate keratotomy to induce astigmatism. This demonstrated the utility of keratoscope analysis of corneal topography to systematic investigation of the response to arcuate keratotomy. Use of PIM information is not a substitute for clinical understanding of prekeratotomy corneal shape characteristics, but measurement of them. General observations of the cornea's response to surgery, such as Rowsey's caveats of keratorefractive surgery, must be applied to surgical design.[17, 18] The selection of useful information from PIM records and the model can translate clinical intuition into specific design strategy.

Objections to the Premises of PIM

Description of corneal topography based on ring shape rather than calculated corneal power has been criticized as naive, simplistic, and misleading. Ring images are reflected from corneal regions at different distances from the line of sight. The central rings of a steeper cornea describe a more central corneal region than do the same numbered rings of a flatter cornea. Some segments of an elliptical or irregularly shaped ring describe the more central cornea, while other segments of the same ring describe the more peripheral cornea. PIM measurements use two points on opposite sides of the cornea connected with chords that do not necessarily pass through a "center."

Many investigators prefer to depict corneal curvature according to the distances from a "center" to a ring, calculated separately along each radial.[1-3] Efforts to improve the precision of corneal charts and maps based on diopter measurements have continued since the introduction of PIM. Newer corneal measurement instruments such as the Corneal Modeling System from Computed Anatomy, Inc. (New York) measure apical regions that previously had to be approximated and include many rings to allow dense measurement of the cornea from center to periphery.[3] Sophisticated software has facilitated measurement of the aspheric cornea.

Although the corneal surface can now be depicted with increased precision, there are problems with the clinical use of the depiction. Diopter calculation from Placido rings assumes that a subject who fixates on a target in the center of a concentric ring pattern will have a keratograph in which the center of the ring pattern in on the line of sight.[19] In truth, the ring pattern will center on the "apex normal," the point at which the cornea is closest to the apparatus, and this point may not be on the patient's line of sight. To the extent that the center used for calculation of diopters differs from the intersection of the line of sight with the corneal surface, the calculated diopter power of the cornea, no matter how precisely or densely computed, will be systematically misrepresented. Thus the accuracy of derived corneal power may not be proportional to the precision of surface measurement.

The interpretation of precise corneal maps presents the greatest obstacle to their clinical implementation. Corneal maps of unusual cases have been presented to show that localized flat or steep corneal regions are neglected by PIM. Although it has been hypothesized that the corneal power of specific, localized areas is important in predicting corneal topographic changes in response to keratorefractive surgery, to our knowledge there has been no clinical trial that demonstrates the effect of local curvature on overall corneal shape change.

Choosing a Corneal Topographic Measurement System

An attentive keratorefractive surgeon is likely to notice corneal topographical phenomena that seem to relate to success and failure. This anecdotal information leads to differing opinions, controversy, and competing surgical and

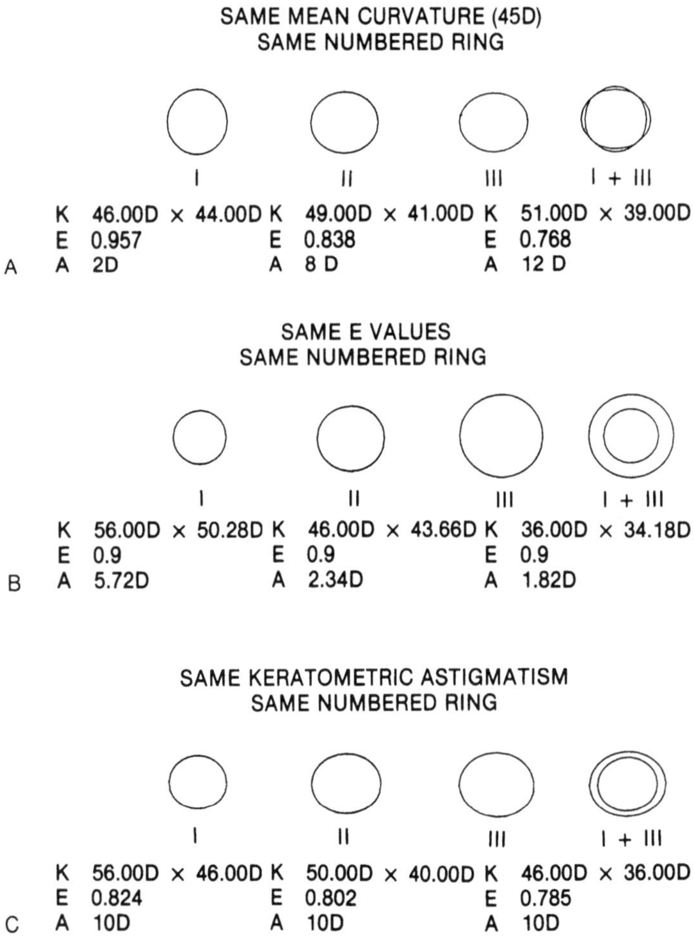

FIGURE 13.11. A comparison of eccentricity (*E*) with keratometric astigmatism. (A) When the mean curvatures of two corneas are the same (45 D), the greater the keratometric astigmatism, the lower the *E* values. The less the keratometric astigmatism, the higher the *E* values. (B) When two corneas have the same *E* values (0.9), the steeper the cornea, the greater the keratometric astigmatism. The flatter the cornea, the less the keratometric astigmatism. (C) When two corneas have the same keratometric astigmatism (10D), the steeper the cornea, the higher the *E* values. The flatter the cornea, the lower the *E* values.

treatment techniques. Maguire et al. recommended the development of a system to prospectively analyze corneal topography which would aid keratorefractive surgery and improve results.[11] Systematic evaluation is needed to discriminate the physical laws that govern corneal shape change from myths based on unsystematic observation. To accomplish this, quantitation of keratoscope data and definitions of specific topography features as metrics must be developed so that corneas can be combined into defined groups and statistically analyzed. At present, PIM is the only published comprehensive astigmatism evaluation method that can be used to analyze the corneal topography of groups of corneas over time. Partial alternatives are keratometric and refractive measurements that can measure only the power and direction of the central principal meridians of the cornea or the eye respectively.

PIM and diopter-based analyses measure different corneal topographic metrics. The aim of diopter topographical depictions is to precisely and accurately quantitate corneal power. PIM aims to provide information based on ring images to describe the symmetry of the corneal surface. PIM eccentricity is a ratio converted to a decimal. Therefore, it has no physical units, and it quantitates astigmatism independent of corneal power. In contrast, keratometric astigmatism is a subtraction of the curvature along the flattest meridian from the curvature along the steepest meridian. If two corneas have the same shaped rings, they will have the same E value. However, the steeper the cornea, the more keratometric astigmatism will be reported. The flatter the cornea, the less keratometric astigmatism will be reported. Two corneas with the same reported keratometric astigmatism will have differently shaped rings depending on their mean curvatures (Fig. 13.11). The steeper cornea will have more nearly circular rings than the flatter cornea. Therefore, the steeper cornea will have a higher E value. The flatter the cornea, the lower the E value.

The selection of an astigmatism measurement system to design keratorefractive surgery for astigmatism is an empirical issue. To do effective keratorefractive surgery, appropriate preoperative feature metrics must be measured and their effect on surgical design and results understood. Keratorefractive surgery results are thought to be related to the amount and nature of preoperative astigmatism. The analysis method that identifies the preoperative corneal shape features that influence postoperative surgical results will become the measurement system of choice.

References

1. Rowsey JJ, Isaac MS. Corneoscopy in keratorefractive surgery. *Cornea.* 1983;2:133–142.
2. Klyce SD. Computer-assisted corneal topography. *Invest Ophthalmol Vis Sci.* 1984;25:1426–1435.
3. Gormely DJ, Gersten M, Koplin RS, et al. Corneal modeling. *Cornea.* 1988;7:30–35.
4. McDonald MB. The future direction of refractive surgery. *J Refract Surg* 1988;4:158–168.
5. Cohen KL, Tripoli NK, Pellom AC, et al. A new photogrammetric method for quantifying corneal topography. *Invest Ophthalmol Vis Sci.* 1984;25:323–330.
6. Duke-Elder S, Abrams D. *System of ophthalmology. Vol. V. Ophthalmic Optics and Refraction.* London: Henry Kimpton, 1970; p 274.
7. Krachmer JH, Fenzl RE. Surgical correction of high postkeratoplasty astigmatism. *Arch Ophthalmol.* 1980;98:1400–1402.
8. Mandel MR, Shapiro MB, Krachmer JH. Relaxing incisions with augmentation sutures for the correction of postkeratoplasty astigmatism. *Am J Ophthalmol.* 1987;103:441–447.
9. Sugar J, Kirk AK. Relaxing keratotomy for post-keratoplasty high astigmatism. *Ophthal Surg.* 1983;14:156–158.
10. Lavery GW, Lindstrom RL, Hofer LA, et al. The surgical management of corneal astigmatism after penetrating keratoplasty. *Ophthal Surg.* 1985;16:166–169.
11. Maguire LJ, Bourne WM. Corneal topography of transverse keratotomies for astigmatism after penetrating keratoplasty. *Am J Ophthalmol.* 1989;107:323–330.
12. Duffey RJ, Jain VN, Tchah H, Hofmann RF, Lindstrom RL, et al. Paired arcuate keratotomy. A surgical approach to mixed and myopic astigmatism. *Arch Ophthalmol.* 1988;106:1130–1135.

13. Tripoli NK, Cohen KL, Holman RE. Corneal topographic response to circumferential keratotomies. *J Refract Surg*. 1987;3:129–136.
14. Cohen KL, Tripoli NK. The application of research data to keratorefractive surgery. *CLAO J*. 1987;13:280–286.
15. Cohen KL, Tripoli NK, Noecker RJ. Prospective analysis of photokeratoscopy for arcuate keratotomy to reduce postkeratoplasty astigmatism. *Refract Corneal Surg*. 1989;5:388–393.
16. Jouve FE, Hanna KD, Waring III GO. Computer simulation of arcuate keratotomy for astigmatism. *Invest Ophthalmol Vis Sci*. 1989;30(suppl):186.
17. Rowsey JJ. Ten Caveats in keratorefractive surgery. *Ophthalmology*. 1983;90:148–155.
18. Rowsey JJ. Review: current concepts in astigmatism surgery. *J Refract Surg*. 1986;2:85–94.
19. Uozato H, Guyton DL. Centering corneal surgical procedures. *Am J Ophthalmol*. 1987; 103:264–275.

Index

MIX
Papier aus verantwortungsvollen Quellen
Paper from responsible sources
FSC® C105338

If you have any concerns about our products,
you can contact us on
ProductSafety@springernature.com

In case Publisher is established outside the EU,
the EU authorized representative is:
Springer Nature Customer Service Center GmbH
Europaplatz 3, 69115 Heidelberg, Germany

Printed by Libri Plureos GmbH
in Hamburg, Germany